The Sinusitis Help Book
A Comprehensive Guide
to a Common Problem

Questions

Answers

Options

M. LEE WILLIAMS, M.D.

JOHN WILEY & SONS, INC.

New York • Chichester • Weinheim • Brisbane • Singapore • Toronto

This book is dedicated to the millions of sinus sufferers
and to my dear wife, Teensa, whose encouragement,
patience, and understanding made it possible.

This book is printed on acid-free paper. ☺

Copyright © 1998 by M. Lee Williams, M.D. All rights reserved.

Published by John Wiley & Sons, Inc.

Published simultaneously in Canada

Previously published by CHRONIMED Publishing

The information contained in this book is not intended to serve as a
replacement for professional medical advice. Any use of the information in this
book is at the reader's discretion. The author and the publisher specifically
disclaim any and all liability arising directly or indirectly from the use or
application of any information contained in this book. A health care
professional should be consulted regarding your specific situation.

ISBN 0-471-34702-7

Printed in the United States of America

10 9 8 7 6 5 4 3 2

CONTENTS

ACKNOWLEDGMENTS

Samuel J. Crowe, MD, former Halsted Appointed Otolaryngologist-in-Chief, Johns Hopkins.

John E. Bordley, MD, former Ancelot Professor and Chairman, Dept. Of Otolaryngology, Johns Hopkins.

Charles W. Cummings, MD, Professor and Chairman, Dept. of Otolaryngology/Head & Neck Surgery, Johns Hopkins.

Thomas E. Van Metre Jr., MD, Professor of Medicine, Johns Hopkins

R. Donald Eney, MD, a former Director of the Pediatric Allergy Clinic, Johns Hopkins and to whom I owe a special thanks for reviewing my material on Allergy and Allergic Rhinitis.

Manuel V. Gatchalian, MD, Chief of Otolaryngology, Head and Neck Surgery at The Union Memorial Hospital, Baltimore, for his interest and support.

A special thanks also to my very special step-daughter, Kathy Kimball, for her editing advice, interest, and encouragement.

Introduction

THIS BOOK ANSWERS the questions most frequently asked by sinus sufferers over the years. I wish I could offer every reader a definite cure for chronic sinusitis, but as you will see, the many complexities of this disease, with its many different predisposing and contributing factors, make such a universal offer impossible. However, a better understanding of sinus disease may make it possible for you to prevent your acute or subacute sinusitis from becoming chronic and may also provide a reasonable chance of reversing chronic sinusitis should it develop. In those cases where it may not be possible to reverse the disease completely, I hope that this book will make coping with chronic sinusitis a much easier task.

By becoming more knowledgeable about sinus disease, you can often tell whether you or one of your family has a sinus problem that requires immediate attention or one that can wait for a routine doctor's appointment. You should also have some idea as to whether a hospital emergency room visit will prove justified (and therefore covered by your insurance). You will find out what effective treatments you can provide at home, as well as what can be accomplished with over-the-counter medications, and even what can be done to prevent you from infecting others.

You will learn how environmental factors such as heating, air-conditioning, humidity, barometric pressure changes, weather, air temperature, air pollutants, dust, and pollen can affect your sinuses both inside and outside the home as well as in the car, at work, and at school, and what can be done to control them.

You will see how both allergic and nonallergic individuals can develop chronic inflammation of the nose, often leading to sinusitis, and what may be done to prevent or treat it. Some of you may have been misdiagnosed as having sinusitis or even allergic rhinitis, and this book should make you aware of this, as well as to whether the so-called sinus headaches you may have been experiencing are really due to sinusitis or possibly to something entirely different.

A better understanding of sinus disease will help you to know if the treatment you or your family receives is proper and responsible. Moreover, your knowledgeable questions and answers regarding the subject may stimulate a greater interest and a more determined study of your case by your physician. All too often, chronic sinusitis patients will leave a doctor's office totally confused about their condition and wishing belatedly that they had asked more pointed questions. Being well informed may even help you, with the guidance of your physician, to decide if and when surgery is necessary, as well as to realize what complications might occur by going ahead with the procedure or what problems could result from waiting too long.

If you have a chronic sinus problem and have, as is so often the case, consulted more than one sinus specialist, you may have also received several different opinions as well as several different recommenda-tions. If so, this book will be useful in helping you make the wiser choice.

Finally, you may become more aware of the possible consequences of allowing a sinus infection to continue untreated for a prolonged period, especially in a child. Parents need to know that any excessive scarring of the sinuses from prolonged infections in childhood may very well invite more sinus problems later in life and may lead to ear problems as well.

With the changes we can expect to see in the practice of medicine over the next few years, it will become more and more important for every prospective patient to have a broader knowledge of the common diseases such as sinusitis, especially with regard to preventative mea-sures, early recognition, and possible complications, as well as a rea-sonable knowledge of the various treatments available and their chances of success. In some instances, this not only may lead to an ear-lier diagnosis but also will permit many patients to participate more effectively in their own treatment and cure.

For those who would turn to the Internet for a solution to their medical problems or those of a family member, it is important to remember that medical cyberspace is not regulated, that there is no computer Medical Board or on-line Food and Drug Administration (FDA), and some of the information obtained could therefore prove misleading or even harmful.

In writing this book, I have tried to avoid any detailed scientific discussion of sinus disease, but I have included certain technical information where I felt it might be helpful. To give complete answers to each question, some repetition has been necessary, but this may also serve to emphasize certain basic facts about this rather complex common disease.

PART ONE

Sinusitis

CHAPTER ONE

What Are Sinuses?
And Why Do We Have Them?

THE SINUSES AND HOW THEY WORK

The sinuses consist of four paired air-containing hollowed-out structures in bone lying mostly adjacent to each side of the nose and connected to it by very small openings, or ducts. Each sinus cavity, like the adjoining nasal cavity, is lined with a mucus-secreting membrane called respiratory epithelium, which is constantly swept clean by very fine microscopic hairs called cilia. Each sinus cavity is identified with the head or facial bone in which it resides, namely, the maxillary, frontal, sphenoid, or ethmoid. Except for the ethmoids, each sinus structure consists of a single cavity on each side and has its own drainage duct or opening. The ethmoids, however, are further divided into anterior and posterior groupings. Together, they total approximately 7 to 15 very small sinus cavities on each side, and each cavity usually has its own drainage opening into the nose as well.

Even though we usually think of our sinuses as 8 separate structures with 4 on each side, when we include the many small ethmoid cavities individually, we could be talking about as many as 30 or more independently draining sinus cavities, each capable of blocking up, becoming infected, and sometimes remaining infected to eventually infect other sinuses nearby. Moreover, each and every one of these individual sinus cavities must be cleared of blockage and any retained infected discharge before you can be considered cured.

To function normally and stay healthy, each sinus cavity not only must drain adequately and continuously but also must contain air and

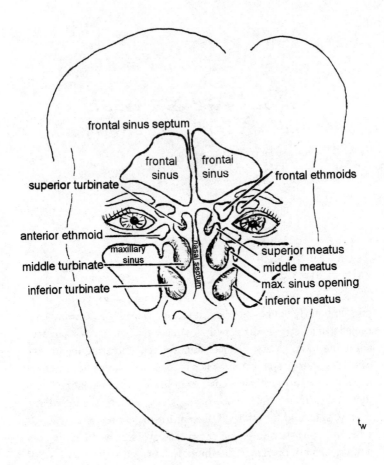

FIGURE 1. The location of the sinuses with regard to the forehead, eyes, and cheeks. The nasal septum is reasonably straight, and the three turbinates on either side of the nose do not appear to be enlarged or pressing against it. The drainage opening from each maxillary sinus into its respective middle meatus is unobstructed, but those leading from the frontal, ethmoidal, and sphenoid sinuses can not be seen in this view. Several frontal ethmoids are visible in the brow areas, and the two frontal sinuses are separated by a thin partition, or septum.

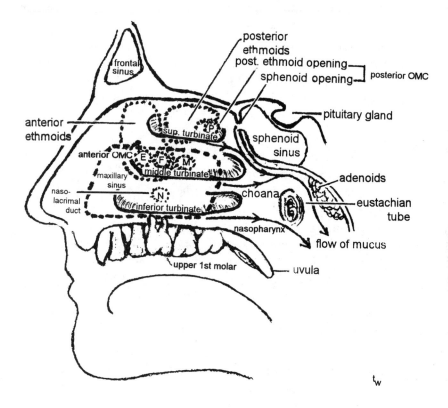

FIGURE 2. A side view of the right nasal passage with the nasal septum removed. The superior, middle, and inferior turbinates appear normal in size and shape. The drainage openings of the anterior ethmoidal (E), frontal (F), and maxillary (M) sinuses forming the anterior OMC are seen as three dotted circles beneath the middle turbinate. Their drainage flow, as well as that from the posterior ethmoidal and sphenoid openings (posterior OMC), is indicated by arrows. The proximity of the eustachian tube opening to this sinus flow and to the adenoid mass is also revealed. The outlines of the right anterior and posterior ethmoidal sinuses as well as the right maxillary sinus, all located on the other side of the nasal wall, are seen as dotted lines and small dashes respectively. The root of an upper first molar can be seen extending close to the floor of the maxillary sinus. The drainage opening of the tear duct (N) is noted beneath the inferior turbinate.

have a free air exchange with the nose. If for any reason a complete blockage of sinus drainage and air exchange should occur, the body will begin to absorb the air trapped within the sinus cavity, causing a partial vacuum to develop. This is usually followed by swelling of the membranous lining of the sinus, retained secretions, and a vacuum-type sinus headache. If the blockage persists, a sinus infection usually develops, which can often be identified by a cloudy nasal discharge or pus.

MAXILLARY SINUSES

The two largest sinuses, called the maxillary sinuses, are located in the cheeks between the eyes and upper teeth. When fully developed, they are usually capable of holding somewhere between a half and full ounce of fluid each. They are often slightly larger in men. They are present, although very small, at birth, and develop very early in life. Along with the ethmoid sinuses, the maxillaries usually play a very important role in infant or childhood sinusitis as well as in adult sinus disease. The maxillary sinus on each side drains into the nose through a small opening in the sinonasal wall beneath the middle turbinate. Attention was first directed to the maxillary sinuses in 1765 when a dentist in Bordeaux first attempted to probe their openings.

FRONTAL SINUSES

The second largest are the two frontal sinuses, which are located in the forehead just above the eyebrows in what is called the frontal bone. They usually appear in the fifth or sixth year of life and continue to develop until the late teens or early twenties. On rare occasions, they may grow larger than the maxillary sinuses. Sometimes one or both frontals may be underdeveloped or even totally absent, especially in someone who has experienced significant and prolonged ethmoid or maxillary sinus infections in early childhood. Some may assume that the absence of a frontal sinus is a good omen, since it could mean one less sinus cavity to become infected. Unfortunately, however, the absence often forecasts more trouble with the anterior ethmoids or maxillary sinus on the same side due to scarring from the same childhood infections that limited the frontal sinus development.

The absence of a frontal sinus may occur in about 4 percent of the population, but absence or lack of development is more common in cleft palate children, who often begin their lives with an almost constant sinus infection due to food contamination of the nose and the sinus drainage openings. Frequent or persistent sinus infections in childhood can and often do lead to further sinus problems in later life, depending of course on the amount of permanent sinus damage, as well as the location and degree of scar tissue formation and whether it interferes significantly with the normal drainage of a sinus, its air exchange, and blood supply.

The frontal sinuses in some 20 to 40 percent of individuals may drain into the nose through a narrow ductlike structure shaped somewhat like an hourglass and measuring from 3 millimeters to three-quarters of an inch in length, possibly making the frontal sinuses more vulnerable to acute obstruction as well as to permanent damage from a facial fracture. In the other 60 to 80 percent, however, the frontals drain into the nose, also beneath the middle turbinates, but in this case through an inverted funnel-like opening called the frontal recess, measuring approximately 3 to 10 millimeters across, which usually has much less chance of blockage. The likelihood of arrested development or complete absence of a frontal sinus would appear greater in the 20 to 40 percent who have the ductlike structure, since its occlusion in early life by a prolonged ethmoid or maxillary sinus infection would seem more likely. Fortunately, frontal sinus infections are usually fairly uncommon before puberty.

SPHENOID SINUSES

The third largest sinuses are the sphenoids, both of which lie in the sphenoid bone just under the brain in the middle of the skull below the pituitary gland and adjacent to the upper part of the back of the nose where the nasal septum ends. They appear as small pits at birth, usually become clinically obvious at five or six years of age, and then gradually enlarge until the middle teens, when they are usually fully developed cavities. Because of their location deep within the skull, the sphenoids are more difficult to examine, and an infection there may sometimes go undetected for a very long time, occasionally with very serious results. Because of this, they were sometimes called "the neglected sinuses." In the past, sphenoid sinus infections were seldom diagnosed in children and often missed in adults, partly because the sphenoid sinuses were very poorly visualized on routine sinus X rays. Now, with lighted telescopes and the increased availability of the CAT scan, doctors are more often able to find infections of the sphenoids, especially in association with a posterior ethmoid infection, since their drainage openings are so closely allied. Fortunately, sphenoid sinusitis rarely occurs in very young children.

ETHMOID SINUSES

The final group is the ethmoid sinuses, which, as previously mentioned, consist of a collection of very small sinus cavities, usually draining separately into the nose through tiny openings just 1 to 2 millimeters in diameter and usually numbering 7 to 15 separate cavities on each side. They are further divided into the anterior and posterior ethmoids, with their posterior cavities being usually larger and fewer in number. The ethmoids lie primarily on the inside of each eye socket, or orbit, but are normally separated from it by a thin wall of bone. Their sinus cavities may extend into the cheek beneath the eye, sometimes behind the eye, and fairly often above the eye into the frontal bone. Those that extend beneath the eye are known as Haller cells and may cause maxillary sinus blockage with infection or sometimes an eye infection. In 4 to 12 percent of the population, an ethmoid sinus may expand into a mucous membrane–covered bony structure inside the nose known as the middle turbinate. Sometimes this condition will make the turbinate swell or balloon out causing a condition known as concha bullosa, which can result in nasal or sinus blockage with headaches.

Although the other sinuses may occasionally infect an eye and even cause blindness, the ethmoid sinuses, because of their presence in very early life, their location, their very thin and sometimes defective bony walls adjoining the orbit, and even because of their sheer numbers, are far more likely to cause an infection of an eye or of the surrounding orbital tissues, producing a condition known as orbital cellulitis or orbital abscess. The posterior ethmoids may also cause an even more serious eye condition directly involving the optic nerve and resulting in blindness. Because of the ethmoids' very close proximity to the eye, their extension beneath the eye in a third of the patients, and in some cases the lack of bone separating them from the orbit or optic nerve (which can't always be determined ahead of time), the ethmoid sinuses offer a much greater risk of eye injuries with sinus surgery.

Some anterior ethmoid sinuses may develop high in the nose near the drainage duct to the frontal sinus, sometimes causing a displacement of the duct and a greater chance of frontal sinus blockage. Some may also extend into the frontal bone above the eyes or even into the partition between the two frontal sinuses in nearly a third of the population. When infected, any of these displaced ethmoid cavities may cause obstruction to the frontal sinus or to its drainage duct and result in a frontal sinus infection.

SECONDARY DRAINAGE OPENINGS

The maxillary sinuses may occasionally have secondary drainage openings into the nose. These apparently sometimes occur naturally but are more often caused by an infection or surgery. Their presence may sometimes be beneficial to a patient should the primary drainage opening become obstructed. However, the secondary openings could also indicate significant maxillary sinus disease in the past and even suggest additional permanent scarring in other sinuses nearby. The secondary drainage openings for the maxillary sinuses are found in about 23 percent of patients and are located inside the nose beneath the protective middle turbinate and just behind the natural drainage opening of the sinus. When present, they usually penetrate an area of very thin membrane in the maxillary sinonasal wall known as the fontanelle, a term also used to identify the very thin membranous soft spots in a baby's skull.

A maxillary sinus infection may sometimes rupture the fontanelle, resulting in a second and sometimes even a third permanent opening. These additional sinus openings may improve sinonasal air exchange, but their help with any mucus drainage is limited because the sinus cilia will continue to sweep the mucus toward the natural drainage opening. The same problem results from surgically creating a separate sinonasal window for better maxillary sinus drainage as opposed to simply enlarging the natural opening for more effective results. Also, more than one drainage opening into a sinus cavity may sometimes cause a recirculation of mucus flow back into the sinus.

The maxillary, frontal, and anterior ethmoid sinuses (located in the front of the nose) each drain into a small channel or groove called the middle meatus, located on each side of the nose and protectively tucked under the middle turbinate. This rather commonly shared sinus drainage area is generally known as the ostiomeatal complex, or anterior OMC to the sinus surgeon, and often represents the main focus for functional endoscopic sinus surgery (FESS), a term used to identify a maximum surgical effort to endoscopically restore adequate sinus function. Inflammation due to an infected discharge into this area from a chronically infected maxillary or ethmoid sinus is the most common cause of recurrent or chronic frontal sinus infection, and its cure may require treatment of all three sinuses.

TURBINATES

The middle turbinate, like the inferior and superior nasal turbinates, is basically a scroll-like horizontal bony shelf measuring approximately 1.5 inches in length in most adults. The superior turbinate is somewhat shorter, and the inferior slightly longer and usually larger. All of the turbinates, like the rest of the nose and sinus cavities, are covered with a ciliated mucus-secreting membrane, although it is much thicker over the turbinates, usually thinner throughout the rest of the nose, and much thinner within the sinus cavities. Both the middle and superior turbinates protect the sinus drainage openings lying beneath them from the drying, irritating, and contaminating effects of the nasal airstream each time you inhale. The inferior turbinate in turn shelters the drainage opening of the tear duct leading from the eye into the nose.

The posterior ethmoid sinuses (located in the back of the nose), along with the sphenoid sinus on each side, ultimately drain into a small cleftlike pocket called the sphenoethmoidal recess, an area now often referred to as the posterior OMC, located near the posterior end of the superior turbinate and protected to some degree by it. Here infection of a posterior ethmoid sinus may initiate swelling, blockage, and infection of the adjoining sphenoid sinus, and the opposite could also occur, although seemingly less often. About 60 percent of individuals may also have a very small rudimentary supreme turbinate higher up in the nose. Unfortunately, almost any of the sinus drainage openings may become blocked by excessive enlargement or deformity of their protective turbinates and may subsequently require surgical correction. A fairly common deformity of the middle turbinate often responsible for chronic sinus obstruction is called the paradoxical turbinate. This is sometimes noted to curve laterally to crowd or obstruct the sinus openings rather than inward toward the nasal septum as it normally does 85 percent of the time.

The superior and supreme turbinates, like the upper margins of the nasal septum, usually contain some of the olfactory end organs of smell on their medial surfaces, and this should be taken into consideration with certain kinds of septal or superior turbinate surgery. All the turbinates in the nose, and especially the middle ones, play an important role in filtering, warming, and moisturizing inhaled air before it reaches the lungs and also in capturing some of the moisture and warmth from exhaled air to be used again. As the name "turbinate" suggests, part of their function is to cause turbulence in the inhaled air, thus creating more mucous membrane surface contact with the airstream, resulting in a more effective filtering, warming, and moisturizing of the air you breathe.

EPITHELIUM

The membranous lining, or epithelium, of the various sinus cavities is very similar to that lining most of the nose, parts of the nasopharynx and larynx, as well as the trachea and bronchi of the lungs, and to a lesser degree the middle ear and eustachian tubes. This epithelium is endowed for the most part with a large number of microscopic mucus-secreting surface cells called goblet cells, which are especially abundant in the nose, trachea, and bronchi but sometimes less abundant in the sinuses. The epithelium also contains numerous deeper glandular secreting structures, known as seromucinous glands, which produce a thinner mucus and are especially prominent within the turbinates, the nose, and lower respiratory tract but are found in greatly reduced numbers within the sinuses. Whereas the largest sinus, the maxillary, may have fewer than 100 seromucinous glands, one of the larger turbinates in the nose may contain 100 times as many. As would be expected, the nose needs an abundance of mucus-secreting glands to avoid drying out and scabbing with bleeding, whereas the sinuses, with their bodily warmth and highly humidified air, are well protected from the very drying effects of the nasal airstream and can function well with fewer glands and secretions.

In healthy sinuses, these mucus-secreting glands and goblet cells, together with those in the nose, provide a constant flow of clear, clean mucus, amounting to a pint or more per day for most adults. Another pint or more a day is produced by the mucous glands lining the walls of the lower respiratory tract leading from the lungs. Three hundred and fifty years ago, the mucus secreted into the nose and throat was called the pituitary, which comes from the Latin word *pituita*, meaning phlegm or thick mucus secretions. At that time, their source was thought to be the pituitary gland, which we now recognize as one of our very important hormonal glands. A seventeenth-century anatomist named Conrad Victor Schneider corrected this misconception, and for the next several hundred years, the mucus-secreting membranes of the respiratory tract and sinuses were known as the Schneiderian membranes. Now we call them respiratory epithelium.

CILIA

To prevent this clear, healthy mucus from accumulating in our sinuses and respiratory tracts, and in order for them to constantly sweep themselves clean, we have fine microscopic hairs called cilia, which arise from the surface membrane cells of these structures. Cilia are approximately 7 microns in length, and they usually average 30 to 50 on the surface of a single cell, although some immature cells, badly scarred cells, or very old cells may have very few or none at all. Cilia are constantly moving back and forth in unison and in a designated direction, usually averaging 10 to 20 full beats per second. Following each beat or sweep, their recovery phase is a bent sideways motion (similar to the feathering of an oar in rowing) so as not to impede the forward flow of mucus. This sweeping action takes place mainly in the inner thinner seromucinous layer, with the pointed tips of the cilia barely brushing the underside of the outer thicker mucous layer so that they can move freely at a very rapid pace and still push the thicker outer layer along. The thicker outer layer of the mucus blanket also helps to protect the thinner inner layer from drying out and stifling cilia sweep.

Their activity may be greatly diminished by inherent abnormalities, by lowered humidity, by any drying out and thickening of the mucous blanket, by cold temperatures, by some acid solutions, by body dehydration, by impaired circulation, by any diminishing of their own cellular metabolism, by cellular aging or immaturity, by tobacco smoke and drug snorting, by glue sniffing, and by inflammation or damage to the epithelial cells from bacterial invasion and scarring as in chronic sinusitis. Their function can also be affected by viruses, by certain bacteria and their toxins, by trauma and irradiation, by prolonged use of irritating nose sprays or certain eyedrops, by exposure to too strong or too weak a salt solution, and by breathing certain chemical compounds, including formaldehyde, ozone, volatile organic compounds (VOCs), and sulfur dioxide or acid rain. Cilia function may also be impaired by certain inherited diseases that cause atypical or irregular movements of the cilia, known as ciliary dyskinesia, as well as by total lack of movement, known as the immotile cilia syndrome. In cystic fibrosis, however, the seemingly inadequate cilia function is mainly the result of their almost futile efforts to propel an abnormally thickened and very sticky mucus, although the usually associated membrane scarring, or fibrosis, from chronic sinusitis and chronic respiratory infections will also impair blood supply and ciliary activity.

The cilia sweep the mucus from the sinuses into the nose and from there through the nose into the back of the throat, where it can be swallowed, usually completing the entire run in less than 30 minutes. Cilia are unique in that their control seems to be entirely within the cell itself and devoid of any central nervous system oversight. They have been shown to beat for 24 to 48 hours after death if they are kept moistened and would appear then to represent the only bodily function still alive. A similar sweeping action propels the mucus from the distant bronchi of the lungs into the trachea, then up through the back of the larynx and into the throat, where it too can be swallowed.

The process of sweeping the nose and sinuses clean will hereafter be referred to as the sinonasal cleansing action, and it is what we try to restore whenever we treat a nasal or sinus infection either medically or surgically. As long as the cleansing action functions well, it will help to protect the entire respiratory tract, as well as the sinuses, from polluted air and even from bacteria, viruses, and fungi in the air you breathe. To take maximum advantage of this air-filtering process, however, you obviously have to breathe through the nose. Even though you don't breathe through the sinuses, if the nose should become grossly contaminated, dried out, swollen, and infected, the sinuses, because of their close proximity to the nose and their need for continuous discharge of their mucous secretions into the nose, will usually become blocked and infected as well.

WHY WE HAVE SINUSES

In answering why we have sinuses, we must consider what useful purposes they may serve and that some reasons for their existence are more relevant than others. It is a question that has been argued for years, and various answers have been offered, including some having to do with evolution. Some say the sinuses are a structural necessity, since solid bone would have made our heads too heavy and put too great a strain on our neck muscles. Having sinus air spaces instead of solid bone does lighten the skull, and for that reason, sinuses would always have been important to some birds and to certain other long-necked creatures. This could also have been important to early humans, who supposedly walked on all fours. Even now, our own maxillary and sphenoid sinuses would drain better if we still walked with our heads tilted downward, since their drainage openings are located well above their cavity floors, and since the floor of the maxillary sinus in the adult also lies below the nasal floor.

The sinuses' built-in capacity to produce a constant flow of warm, well-hydrated, free-flowing, unpolluted, and relatively bacteria-free mucus not only provides a protective coating and a means for cleansing themselves but also contributes close to 10 percent of the protective mucous coating of the nose and throat. In this, their seemingly most important role, the sinuses also provide the nose with a continuous supply of fresh antibodies, immunity-producing proteins, and bacteria-destroying enzymes, all mostly uncompromised by the bacterial contamination constantly experienced by similar secretions within the nose itself. With the aid of this additional supply of mucus from the sinuses, the nose is better able to bathe itself; collect, neutralize, and flush out invading organisms and pollutants; cope with excessive temperature changes; and adjust to fluctuations in environmental humidity. This mucus flow, as it continues from the nose and sinuses into the back of the throat, where it can be swallowed, also serves as a major bulwark in protecting the lower respiratory tract and lungs from inhaled air pollutants as well as the body itself from invasion by airborne diseases. If this protective mucus blanket in the nose should dry up completely, it would be much more difficult to restart the process without the backup and assistance of the free-flowing mucus provided by the sinuses; and any excessive drying up of the mucus in the nose would soon result in scabbing, mucous crusts, bleeding, rhinitis, and, of course, sinusitis.

In discussing the protective role of the sinuses, it should also be mentioned that they, along with the nasal and other facial bones, afford considerable protection to our brains from possible anterior or basilar skull fractures. The ability of these structures to give or crush inward to soften a blow may prevent a skull fracture and greatly reduce the chances of a more serious or sometimes fatal brain injury from a blow to the face. I have thankfully observed this protective mechanism on numerous occasions, and some automobile manufacturers have employed similar ideas with their frame and engine collapse points, thus reducing the force of the blow to the occupants of the car. Even the prominent brow structure over the eyes, accentuated by the large frontal sinuses and especially impressive in early humans, not only protected the brain and eyes from an external blow but also may have improved vision by shading the eyes from the very bright and sometimes damaging rays of the sun.

Another useful purpose provided by the sinuses is to give resonance to the voice. The nose, nasopharynx, throat, lower respiratory tract, and sinuses, all acting as resonating air chambers, provide resonance to our voices, thus improving the sound quality of speech and singing. This is often dramatically demonstrated when you have a very bad cold or an attack of hay fever, and the nose and sinuses are completely blocked. We then say that you sound "nasal," and it is especially noticeable if one or both of the large maxillary sinuses are blocked. Therefore, without the larger sinuses, our speech and singing might lose some of their pleasant and melodious ring. Just how much the sinuses would be missed in this respect is hard to say. Singers and professional speakers do find their tasks made easier by good resonance. Communication among ourselves (as well as between most birds and animals) is often more rewarding for the same reason. Resonance assists in the variations of animal and bird calls, often signifying changes in emotions, such as from fright to contentment. Our own ability to gain attention is definitely enhanced by good resonance in our voices. For the same reason, prolonged sinus blockage from chronic infection, persistent allergies, or recurrent nasal and sinus polyps could mean the downfall of the TV commentator, sports announcer, public speaker, stage actor, and even the minister.

WHAT IS MUCUS, WHAT DOES IT DO, AND WHAT IS POSTNASAL DRIP?

Mucus is a clear, rather slippery, and sometimes sticky fluidlike coating of certain delicate membranes found in nearly every part of the body where there is a tubular structure or opening connecting the inside of the body with the outside world. Mucus is composed of a protein material called mucin, white blood cells, various salts dissolved in water, digestive enzymes, plasma exudate, immunity-producing proteins, antibodies, dead tissue cells, cellular debris, bacteria and other organisms, as well as many foreign pollutants; and like the rest of the body, it is mostly water. Since its main purpose is to form a moist protective coating to underlying membranes, its salt concentration must resemble that of body tissue fluid so as not to irritate and inflame the delicate tissues beneath it. This always presents a good argument for using manufactured and specifically formulated saline nose drops and sprays rather than mixing your own salt solution, which may irritate the tissue of your nose.

We recognize normal mucus as saliva, drool, spit, or the clear discharge we blow into a handkerchief. It coats the entire alimentary canal from the mouth to the rectum, the entire respiratory tract from the nose and sinuses to the lungs, and the genitourinary tract from the kidneys to the organs of reproduction. Mucus even coats a few side tracts of these channels to the outside world, such as the eustachian tubes draining from the ears into the nasopharynx, the tear ducts entering the nose, and the saliva ducts emptying into the mouth. It provides a continuous coating to all of these areas and helps to keep them moistened, healthy, and protected. Mucus even plays a significant role in reproduction by maintaining a moist, free-flowing surface to hasten the sperm through various body tubes and ducts to its anticipated union with the ovum. Once the egg is fertilized, mucus also provides it with a slippery passage down the oviduct to the womb. It likewise helps to protect the developing fetus from any bacterial, viral, and fungal intrusions from the vagina by creating a cervical mucous plug, which usually remains in place until just before delivery.

Within the GI tract, mucus adheres to the walls and coats food particles, affording them a slicker surface and easier passage as well as protecting the walls from injury by any coarse food or foreign material. Along with the pancreatic secretions, mucus also acts as a protective buffer to neutralize food and stomach acid.

Mucus secretions within the body are affected by local stimulation and trauma, by release of histamine, by diseases and congenital abnormalities, by nerve impulses, by body hydration, by temperature and humidity, by adequacy or inadequacy of local circulation, by chemical irritants and pollution, by infections and allergies, by hormonal activity, and even by various local and systemic medications.

The mucous membranes of the respiratory tract and sinuses are constantly fed by millions of microscopic mucus-secreting glands on or just beneath their surfaces. To prevent stagnation or pooling, which can lead to bacterial overgrowth, these mucous secretions are constantly moved along by the sweeping effect of the fine microscopic hairs called cilia. Any slowing down of this mucous flow allows bacteria and viruses a greater opportunity to attach themselves to the underlying membranes and to penetrate their linings. Some bacteria even have special hairlike projections, or pili (from the Latin word for hair), by which they attach themselves to healthy respiratory membranes once the bacteria penetrate a slow-moving, defective, or dried-out protective mucous blanket. A good analogy for the need to maintain this healthy mucus flow from the sinuses into the nose and down the throat is a stream flowing down a mountain: As long as that stream flows freely, it usually remains clean and clear, but if you dam it up, it may quickly become murky and contaminated.

In some of the other areas of the body, mucus flow may be further aided by peristalsis, by the pull of gravity, by cohesion (or sticking together), and sometimes simply by the accompaniment of liquids and solids passing through the body's tubelike structures. Mucus does for most of these body parts what a very fine oil does for a machine; the main difference is that mucus has a very high water content (96 percent), and whenever it begins to dry out, it tends to lose some of its slippery nature, becomes very sticky, doesn't flow well, may become contaminated by bacterial growth and dead cells to turn cloudy, and may even form crusts or scabs, especially in the nose. This only emphasizes the point that mucus must be kept well moistened to do its job. If you have ever tried to remove spittle, saliva, expectorant, or ordinary spit from a sink, basin, floor, or deck after it has dried, you know that it can be almost like hardened glue. Some of the rather annoying problems of old age are no doubt related in part to the diminution in the amount and quality of the body's free-flowing mucus, including dry mouth, dry eyes, occasional difficulty swallowing, and constipation.

The respiratory tract and sinuses contain several different kinds of microscopic mucus-secreting structures. Some lie beneath the surface and are known as the seromucinous glands. They secrete a thin watery serous liquid. Others, known as goblet cells, are located on the surface and produce a thicker mucous covering. This thicker outer layer picks up a large part of our inhaled particle matter, viruses, and bacteria, including any infected sinonasal discharge, and moves it all along on the surface of the inner thinner layer very much like debris floating down a stream. The seromucinous glands that are mainly responsible for the inner thinner layer are plentiful in the trachea, larger bronchi, nose, and especially the turbinates but are somewhat diminished in the thinner and more delicate mucous membranes of the sinuses. Their seromucinous-secreting cells are surrounded by contractile tissue that squeezes their secretions through very small ducts to coat the surface membranes of the nose, sinuses, and lower respiratory tract. Some believe that these cells can even vary their mixtures of serum and mucin, thereby making their secretions thicker or thinner. These glands are microscopic in size and are occasionally referred to as secondary salivary glands, structurally resembling the large saliva glands that drain into the mouth.

Unfortunately, these secondary salivary, or seromucinous, glands may sometimes cause an annoying condition in older people in which the taste or smell of food, or even just the anticipation of food at mealtime, may cause a clear very thin watery nasal discharge to run down the upper lip. This is sometimes referred to as the nasogustatory reflex, and it can at times be very embarrassing. A mucus-drying medication such as a short-acting antihistamine or a mucus-drying nasal spray such as ipratropium bromide preferably administered at least 30 to 40 minutes before mealtime may sometimes help. If drowsiness from taking an antihistamine is a problem, then you should only use the nasal spray, unless you are allergic to atropine or its related products. When spraying the nose, always take great care to avoid spraying the eyes. Also, nasal spray should be used with caution if you have certain types of glaucoma, or prostate and urinary problems. Inhaling cold air or consuming certain hot spicy foods, especially those containing capsaicin, may also produce an excessive and sometimes embarrassing clear watery discharge from the nose, even in younger individuals.

The sinonasal mucous glands also tend to secrete excessively in the first few days of a cold, probably partly because of viral irritation and tissue trauma with the release of histamine as well as other mediators, and partly as an effort by the body to wash away a harmful substance. For this reason, you should generally avoid medications that would tend to dry mucus secretions up. In such instances, it is often wiser to keep the nasal passages open with a decongestant and allow the excess mucous secretions to drain down the throat.

The mucus-secreting goblet cells are also very plentiful throughout the upper and lower respiratory tracts but are likewise noted to a lesser degree within the sinuses, often appearing more numerous near their drainage openings. Together, these mucus-secreting structures form a double-layered mucous blanket, or protective covering, to the respiratory tract and sinuses, with the heavier thicker secretions on the surface and the thinner serous secretions beneath. Located within this thinner inner layer are millions of microscopic hairs called cilia, which sweep back and forth on the average of 10 to 20 complete beats per second, pulling and pushing the mucous blanket along its way with their sharp clawlike tips. In doing so, the cilia can clear all the sinuses of their mucous secretions in less than 10 minutes and then propel the entire sinonasal mucous contents of the nose into the throat in 20 to 30 minutes at an average speed of about 1 inch every 2 to 3 minutes.

Although this mucous flow may take a somewhat circuitous route within the nose and sinuses themselves, especially in the frontal sinuses, where the flow is often upward across the roof and down, the general direction is from the sinus cavities toward their natural drainage openings into the nose and from the front part of the nose to the back, with the principal nasal flow there concentrated along the three main routes leading past the sinus openings themselves. In instances where there is more than one drainage opening from a maxillary sinus into the nose, either naturally or as a result of infection or surgery, mucus may recirculate out of one opening and back into the sinus through the same opening or through another, sometimes causing mucous stasis with a persistent sinus infection. Another exception to the usual posterior flow of mucus within the nose is a small area in the front of the nose on both sides of the nasal septum where the cilia sweep and mucous flow is forward toward the nasal openings possibly to barricade and neutralize contamination there. Because of this reversal of mucous flow just within the nostrils, plus the snaring of dust particles there by the nasal hairs, or vibrissae, scabs and crusts tend to form in this area, and attempts to remove them may sometimes result in avulsion of hairs, occasionally followed by a very serious and dangerous infection, since part of the venous blood flow from this area is toward the brain.

The mucous secretions of the nose, sinuses, and nasopharynx, as well as those of the larynx, trachea, bronchi, and lungs, contain various substances that are capable of inhibiting or destroying bacteria and viruses. Some are specific antibodies for viruses as well as for certain bacteria, especially *Streptococcus, Staphylococcus, M. catarrhalis,* and *H. influenzae,* any of which may frequent the respiratory tract, ears, and sinuses. These antibodies, which are also called immunoglobulins, are produced mainly by the immune system's B cells with the help of cytokines and other mediators. Some are produced locally by the respiratory and sinus membranes themselves, and some may reach the areas and their mucous secretions through the circulating blood.

Other bacterial and viral inhibitors in mucus include various white blood cells, including the now well-known T cells, which play such an important role in HIV infection, as well as certain proteolytic or protein-destroying enzymes, and especially one called lysozyme or muramidase, which is capable of eliminating bacteria by digesting their walls and can even attack a fungus such as Candida. Another antibacterial substance found in the mucous secretions of the sinuses is salivary nitrite. It is converted to nitric oxide, a powerful antimicrobial agent, which also acts as a vasodilator and a messenger in nerve transmissions. In addition to being found in the respiratory tract, nitric oxide has also been demonstrated in the salivary secretions of the mouth, where it is credited with the healing successes of wound licking in both animals and humans. Fiji Islanders are said to allow their dogs to lick their wounds to reduce bacterial contamination and to promote healing. An antiviral substance known as interferon is also present in sinonasal mucous secretions and is especially prevalent during viral respiratory infections.

Studies have shown that when you bring a contagious respiratory virus into a household, the virus can be found in the nose and throat of most, if not all, of the occupants. However, the virus still may not clinically infect anyone else, thanks to this protective mucous blanket, its viral inhibitors, and the antibody response of the individual. A similar protection is afforded the sinuses and respiratory tract from most bacterial and fungal infections, which are usually much less contagious than respiratory viruses, often requiring a more prolonged or more intimate exposure, as well as the presence of some already existing membrane irritation or damage, such as may follow an allergic or nonallergic rhinitis or a viral respiratory infection such as a cold or flu. On entering the nasal airway, most of these microorganisms become ensnared in the mucus, coated with its sticky material, neutralized by antibodies, and their walls dissolved by enzymes. Those that escape are swept down the throat to their doom in the waiting stomach acid, with the mucus bathing the tissues as it moves along. For those organisms and fine pollution particles that happen to travel through the nose in the center of the airstream, undeflected by the turbinates, and eventually reaching the lower respiratory tract or lungs, a similar sweeping action and elimination process takes place, mainly from within the trachea and bronchi.

However, if your body's immune defenses are depressed because of insufficient antibodies, which can occur if you haven't had flu or pneumonia shots; if there is damage to the respiratory membranes or breaks in their protective mucous blanket from injuries such as finger trauma, from a virus such as a cold or flu, from drying out or from exposure to cold, as well as from breathing membrane-irritating allergens, chemicals, sprays, or pollutants; if there is inadequate production of healthy mucous secretions due to chronic infection, dehydration, diminished circulation, scarring, or improper mucus formation due to a disease such as cystic fibrosis or Sjögren's syndrome;

if there is insufficient cilia movement from breathing cigarette smoke or inhaling certain pollutants, from physical or chemical injury, from allergic rhinitis or chronic sinusitis, from radiation damage or impaired circulation, from sniffing drugs, or from certain illnesses; or if the invaders are particularly powerful and attack in overwhelming numbers, then these body defenses may be breached and the disease contracted.

Although the nose provides slightly better than 90 percent of the mucus needed to protect the upper respiratory tract, the sinuses, by providing the other 8 to 10 percent, offer the nose a fresh, continuous supply of relatively uncontaminated mucus, well hydrated and warmed to body temperature, also containing additional immunity-producing proteins and bacteria-dissolving enzymes, all untested and ready to join the fray. With the entire mucous contents of the nose being swept away into the throat every 20 to 30 minutes, it's no wonder that the nose needs all the additional mucus it can obtain from the sinuses. Here the sinuses act very much like underground springs supplying a pond. The pond can't dry up completely because of the continuous flow from the well-protected springs deep beneath its surface. This sinus mucus, also having been warmed to body temperature, on reaching the drier and often cooler nose, helps to maintain a more active mucociliary flow on the nasal side of the sinus drainage openings, especially in cold weather, when the nasal mucociliary flow within the front part of the nose may tend to slow down.

A successful breach of these body defenses by an invading head cold or flu virus often temporarily destroys up to 90 percent of the ciliated hair cells within a fairly large portion of the respiratory tract, thereby stopping or greatly reducing the mucus-sweeping action and causing temporary stasis, or stagnation, of the mucous flow. This provides an open invitation for the ever present bacteria in the nose to invade these viral-damaged membranes and to multiply. By the third or fourth day following the onset of the head cold or flu, the sinonasal discharge will usually have turned cloudy, often indicating the beginning of a bacterial rhinosinusitis. Fortunately for us, with most of these viral respiratory infections, the damaged or destroyed ciliated hair cells will begin to regenerate in just a few days and gradually resume their coordinated sweeping action even in the presence of the thickest and most profuse infected cloudy discharge or pus. If the infection is not overwhelming—if the body resistance is adequate and the sinus openings are not completely obstructed—then the healing process will usually proceed on its own with little or no outside help, and the membranes will be restored to their relatively normal state within 10 days to two weeks. However, patchy, raw areas, especially in the larynx, trachea, or bronchi, that may be slow to heal are often responsible for a lingering cough, which usually won't go away until these areas are completely healed and again covered with ciliated cells as well as the protective mucous blanket. Just the passage of air over these raw exposed areas when breathing is often enough to initiate a cough.

POSTNASAL DRIP

Since the flow of mucus from the nose and sinuses amounts to a pint or more every 24 hours, and possibly 2 pints or more at various times in some allergic individuals, you must realize that all of us have post-nasal drips. Fortunately, most of the time, we are unaware of this small river flowing down the back of our throats. It may only become obvious and annoying when your throat is very dry from prolonged mouth breathing; body dehydration; lowered environmental humidity; working, living, or sleeping in a cold or overheated area; or continuous mouth breathing with vigorous exercise, excessive talking, or singing. Anything contributing to nasal blockage, such as irritating pollutants, head colds, sinus infection, polyps, nasal packing, septal deviations, congenital abnormalities, enlarged turbinates, trauma, growths, and nasal allergies, may also cause prolonged mouth breathing, especially at night, and further aggravate the problem. You may not realize it, but when you sing or talk continuously, you must breathe through your mouth to obtain enough oxygen. Consequently, your throat tends to dry out, and you feel the need for a drink of water. A similar problem occurs with the elderly, especially when they sleep on their backs and their sagging jaw muscles allow their chins to drop. They may then breathe through their mouths all night and often awaken with a very dry throat. The diminished salivary secretions normally occurring during sleep, as well as those developing with age, will usually exacerbate the problem.

Under most of these circumstances, you may at any time become aware of your normal postnasal drip from a glob of rather sticky mucus trying to work its way along a temporarily dried-out membrane in the back of your throat so that it may be swallowed. Unfortunately, in the back of the throat, there are no cilia to propel the mucus along, so we have to depend on gravity, the swallow reflex, the curling back of the tongue, and the peristalsis-like action of the lower throat, along with the squeezing down or milking effect of the soft palate and uvula to accomplish this. To dispose of this mucus constantly collecting in the throat, you normally swallow approximately every 30 to 40 seconds when awake and, as would be expected, less often when asleep and much less often in deep sleep or in a very weakened condition. It was the accumulation and gurgling of this thick mucus in the throat and larynx of a dying patient, usually dehydrated and too weak to swallow, that years ago was referred to as the "death rattle" and was often considered to signal impending doom.

The drying out of mucus in even a small area of the throat can make the flow more difficult, since it interrupts its cohesive action as a single unit, namely, when the flowing mucus in front tries to pull the dry, sticky mucus from behind along with it. For people who have very sensitive throats, an awareness of this thickened mucus collecting there may make them gag repeatedly and even vomit in an effort to disrupt the sensation of something caught in the throat. Often it is a reflex that can't be controlled. It may be especially noticeable on awakening in the morning and can be helped immediately by repeatedly sipping water, trying to avoid gagging, using a manufactured saline nasal spray or drops, improving nasal breathing by the upright position or sometimes by temporarily using a nasal decongestant spray at night, especially with a cold, as well as ingesting a cup of hot coffee, juice, or food to increase the flow of saliva first thing in the morning. Also, if you normally get up frequently during the night, taking a sip of water each time should reduce and help prevent dryness in the throat. The most important thing is to understand what a postnasal drip really is, to know that the unpleasant sensation in your throat will usually correct itself shortly, and to try to ignore it. The next most important thing is to observe the character of this mucous drainage from the nose and throat. If it is cloudy, it nearly always means sinusitis and therefore should be treated until it becomes clear and stays clear. Again, it is very important to realize that normal mucus is perfectly clear, although some may describe it as foamy and grayish in appearance, whereas infected mucus is cloudy and may vary in color from yellow to green to milky white with various shades in between. Even mucus that appears to be a very pale white, resembling skim milk, should be considered infected. Repeated gagging or vomiting even when a postnasal drip is perfectly clear can irritate the throat and make matters progressively worse. Repeated efforts to clear the throat of mucus can also become a habit and may be particularly disturbing to those around you. When postnasal drip is very troublesome, preventative measures such as drinking more water during the day and adding humidity, preferably hot steam, to the bedroom environment at night, especially in dry, cold weather, will help to keep the throat membranes moist and less sensitive to the mucous flow. Avoiding the draft from an air conditioner, heating duct, or fan, as well as too cold a temperature in the bedroom at night, will help in keeping the membranes moist and the mucus flowing freely.

As previously noted, the nose is your own built-in humidifier. When you breathe through it, and only then, you add a pint or more of moisture to the air you breathe every 24 hours. Therefore, for anyone who regularly experiences nighttime nasal blockage and a dry throat, sleeping elevated on a 7-inch foam wedge with a pillow on top of that should improve nasal breathing and thereby add moisture to the throat and lungs. Sleeping in this position will also lessen gastroesophagial reflux (GER) if you have that problem as well. Sleeping only on an extra pillow or two is usually not adequate to keep the nose open, since a pillow doesn't elevate the chest along with the head. It may also cause too much neck flexion, and you may develop some neck discomfort later. Decongestant pills and decongestant sprays sometimes tend to dry the throat out, but by permitting better nasal breathing with occasional usage, they may indirectly provide additional moisture. The same is true for nasal blockage from allergic rhinitis, where the use of a steroid nasal spray, sometimes along with an antihistamine, should diminish the allergic response and thereby improve nasal breathing with a resulting increase in respiratory humidification. It should be emphasized again, however, that antihistamines, especially the conventional sedating kind, when used for more than a very short period may dry out mucous secretions and respiratory membranes, which could unfortunately be detrimental to the sinus or lung patient. Antihistamines will not reduce nasal swelling, but steroid nasal sprays can, although they may take a few days to accomplish it.

If you experience nasal blockage at night followed by a dry throat and a subsequent awareness of a postnasal drip on awakening, following some of these suggestions should help to keep the throat and its mucous blanket moist and free-flowing, often with a reduced or totally absent awareness of any postnasal drip.

Again, it should be emphasized that everyone has a postnasal drip amounting to a pint or more of mucus every 24 hours, but to be normal, the mucus should be clear. If it is cloudy white, yellow, green, tan, or dark grayish—in other words, not clear or transparent but fairly opaque—it is an infected postnasal drip, and this nearly always means sinusitis. Except for some chronic mouth breathers and a few individuals who have very sensitive throats, most people are generally unaware of having constant postnasal drips, even when infected. You may only notice it when your throat is very dry, and then usually as a result of nasal blockage, dehydration, low humidity, or excessive mouth breathing.

HOW DO THE NOSE AND SINUSES WORK TOGETHER, AND HOW DO THEY RELATE TO OUR LUNGS?

The sinuses as well as the entire respiratory tract from the nose to the lungs are very closely related, especially when it comes to an infectious or allergic process. To begin with, they all have the same type of membranous lining, known as respiratory epithelium, which constantly secretes mucus and is consistently swept clean by microscopic hairs called cilia. This continuous flow of mucus from the sinuses, nose, and lungs eventually reaches the lower throat, where the mucus is regularly swallowed and, together with its many respiratory contaminants, finally ends up in the stomach. A viral respiratory infection such as a head cold or flu can involve all three areas, and a bacterial infection, if it lasts long enough, nearly always will. Most patients with chronic lung infections will eventually develop chronic sinusitis, and most chronic sinusitis patients will usually develop chronic bronchitis. All three areas may also interact in an allergic way with an allergic rhinitis attack involving the nose and sinuses and an asthmatic attack involving the bronchi and lungs, and both can occur at the same time from the same exposure to the same allergen.

The nose, sinuses, and lungs are further connected with each other by nerve reflex arcs that pass through the brain. Through them, a stimulus in one side of the nose may cause swelling and blockage on the opposite side through the nasonasal reflex. Moreover, a stimulus to the inside wall of a maxillary sinus can cause swelling of the nasal turbinates on the same side, presumably due to a sinonasal reflex. I have also seen sudden blockage of a maxillary sinus due to flying or diving, or from a drop in barometric pressure due to an approaching storm, cause rapid congestion of the nose on the same side. A stimulus in the nose or sinuses may also cause bronchial constriction with asthmatic wheezing and coughing, presumably through the rhinosinobronchial reflex. This particular nerve reflex may also be a factor in some people who have acute frontal sinusitis and subsequently develop rather severe asthma for the first time, as well as in the sometimes complete relief of wheezing experienced by some asthmatic patients on clearing up their obstructive sinusitis.

Since the rhinosinobronchial reflex is considered to have a cardiac component as well, it has occasionally been blamed for the sudden death of glue sniffers and possibly for an occasional case of sudden infant death syndrome (SIDS). Also suspected of acting through the rhinosinobronchial reflex is the diver's immersion, or drowning, reflex, sometimes referred to as the mammalian diving reflex. Immersion of the head beneath the surface, especially of cold water, may cause an immediate cessation of breathing with closing of the larynx to prevent aspiration, bronchial constriction, a slowing of the heart rate, and a contraction of the peripheral arteries with an increase in arterial blood flow to the brain. This nerve reflex can be of considerable help to deep divers and is credited with preventing many near drownings, especially in small children.

Various theories have been advanced in an effort also to explain the reflex swelling and blockage of the nose often noted in the recumbent, or lying down, position, especially the tendency for it to be much worse on the down side next to the pillow. A change of position by rolling to the opposite side during the night will usually cause a reversal of this nasal swelling and sinus blockage in the normally unobstructed nose. The longer you remain on one side, however, the more persistent the nasal and sinus blockage will be, and the longer it will take for that side to open up following a change of the sleeping position. People who have wide-open nasal passages may be totally unaware of this positional effect. However, if you have an existing partial nasal obstruction of one or both sides due to a septal deviation, an infected sinus discharge, an enlarged turbinate, allergic rhinitis, or nasal polyp formation, you may become very much aware of this phenomenon, since lying down and any change of position during the night will cause additional swelling with further airway blockage, possibly aggravating a sinus problem as well. Often this condition will subconsciously dictate which side you choose to sleep on for easier breathing, less snoring, and a more comfortable night. After going through a careful nasal examination, some people are often very surprised to learn from the doctor which side they prefer for sleeping.

Several factors play a role in this nose and sinus swelling when lying down, especially for the increased swelling noted on the dependent, or down, side. One is apparently due to a fast component, and the other has a much slower and more sustained response. The fast component, sometimes apparent within a minute or two of rolling onto one's side, is generally considered to be the result of a nerve reflex supposedly initiated by pressure stimulation of skin receptors from the weight of the body parts, especially the chest, hip, and shoulder, against the bedding. However, proof of this reflex has not always been entirely consistent. Such a rapid response would strongly indicate a nerve reflex, but one has to wonder why it is not carried out within the respiratory system itself by the restriction placed on the down side of the chest or rib cage, resulting in limited bronchial and lung expansion of that side during inhalation. This could then conceivably cause a reflex blockage of the nose on the same side through the bronchonasal reflex.

The slow component in the nasal swelling resulting from the lying down position, especially when you are lying on your side, takes a while longer to develop and may require several hours, rather than seconds or minutes, to disappear when you change position. This prolonged swelling and blockage, which very likely plays a role in early-morning ethmoid sinus congestion and headache, may be initiated by positional reflexes but further sustained throughout the night and into the early-morning hours by the gravitational flow of tissue fluid to the head when you're in the lying down position. This position causes venous congestion in the head with some subsequent swelling of the nasal and sinus membranes. If you lie on your side, this effect will be more pronounced on the down side also because of the gravitational flow of blood and tissue fluid.

Further contributing to this sluggish venous blood flow in the head, nose, and sinuses from the lying down position at night is the resting state of the heart and lungs during sleep, characterized by a diminished pulse, respirations, and blood pressure, as well as the crowding of these intrathoracic structures by the elevated diaphragms from upward shifting of the abdominal contents. Added to this is the downside splinting or limited expansion of the rib cage with further compression of the chest and lungs on that side. If you are a sinus patient or are troubled by nasal congestion with early-morning headaches, improving this flow of venous blood from the head back to the heart by sleeping elevated on a 7-inch wedge with a pillow on top of that can usually make a significant difference and is often worth trying. This means elevating the upper body as well as the head, which cannot be accomplished very effectively by sleeping on just an extra pillow or two.

When you are lying on your side, the 12 intercostal nerves running along the ribs of the down-side splinted chest wall and supplying the skin of the chest, abdomen, buttocks, armpit, and shoulder on that side, as well as the abdominal and rib muscles, could conceivably serve as nerve relay stations between skin pressure stimulation and the lung or bronchi on that side and could very well initiate the reflex nasal swelling directly through the bronchonasal reflex. Supporting this is the finding that blocking the intercostal nerves with an anesthetic injection can interrupt the nasal response to the lateral body pressure stimulus, but anesthesia of the skin does not. Of special interest to some may be the finding that the pressure of a crutch in an armpit can cause congestion of the nose on the same side as well.

THE NASAL CYCLE

This swelling and congestion of the nose, normally caused by the lying down or side position, if sustained, may tend to override the spontaneous alternating nasal congestion and decongestion (known as the nasal cycle) occurring every few hours in most people. This cycle may often go unnoticed as well. It, too, depends on the alternating constriction and dilation, or engorgement, of special blood vessels called venous sinusoids located in the nasal membranes, turbinates, and especially the erectile tissue in the front of the nose. Most people are totally unaware of this phenomenon, especially if you have normal unobstructed nasal air passages. Since the nasal cycle does move back and forth from one side of the nose to the other, a permanently narrowed nasal passage on one side may call attention to it. This cycle is unaffected by sleep or by occluding both nostrils but may be suppressed or modified by certain superimposed changes in the nasal airway such as sleeping on your side or by using a decongestant nasal spray. Even though the cycle seems to be tied to our biological rhythms, no one is really certain as to what useful purpose it may serve. During this nasal cycle, when one side of the nose decongests, there is usually an increase in nasal secretions, especially from the turbinates, on that side, which in some instances of excessive nasal dryness might be beneficial. There is no evidence to date that the nasal cycle plays any role in the rebound swelling of the nose sometimes noted from the use of decongestant nasal sprays.

To understand how the nose and sinuses work together, we must be aware of the many functions performed by this rather specialized organ called the nose and how it relates to the body's health as well as to our enjoyment of life.

TASTE AND SMELL

First of all, we know that the nose houses one of the five sense organs of the body, namely, the sense of smell. When a wine expert sniffs the cork or glass of wine before finally tasting it, he or she does so because the sense of smell is far more discerning than the sense of taste, which can tell us only four things: whether something is bitter, sweet, salty, or sour. Your sense of smell, by complementing your sense of taste, will usually tell you whether you are eating broccoli, cauliflower, chicken, turkey, or fish, and many times even what kind of fish. The well-known Pepsi ad in which the blind piano player can supposedly tell that he is drinking Pepsi and not Coca-Cola would be no thanks to his sense of taste, which can tell him only that both drinks are sweet, but rather to his more discerning sense of smell.

Since the sensory end organs of smell are located in the vault, or top, of the nose, any temporary swelling in that area from a bad cold, a flare-up of sinusitis, or an attack of hay fever may temporarily block your appreciation of food as well as your perception of any good and bad odors in the environment. People who have completely lost their sense of smell from a head injury, skull fracture, nasal polyps, nasal medications, brain injury, viral infections, the aging process, chronic sinusitis, allergic rhinitis, caustic inhalations, tumors, or in some cases extensive nose and sinus surgery can of course be in mortal danger from fire, smoke, or gas leaks. Animals in the wild that lose the sense of smell will not survive very long, since they depend on it for finding safe food and avoiding predators. The taste buds on the tongue will not even warn a scavenger that has lost the sense of smell that food is spoiled, rotten, or deadly even after chewing and swallowing it. The stomach may sometimes be more revealing by rejecting spoiled food. During our lifetime, by using our sense of smell and our brain, we learn to distinguish and to memorize many different odors and what they mean, and even to separate the pleasant from the unpleasant, the mild from the strong, and sometimes even the safe from the toxic.

The diminishing sense of smell brings many older people (more men than women) to the physician's office complaining that their sense of taste has gone or that things don't taste the same anymore. Some say that they have to add more and more seasoning to their food to appreciate it at all. Heavy seasoning with garlic, onion, chives, chili, pepper, and salt does make you more aware of food but also alters the food's taste—or, more significantly, its smell—from the way your brain remembers it, and therefore the food will not taste the same. The heavy use of salt (which has no smell) may stimulate your 2,000 to 5,000 taste buds—but only for the appreciation of salt. For older people, it's mainly the sense of smell that has deteriorated, and that is what they miss the most.

By being more aware of this highly specialized function of the upper nose that is so often taken for granted, you should realize how important it is to have an open nasal passage all the way up to the nasal vault, and to be able to breathe through it, unobstructed by swelling or blockage, if you are to fully use your sense of smell and fully appreciate your sense of taste. Another good thing to remember is that chewing food slowly and thoroughly will release more food aromas into this open area of the nose, often enhancing your sense of smell, as well as making your food more enjoyable.

MOUTH BREATHING
The nose is also the premier upper air passage. From the time you are born, you are programmed to breathe through the nose and not through the mouth. When it comes to breathing, the mouth is more of a safety valve, mainly to be used when the nose is blocked or when you cannot obtain enough air through the nose, as when vigorously exercising, talking constantly, or singing. A few individuals without nasal blockage may constantly breathe through their mouths because their teeth and jaw structures are so arranged that the relaxed position of their mouths is open and with the lips parted. However, even some people who have all the appearances of mouth breathers may still continue to breathe almost entirely through the nose. Mouth breathing, as well as snoring, is more common in males than in females.

THE INFANT AIRWAY
Unfortunately, most newborn babies have serious difficulty breathing through their mouths during the first four to six weeks of life. Some may even asphyxiate if both nasal passages are totally blocked even for a very short period. Asphyxiation may also occur at birth or very shortly thereafter from a congenital bony or membranous partition across the back of the nose known as a choanal atresia, or sometimes from the presence of large bilateral congenital tear duct cysts in the nose. Momentary obstruction of the nose at birth may occur from a

large plug of the newborn's own intestinal discharge, known as meconium. However, this can usually be suctioned away immediately, but large congenital cysts or a partition completely sealing off the back of the nose would have to be surgically removed or perforated, usually on an emergency basis, for the infant to survive. It could be very serious indeed for any parent to assume that a newborn infant can just as easily breathe through the mouth if the nasal airway should become totally blocked. An infant also needs an adequate nasal airway to nurse or to take a bottle properly, and any obvious difficulty in doing so could be a warning of a nasal obstructive problem. It's no easy task even for the older infant to breathe through the mouth and suck at the same time, so an adequate nasal airway is essential for proper breast or bottle feeding.

Some blockage of, or resistance to, nasal airflow, especially in the front of the nose, or valve area, is important to the proper exchange of oxygen and carbon dioxide in the tiny air sacs of the lungs. Approximately 50 percent of this needed resistance to airflow to the lungs is caused by the narrowing in the nose, and the rest is due to the very narrow larynx, the trachea, and the tapered bronchi. However, a continuous upper-airway obstruction, as sometimes noted with very large tonsils or adenoids, large nasal polyps, severe rhinitis, cysts, or other congenital abnormalities, may depress the lungs' ventilating capacities and lead to chronic cardiopulmonary problems, particularly right-sided heart enlargement, especially in a child.

FILTERING, WARMING, AND MOISTENING

The nose, as the premier upper airway, also becomes the main portal of entry to the lower respiratory tract and lungs for air pollutants, noxious gases, bacteria, fungi, and viruses, including those related to head colds and flu. Even some of the more deadly viruses that cause polio, herpes, rabies, and encephalitis may enter the brain through the exposed nerve endings of the sense of smell in the top of the nose. The lungs, on the other hand, are two of the body's most vital structures. They need to work constantly and for a very long time, so they must be protected not only from airborne infectious invaders and pollutants but also from very dry or very cold air. To accomplish this, the nose has the ability not only to filter the air you breathe but to moisten and warm it as well. The filtering process, which can be a very important function in a badly polluted environment, begins in the front of the nose with the coarse hairs, called vibrissae, just inside the nostrils. Any coarse particles that we breathe may collect in these hairs along with dried mucous secretions and be blown or sneezed out.

THE SNEEZE REFLEX

This again emphasizes the sneeze reflex as an important respiratory protective mechanism for all of us, and especially for those who work in heavy dust or for children who enjoy putting things in their noses. Even animals that root and grub in the ground need to snort and sneeze to clear their nasal passages as well as their sinus openings of dirt and mud. Some monkeys have learned to tickle their nostrils with a twig or straw to evoke a sneeze, thereby relieving nasal blockage and temporarily improving their sense of smell. The sneeze reflex is a good example of how a stimulus in the nose can initiate an explosive response from the lower respiratory tract and thoracic cage, and at the same time can retract the palate and uvula for a sudden rapid expulsion of lung air through the nose. By contrast, the explosive burst of the cough reflex is usually initiated by stimuli in the lower respiratory tract, followed by closure of the palate opening and expulsion of air, including any foreign matter, in this case through the mouth.

It has been variously estimated that vigorous sniffing or blowing can move air through the nose at greater than hurricane force, especially through the narrow valvular area in the front of the nose, which is also an area of major resistance to airflow. A sneeze, on the other hand, may expel a mucous droplet from the nose at the speed of a bullet, and a sudden cough may eject foreign matter or vapor droplets at close to 100 miles per hour. In all such expulsive acts by the body, including crying, laughing, vomiting, urinating, defecating, and giving birth, a sudden deep inspiration immediately followed by a vigorous contraction of the muscles of the chest wall, abdomen, larynx, throat, and sometimes the palate is usually required.

If you suffer from allergies, you are usually well acquainted with the sneeze reflex, since it may sometimes reduce your nasal contamination from pollen and other inhaled allergens. If inhaled dust, molds, pollen, bacteria, fungi, viruses, or any other particle pollutants are successful in bypassing the vibrissae, or nasal hairs, in the front of the nose and manage to avoid the sneeze reflex as well, most of them, especially the larger particles, will then become entangled in the protective mucous blanket. Mucus coats the entire membranous lining of the nose, as well as that of the sinuses and lower respiratory tract, and is constantly swept along by the cilia into the back of the nose and throat, where the mucus is swallowed. Some of the very fine particle pollutants or microorganisms traveling in the center of the airstream that manage to avoid being caught by the protective mucous blanket of the nose, as well as some that enter through the mouths of chronic mouth breathers and likewise avoid capture, may subsequently be caught up in another cilia-propelled blanket of mucus moving up from the trachea, bronchi, and lungs and into the throat, where it too may be swallowed along with its contaminants. Some very fine particle matter will always make it through all of this to the very smallest bronchi or bronchioles of the lungs, where cilia and mucous glands are lacking, but a simulated peristaltic action there or sometimes just a good cough will usually expel these particles forward into the nearest mucous flow, and thence up from the lungs by the cilia sweep. In such instances, and for obvious reasons, a cough syrup that entirely suppresses a cough for long periods is not always a wise choice.

THE PROTECTIVE MUCOUS BLANKET

All of this mucus from the sinuses, as well as that from the nose and lower respiratory tract, amounting to a quart or more a day, eventually ends up in the stomach, where any microorganisms and particle matter traveling in the mucus can be detoxified or destroyed by the stomach acid and enzymes. The mucous protein itself is continuously digested, absorbed, and in a sense reused by the body to manufacture more mucus. This recycling process replenishes the continuous loss of mucous proteins from millions of mucus-secreting glands and goblet cells lining the membranes of the sinuses, nose, nasopharynx, larynx, trachea, and bronchi, as well as the GI and genitourinary tracts. The protective mucous blanket with its cilia propellants not only sweeps the entire respiratory tract and sinuses clean but also contains antibodies, digestive enzymes, and immunity-producing proteins, capable of destroying or neutralizing certain bacteria and viruses caught up in its flow.

In addition to its efficient filtering and mucus-cleansing action, the nose also provides humidified air to the fragile lung tissues by adding as much as a pint of water a day to the air you breathe. Both heat and moisture are recovered by the nose each time you exhale and are then added to the inspired air with the very next breath, provided of course that you breathe through the nose. With its turbinates and narrow, convoluted spaces, the nose is far better adapted to capturing this heat and moisture, as well as to filtering the inspired air, than one could possibly expect from the mouth or throat. The trachea and bronchi of the lower airway also play a significant role in moisturizing, warming, and filtering the inspired air thanks to their extensive membranous linings and tapered, branching passageways. If you live in a cold climate or work in a cold environment, this warming of the air you breathe can be particularly helpful in protecting the lungs from the shock of suddenly inhaling very cold air, which can cause bronchial spasm with wheezing, especially in an asthmatic as well as in someone with chronic lung disease or with an allergy to cold. Cold air can also thicken mucus and reduce cilia activity, thereby interfering with the normal flow of mucus within the respiratory tract. Mouth breathing will provide some warming and some humidifying and filtering of the air, but not nearly so effectively as nasal breathing.

THE FIRST LINE OF DEFENSE

Since the nose is the bulwark and first line of defense for the respiratory tract and lungs, it receives its share of punishment. On cold days, since cold air doesn't hold much moisture, the mucous membrane lining of the nose tends to dry out, sometimes forming crusts or scabs and occasionally bleeding. It is also frequently exposed to many irritating substances in the air you breathe, including a variety of potential allergens, viruses, bacteria, irritating chemical dusts, vapors, and fungi or molds. To counter this drying out of mucus, as well as to dilute and sweep away all kinds of air-polluting irritants, particularly from the areas of the sinus openings, the nose needs the additional help of the warmed, free-flowing mucus supplied by the sinuses. Many of the nasal mucus-secreting glands are incorporated into the turbinates, which consist of very vascular soft tissue draped in three longitudinal folds over the three horizontal bony ridges within each nasal passage. The turbinates, as well as certain erectile tissues in the front of the nose, may swell and contract in response to various stimuli such as breathing cold air, allergens, polluting irritants, nose sprays, emotional disturbances, exercising, stress, breath holding, psychic stimuli, and hyperventilating may cause either a narrowing or an enlargement of the nasal passages.

It was recognized years ago that placing your feet in cold water or cooling them down by getting them wet would cause a significant drop in nasal temperature from reflex blood vessel constriction within the nasal membranes and erectile tissue. At first, this causes the nasal breathing passages to open up, but they may then become congested and tend to block up, especially if you enter a warm environment such as the home. This subsequent congestion of the nose may have given rise to the old idea that wet feet cause a head cold; and they still might, if the impaired circulation in the nose persists long enough, but only if the cold virus is present in sufficient numbers and has ample opportunity to invade the protective mucous blanket and underlying nasal membrane. Exercise or decongestants are also very effective in opening up the nose, and so is the feeling of fright or terror. However, breathing cold air, allergens, irritating sprays, or dusts, or experiencing certain emotional situations such as anxiety, resentment, remorse, sadness, and frustration are usually very effective in closing the nose.

THE TURBINATES

Inhaled air passes mostly along the nasal septum and over the turbinates, especially the middle ones, to pick up some of its warmth and moisture as well as to deposit its particle and vapor pollutants. As previously mentioned, the turbinates create turbulence or deflections in the nasal airstream. This turbulence exposes more inspired and expired air to more nasal membrane surfaces, thus aiding in the deposit of more pollution particles within the nasal mucous blanket and also permitting more pickup of warmed moisture vapor to and from the lungs. The abundant mucous secretions of the turbinates, as well as their protective shielding of the sinus drainage openings beneath them, is of great help not only in maintaining a constant flow of nasal and sinus secretions but also in keeping the sinonasal drainage openings swept clean and moist.

It is also here that the sinuses are able to fulfill their important task of helping to maintain this nasal mucous blanket by providing a continuous additional flow of warmed, thin, well-hydrated mucus from a fairly large combined secretory area and propelling it by means of cilia through the small sinus openings and into the nose beneath the middle and superior turbinates. Even though the sinuses are not nearly so rich in mucus-secreting glands as the nose, their combined fairly extensive secreting surfaces are tucked away well out of the nasal airstream, where there are usually no drying or dehydrating effects and where their warm air content will also retain more moisture, thus keeping their secretions thin and free-flowing.

A healthy nose in turn must help in sweeping away any infected sinus discharge that might collect on the nasal side of the sinus drainage openings, thereby preventing any blockage there. By creating an alternating negative and positive pressure in the nose by breathing in and breathing out through your narrowed, flow-resistant nasal valves, and also by sniffing and swallowing, you can often move a blocking plug of mucus from a sinus opening into the nose, to be further propelled into the throat by cilia action and then swallowed. This process should provide some reasoning as to why a nose specialist will try to discourage too vigorous blowing of the nose and even encourage you, if you have to blow, to do so with both nostrils open. It's not very satisfying to blow in this fashion, but it might keep you from forcing a soft plug of infected mucus back into a sinus cavity that has been struggling for some time to sweep it out. Moreover, it may also prevent forcing infected sinus discharge into the eustachian tube of the ear or from the nose into another sinus cavity that until then may have avoided infection altogether. From this, you may realize that sniffing may be safer and more effective in most instances than very forceful blowing, especially as far as the sinuses are concerned.

SINONASAL AIR EXCHANGE

Although there is normally very minimal air exchange between the nose and sinuses with breathing, sniffing, blowing, and sneezing, the presence of an unobstructed sinus drainage opening means that any air pressure difference between the nose and sinuses, whether it be from flying or diving, from air absorption within the sinus cavity itself, or from a barometric pressure drop due to an approaching storm, will be immediately corrected and equalized. This will usually prevent the development of a sometimes painful partial vacuum within the sinus cavity, which, like a blocked eustachian tube to an ear, can lead to fluid accumulation and infection. The constant opportunity for this sinonasal air exchange to take place when needed and the presence of a continuously flowing sinus drainage are both essential to normal sinus function.

From this discussion, it should be apparent that there is a working commitment between the nose and sinuses that not only benefits them mutually but in turn provides a much healthier environment for those two vital organs known as the lungs.

CHAPTER TWO

What Is Sinusitis?

How Does Acute Sinusitis Differ From Chronic Sinusitis?

How Does Sinusitis in Infants and Children Differ From That in Adolescents and Adults?

IN MEDICAL LANGUAGE, "itis" means "inflammation of" and may be attached to a word identifying any part of the anatomy to mean inflammation of that particular organ or body structure. Although there are more than 60 different sinuses distributed throughout the body, the word "sinusitis" has come to mean inflammation of the paranasal sinuses, or those beside the nose.

INFLAMMATION

Inflammation is a fairly localized tissue reaction to an abnormal stimulus and may result from a physical injury, a chemical irritation, a hot or cold burn, or an invasion of the tissue by microorganisms such as bacteria, viruses, yeast, and fungi. The resultant redness and swelling is mainly damage control on the part of the body, namely, to bring in more blood with its disease-fighting components, to wall off the area, and, if there is a foreign intruder, to neutralize its ability to do more damage, hopefully to cast it out, and finally to set about the tissue repair or healing process. An allergic reaction may also cause inflammation with redness and swelling, but it is mainly due to the release of histamine from mast cells as a result of an allergen-antibody reaction in a previously sensitized individual. With an allergic reaction, however, the site of the inflammatory response may, in many instances, be far removed from the source of the stimulus. This is essentially a sterile reaction, but it can become secondarily infected, especially when it is prolonged and involves the delicate mucous membranes of the body.

In either case, the redness, swelling, and increased heat are mainly due to increased blood flow to the area as part of a defensive mechanism and healing process on the part of the body. The associated swelling may also cause pressure on a nerve or nerve endings, resulting in pain or headache. Unfortunately, for the nose and sinuses, this normal inflammatory response to infection or allergies and the body's effort to heal by scar formation can encourage even more sinus blockage with further progression of the disease. To prevent more scarring, it is important to reduce sinonasal swelling, relieve sinus blockage, and treat the infection as soon as possible.

Sinusitis is primarily an infective disease, often initiated by a virus such as with a head cold or flu, but sustained by bacterial invaders, or occasionally by a fungus, and persisting mainly because of inadequate or obstructed sinonasal drainage. Inadequate sinus drainage may result from blockage of the sinuses, small drainage openings, diminished or altered secretions within the sinus cavities themselves, sinus obstructive problems within the nose, or inadequate ciliary propulsion of the mucous secretions from the sinus cavities into the nose and down the throat. The latter is frequently referred to here as the sinonasal sweeping action, or cleansing action. Any one of these inadequacies or deficiencies, if sustained, can lead to stasis or pooling of mucus within a sinus cavity, and then certain harmful bacteria often found in the nose may seize this opportunity to multiply and invade. There is even some suggestion that when exposed to viral-damaged membranes, usually harmless bacteria, also present in the nose, may grow rapidly enough that possibly through sheer numbers they may initiate or prolong a sinus infection. Any time the flow of sinonasal mucous secretions is interrupted or even slowed down for very long, bacteria may attach themselves to the underlying membranes of the nose and sinuses to cause infection. With this disease process, however, the normally clear uninfected sinonasal drainage will be replaced by a cloudy and infected one.

If the mucus secreted by the sinuses is of a good quality, in adequate supply, free-flowing, devoid of irritating contaminants, free of allergens, and rich in immunity-producing proteins, antiviral agents, and bacteria-digesting enzymes; if the membranes lining the sinuses have minimal scarring and therefore a good blood supply and are not constantly swollen; if the microscopic hairs called cilia are plentiful and performing their sweeping action properly; and if the small drainage openings of all the sinuses are sufficiently open so that they not only drain well but also allow a free exchange of air between the nose and sinus cavities; then symptomatic sinusitis may seldom develop to the point of requiring medical treatment, and most head colds will usually clear up on their own.

SINUS BLOCKAGE

Blockage of a sinus opening, the basic problem in most cases of sinusitis, may occur either directly within the sinus drainage opening itself from membrane swelling or scarring or on the sinus side of the opening from polyps, cysts, tumors, swelling, and scarring, or on the nasal side of the sinus opening, also from swelling and scarring as well as from polyps, cysts, and tumors. Sinus blockage can also result from enlargement or deformity of a nasal turbinate or even a badly deviated nasal septum. Sinus blockage due to swelling alone may frequently occur as a result of a viral or bacterial infection, but it can also develop from allergy, from trauma, or from applying or inhaling almost any membrane irritant. Sinus blockage due to scarring may occur as a result of prolonged infections, prolonged irritant exposure, injury, surgery, or whenever an inflammatory swelling is allowed to continue untreated for weeks or months.

Within the sinus cavity itself, the fundamental cause of the irritation and inflammatory swelling is usually infection due to bacteria, viruses, or occasionally a fungus, as they attack the lining membranes of the sinus cavities. Nasal allergies may cause some sinus swelling as well. Infectious organisms are not normally found in the nose and sinuses in significant numbers but when present should still be viewed as potential invaders even though the total number of bacteria required to initiate an infection probably varies immensely. Bacterial and viral invaders from the nose can breach even a totally blocked sinonasal drainage opening and introduce infection into a sinus. An invading organism capable of causing infection or disease is called a pathogen. Pathogens may pass through, or come to rest in, the nose in small numbers fairly often and are usually easily handled by the sinonasal mucus-cleansing action. If, however, they should arrive in larger numbers, and especially if the nose or sinus defenses are depressed or damaged, then pathogens may invade.

When inflammatory swelling of the nose is initiated by breathing a noninfectious but very irritating inhalant such as a chemical powder, smoke, various sprays, dust, perfumes, and other strong pollutants, the sinuses, which are tucked away and well protected from the nasal airstream, can usually avoid any direct contamination. However, they may become secondarily involved when their drainage openings become blocked by the nasal swelling. The nose, on the other hand, having received the full brunt of an irritating inhalant, may as a result have its tissues so badly irritated and inflamed that it is unable to ward off an invasion by the ever present bacteria. The inflammation and swelling of nasal membranes that follows is called rhinitis, and when it includes the sinuses, it is known as rhinosinusitis. In general, if the nose doesn't drain well because it is inflamed and swollen, then the sinuses can't be expected to drain well, either. Any significant obstruction to drainage flow from almost anywhere in the body, whether in the nose, sinuses, ears, saliva glands, tear ducts, lungs, esophagus, gallbladder, intestines, kidney, or bladder, if sustained, will usually lead to infection, often fairly rapidly. In such instances, it is the constant flow of mucus being swept away at a fairly rapid pace that prevents an infection from developing. Therefore, a reduction in mucous flow will not only encourage the development of a sinus infection but can also make it much more difficult to cure should it develop.

The sinonasal mucous flow, as previously stated, is also diminished by inadequate cilia function such as seen in certain congenital diseases, in chronic sinusitis, in heavy smokers, or from temporary cilia destruction by respiratory viruses, from breathing certain chemical inhalants, the use of cocaine, snuff, local adrenaline, caustics, and even by the repeated use of strong salt solutions in the nose. I have seen cocaine users with deep destruction of nasal tissues and even destruction of the underlying nasal cartilage. I have also examined prizefighters and other contact sport athletes who showed considerable damage to their ciliated nasal membranes as a result of scarring from caustics used to control nosebleeds in the ring and on the field of play so that the participant may continue, which of course can lead to chronic rhinitis and chronic sinusitis. Fortunately, with certain respiratory viruses that cause colds or flu, most of the destroyed or damaged cilia, which can sometimes be rather extensive, will regenerate in 48 to 72 hours and be completely replaced in 5 to 10 days, but the damage to cilia and their basal cells from some of the above mentioned may be permanent, especially if continued until significant scarring results. The formation of scar tissue, or fibrosis, as a result of prolonged inflammatory swelling and ulceration within the nose or sinuses can cause reduction in blood flow and oxygen supply to the nasal and sinus membranes and further reduce their glandular secretions as well as their cilia function. The question is how long a sinus infection has to be present to cause obstructive scarring, and how long obstructive sinus swelling will persist after the infection has cleared.

OBSTRUCTIVE SINUS SCARRING

CAT scans have revealed that sinus membrane swelling may persist for as long as six weeks after the infection has cleared, but most of the time, adequate sinus drainage may recover well before that. However, the longer sinonasal membrane swelling is allowed to persist, the longer it will take to go away and the more scarring or fibrosis may occur. Also, if any sinonasal membrane irritation is allowed to continue, the inflammatory swelling and sinus blockage will usually persist.

As to how long a sinus infection must be present to produce enough scarring to cause persistent obstructive sinus disease is difficult to say. It would depend on how much previous scarring existed, as well as its location, the virulence of the bacteria, whether there is sinus membrane ulceration near a sinus drainage opening, whether you were treated with an antibiotic at any time during the infection and for how long, whether there are any contributing sinonasal obstructive abnormalities already present, the status of your immune response, the effectiveness of the sinonasal sweeping action, and finally the degree of tissue reactivity, since some people swell and scar more than others. Taking all of this into consideration, a reasonable estimate as to the length of time a sinus infection would usually have to be present to cause significant scarring and possibly permanent functional damage would probably be at least 6 to 8 weeks and possibly as long as 10 to 12 weeks before truly chronic disease might develop. Fortunately, medically irreversible chronic sinusitis in many instances may take even longer than that.

This would seem to compare fairly accurately with the duration of the usually reversible subacute stage of sinus disease. These estimates also match up with a number of patients I have treated who have had foreign bodies in their nasal passages and who carried an associated sinusitis for a specific length of time before removal and treatment. Many of those with previous sinus problems whose nasal foreign bodies and associated sinusitis had been present for as long as 6 to 8 weeks would, even after foreign body removal and adequate treatment, tend to have a lingering sinusitis on that same side following a head cold. They would also usually require antibiotics each time to get well, both of which would be highly suggestive of persistent obstructive sinus drainage problems due to previous infectious scarring.

MECONIUM SINUSITIS

In further support of this estimate, I once saw a case of infant sinusitis that showed up several weeks after birth and was apparently caused by a meconium plug lodged in the right nasal passage. Meconium is normally the first intestinal discharge of a newborn infant, but it may sometimes be released just before birth and sucked into an infant's nasal airway to block the respiratory tract, sometimes resulting in lower-airway distress or, as in this case, sinusitis. Here it was not noted in the nose at birth; nor was it visible 3 weeks later when the infant was examined for a cloudy, infected nasal discharge from the right side. The plug was subsequently sneezed out about 10 days after that and identified as meconium. The associated ethmoid sinusitis and infected nasal discharge finally cleared up after 6 weeks of antibiotic therapy, but over the next 3 or 4 years, it would recur and persist only on the right side following a head cold. Several weeks of antibiotic treatment would be required each time to make it go away. This case is particularly supportive of the 6 to 8 week estimate for damage control, especially since there couldn't have been any previous sinus scarring in this patient before this episode.

So far, I have been unable to find any reports in the literature of a meconium-induced sinusitis, but it probably occurs more often than we realize and could be responsible for an occasional case of chronic sinusitis in children. This case might also be considered a prime example of how a prolonged sinus infection in infancy or childhood, if not thoroughly treated, might continue to recur and to cause chronic sinusitis persisting throughout adolescence and into adulthood.

ACUTE VERSUS SUBACUTE

Sinusitis patients, for the sake of simplicity, are often divided into those with acute and those with chronic disease. Many of the chronic cases may also experience periodic acute flare-ups. If a person who has an acute sinus infection, such as that which nearly always accompanies a viral head cold, recovers almost completely from the very active acute stage of the disease, usually within the first week or two, but then continues to show minimal evidence of a low-grade sinus infection, often with a cloudy nasal discharge or cloudy postnasal drip, possibly a mild morning sore throat, intermittent nasal congestion, and sometimes a slight daytime headache usually in the morning, and if these symptoms should continue during the next 6 to 8 weeks, this stage should be recognized and referred to as subacute sinusitis. This is very important, since it represents an in-between category indicating that the condition has gone beyond the very active and sometimes distressing symptoms of the acute phase but hopefully hasn't produced enough permanent damage, such as scarring, to label it as chronic disease. Unlike the acute sinusitis usually accompanying a head cold or flu and usually involving sinuses on both sides of the nose, subacute sinusitis will more often settle on only one side and in one particular sinus or group of sinuses. Following a head cold or flu, most of the sinuses will usually throw off the infection, but one or two may remain diseased because of impaired drainage from previous scarring or from a deviated nasal septum, an enlarged turbinate, an obstructive polyp, or sometimes just from sleeping consistently on one side, resulting in more swelling and sinus blockage on that side. Once chronic sinusitis develops, a diseased sinus may act as a reservoir to infect other sinuses on that side and later on both sides. In the subacute stage, however, the condition is still considered reversible, which makes it doubly important to recognize it and to treat it vigorously, thereby preventing the development of a chronic condition. So often it is the failure to recognize and completely cure a subacute sinusitis that is mainly responsible for the development of chronic sinusitis. The doctor's task, with your help and cooperation, is to identify this subacute stage early enough and to prevent this from happening.

CHRONIC SINUSITIS

There are varying degrees of chronic sinusitis, and some early cases with minimal scarring can also be reverted with intensive medical therapy. Some people with chronic sinusitis, however, have so much permanent damage, with so much scarring causing so much blockage, impairment of mucous secretions, and diminished cilia activity, that they may experience only temporary clearing of their infected discharge and sinus symptoms even after very prolonged antibiotic therapy. Antibiotic therapy may eventually allow the infected sinus discharge to become clear, but it may be only very temporary, and the sinonasal discharge may cloud up again within a week or two of discontinuing the medication. In such cases, endoscopic sinus surgery (ESS) can often be effective.

CHRONIC SUPPURATIVE SINUSITIS

This state of a persistent infected sinonasal discharge is sometimes referred to as chronic suppurative sinusitis, indicating that the sinus discharge is always cloudy, except possibly when temporarily relieved by antibiotic therapy. If most or all of the sinuses are involved on both sides of the nose, then the condition may be referred to as a pansinusitis. People who have chronic suppurative pansinusitis, with their continuous infected discharge, rarely seem to have acute flare-ups and very rarely to contract head colds. Whether the cold virus just doesn't like this suppurative media, or whether it's just hard for the patient to tell when a cold is present, is sometimes difficult to determine, but generally speaking, they seldom seem to experience the profuse clear nasal discharge, nasal swelling, and marked congestion of an acute viral head cold.

RECURRENT ACUTE SINUSITIS

Another large group of people with sinusitis may fail to reveal any evidence of chronic disease and seem to remain free of cloudy discharge most of the time. Their defenses against sinus flare-ups might be considered borderline. The mucus-cleansing action of their nose and sinuses may be barely adequate, and then only under the best of circumstances. Their drainage openings may be somewhat narrowed from scarring but again adequate under perfectly normal conditions. Their antibody formation and other immune defenses may even function reasonably well. The problem is that any setback in the body systems may push such an individual, who may just barely be holding his or her own, over the brink and cause a flare-up of acute sinusitis with an infected cloudy discharge. Typical triggers include anxiety and depression, loss of sleep, stress, hormonal changes such as in PMS and pregnancy, excessive alcohol intake, an allergic rhinitis attack, too much smoking, dehydration, body fluid retention, and gastrointestinal upset; any abnormal changes in the environment adversely affecting the body, such as getting chilled, being caught in the rain, breathing a heavy dose of pollen, getting your feet wet, sleeping in a draft or in front of a window, being overheated and then going outside in the cold, going to bed with a damp head, breathing irritating dusts, sprays, or paints, inhaling drugs, scuba diving or flying, swimming in a chlorinated pool, especially in the wintertime, going outside without a hat or head cover in cold weather, being exposed to too much humidity or too much dryness, breathing secondhand cigar or cigarette smoke, washing your hair and not drying it thoroughly, and sleeping in or near a freshly painted room.

Here we are speaking of the sinusitis-prone adult who, because of some impairment of normal resistance to infection, or possibly because of an excessive exposure to infection (for example, by a close companion), or perhaps because of some seemingly minor dysfunction on the part of the sinuses themselves, will experience more than the usual two or three acute sinusitis flare-ups a year. Under these circumstances, the acute symptoms may sometimes be fairly mild but are occasionally moderate to severe. These episodes may be referred to as recurrent acute attacks of sinusitis and often occur in addition to any acute flare-ups from head colds or flu. In such cases, the potential for a sinus flare-up is always there, but it seems to be in a delicate balance with the body's resistance much of the time, or until some seemingly minor occurrence trips it up. These episodes will usually last a week or two, but if they persist, they could require antibiotic therapy to avoid more chronic damage.

BACTERIAL FLORA

People who have chronic sinusitis will often show a somewhat different bacterial flora or infestation than that usually found in acute or subacute cases. They are more often infected with anaerobic bacteria that grow in the absence of oxygen and with antibiotic-resistant organisms due to repeated antibiotic treatments, as well as with some of the less common bacteria and often with several different organisms present at the same time. Occasionally one of the bacteria commonly found in acute and subacute sinusitis such as *Strep. pneumoniae, H. influenzae,* and *M. catarrhalis* may be found in chronic sinusitis, especially in children, and particularly during an acute flare-up.

Primary acute episodes of sinusitis are nearly always the result of a viral respiratory infection such as a cold or flu and usually involve healthy, relatively undamaged sinuses. Despite the presence of a thick, cloudy discharge on the third or fourth day of the cold, such infections will usually clear up on their own or with very minimal treatment. Acute episodes in healthy sinuses usually occur only two or three times a year, since that is the usual frequency for head colds or flu in most healthy adults. Some adults who have large families, as well as schoolteachers, carpoolers, nursery school supervisors, and certain medical personnel, may have colds and sinus infections more frequently, but a few lucky individuals may go for years without any head colds or sinusitis at all. If you should have acute episodes of sinusitis more than three or four times a year, mostly unrelated to head colds or flu, and especially if you nearly always require antibiotics to get well, then you very likely have an underlying chronic sinus problem. Children, of course, may have viral respiratory infections two or three times as often as adults, which can mean six to eight head colds a year, and six to eight episodes of associated sinus involvement as well. This is particularly true of children who have excessive exposure to other children in confining areas such as day care centers, carpools, school buses, and classrooms.

With most acute episodes of sinusitis, unless they are precipitated by a viral infection, their onset can be fairly subtle and rarely so dramatic as the acute sinusitis accompanying a head cold or flu, and seldom is any fever associated. Your white blood count may be normal or low, especially if there is an accompanying viral infection, or occasionally only slightly elevated. A significant fever or white count elevation might indicate possible complications of the sinusitis or an associated infection in the lungs, tonsils, or ears, especially in children. Since the paranasal sinuses are surrounded by bone, somewhat separated and walled off from the very vascular soft tissues of the body, bacterial toxins emitted by the sinus-infecting organisms may remain fairly localized and are mostly swept away in the mucous flow, with limited absorption into the body system. Consequently they seldom produce much in the way of a systemic response such as fever, chills, or an elevated white count, even when infected with the most virulent types of bacteria.

People who have chronic sinusitis cover a wide span, from those with minimal sinus damage who may be reverted to a more permanently healthy sinus state by vigorous treatment to those at the other end of the spectrum, who may have stopped responding to medical treatment and who may then proceed to a permanent state of chronic suppurative sinusitis possibly involving all of their sinuses. Even in such a case, you should not give up if you suffer from chronic sinusitis. I recall a young lady of 13 years who had had chronic suppurative pansinusitis for at least three years and finally cleared up and stayed healthy after receiving variable antibiotic treatment continuously for a year. In between, there are a large number of people who have rather subdued chronic disease, many of them with periodic acute episodes, who will remain much the same provided that their acute flare-ups are thoroughly treated each time they occur and are not allowed to cause further permanent damage with scarring. If each flare-up is treated and cleared up promptly, many of these people, even though they have chronic sinus damage, may feel reasonably normal and symptom free most of the time. They gradually learn from experience what brings on their acute attacks and usually how to avoid such situations whenever possible. Nevertheless, there is a certain amount of subtle anxiety as to when the next episode will occur, what will precipitate it, and whether it will occur at a very inconvenient time. Some of these may also benefit from endoscopic sinus surgery.

Some sinusitis sufferers, perhaps with more permanent sinus damage or maybe in some instances just more sensitivity, may never feel good from the time they get up in the morning until they go to bed at night. Although they may be unable to specifically identify the problem, and may be mostly unaware of any cloudy nasal discharge, they will usually admit that they seldom feel good. In addition to an occasional awareness of a postnasal drip, intermittent nasal congestion, morning sore throats, and an occasional headache, they are usually tired much of the time, may have difficulty concentrating, find themselves falling behind at work or in school, are often irritable, sometimes short-tempered, even forgetful, and usually have a rather constant sensation of feeling weak in the legs. They may intermittently experience sinus headaches, especially in dampness or cold weather and sometimes with barometric pressure changes, but their headaches are usually not so disturbing as with an acute flare-up, and can be totally absent. These headaches, when present, are usually dull, occasionally pressure-like, and often of only 2 to 6 hours in duration, nearly always absent during the night, but usually recurring again the very next day and at about the same time. Headaches may be present without any obvious signs of a cloudy discharge, at least to the patient and sometimes not even to the doctor. Yet if one had to choose a single sign or finding that should be present or evident in diagnosing an active sinus infection, it would have to be the presence of a cloudy discharge in the nose or throat.

You must remember, however, that it may be difficult, even for the physician, to determine exactly where you stand regarding the duration and extent of your disease or even the possibility of a complete cure, until every effort has been made to reverse the disease process. Fortunately for you, as well as for your doctor, the sinuses have an amazing ability to recover, even after a rather intensive infectious insult over a fairly extended period of time, and to return, even with some permanent scarring and some chronic changes, to a fairly normal functioning state, provided, of course, they are given sufficient help.

From these discussions, it should be evident that acute, subacute, recurrent acute, and chronic sinusitis represent different stages of the same disease; and even though they may tend to run together, they may vary considerably in the intensity of their symptoms, their treatment, and unfortunately even in their prognosis.

HOW DOES SINUSITIS IN INFANTS AND CHILDREN DIFFER FROM THAT IN ADOLESCENTS AND ADULTS?

Both the maxillary and ethmoid sinuses are present at birth, and even though they are quite small, the possibility of their becoming infected anytime thereafter has to be considered. Fortunately, thanks to some maternally transferred immunity to the newborn for colds and other respiratory viruses, episodes of sinusitis in the first few months of life are rare.

Not many years ago, a child who had a runny nose all winter, even when the drainage was obviously cloudy and infected, was regarded by most people and even by some doctors as being a normal condition, since so many children in the neighborhood, nursery, and classroom had it. This cloudy, infected sinus drainage, which may well have been present all winter and even held over from the winter before, would gradually clear up or rather become much less obvious by early summer with the advent of better sinonasal mucous flow due to increased warmth and humidity, sometimes aided by the nasal flushing effects of swimming pool water. This thinner, freer-flowing warm-weather mucus, although still infected, would be more inclined to drain unobserved down the throat rather than to collect in the nostrils or to drain down the upper lip, as would so often occur in the drier winter months. Because of this, it was not too unusual for a doctor to assume and even advise the parents that the runny nose would clear up in warm weather. Some did, but others, less fortunate, who had perhaps gone through several winters like this and thereby developed permanent sinus scarring, would carry their chronic sinus infection, mostly unobserved, throughout the summer only to have it become obvious again in the fall with the advent of the cooler, drier air and the starting up of the home, school, or workplace furnaces.

Now, fortunately, medical personnel, teachers, and parents have become much more alert to the signs and symptoms of a persistent nasal or sinus infection in children. Many adults now realize that their own respiratory tracts could also become infected by contaminated discharge sneezed and blown into the air in carpools and classrooms, as well as by hand contact with contaminated pencils, chalk, light switches, doorknobs, spigot and toilet handles, water fountains, books, and toys. This increased awareness of an infected nasal discharge has resulted in earlier treatment with less chance of contaminating other children who like to share their playthings and who spend long hours together in such close quarters.

Children themselves may rarely call attention to their sinus problems, and working parents may not be around often enough to recognize them. Parents may also be reluctant to take time off from work to stay home with a child who has no fever, or to spend the money to see a doctor for something as mundane as a runny nose. With children, it is sometimes difficult to separate sinusitis from allergic rhinitis, and consequently many cases of sinusitis are overlooked or go untreated on the assumption that it is an allergy and will therefore probably go away. Of course, both may be present at the same time, and both may have to be treated to clear up the sinus infection. This is especially true because allergic rhinitis can be an important factor in someone developing chronic sinusitis and for children in particular. However, it should be emphasized that untreated or inadequately treated subacute sinus disease is responsible for most of the cases of chronic sinusitis in both adults and children.

Even though infants' and children's sinuses are still in the process of developing, and therefore may be fewer and definitely smaller, the infectious involvement of their sinus cavities is similar in many ways to that of adolescents or adults. They both represent infectious inflammatory processes involving the sinus cavities, including their membranous linings and drainage openings, usually accompanied by a corresponding involvement of the nasal membranes on the same side of the nose as well. In both instances, they are usually bacterial infections producing a cloudy discharge, although initially they may have started with a viral infection and clear discharge, as in the case of a head cold or flu. In both the child and adult, sinus problems may begin as an acute sinus infection, progress untreated to the subacute stage, and finally end up as chronic disease. Although sinusitis usually begins with a nasal or upper respiratory infection, some episodes may start primarily in a sinus cavity, especially in the adult, and subsequently infect the nose. This may occur if a sinus cavity is already partially blocked by a cyst, polyp, or tumor, has previously been badly scarred or damaged, contains bone fragments or a foreign body, or if the sinusitis is initiated by an infected upper tooth, usually a more common finding in the adult, especially after age 30. The ethmoid and maxillary sinuses are the ones most commonly infected in both adults and children and usually the only ones involved in very young children. In both children and adults, most of the time, a sustained inflammatory swelling of the nasal membranes and sinus openings with obstruction to sinus drainage encourages the development and persistence of a sinus infection. However, from this point on, some divergence of the two conditions seems to follow, especially with regard to the diagnosis and treatment.

In the older adolescent or adult, the history may play a major role in the diagnosis, especially when there is no infected discharge to be seen on examination. After careful questioning, a doctor can frequently make the diagnosis of sinusitis over the telephone when dealing with a mature and very observant patient. However, an examination by the doctor would then be necessary to determine what caused the sinusitis, which sinuses are involved, and whether there are any contributing factors or complications. With the infant or child, however, the history, even from a parent, may be of little or no value, since both parents may have full-time jobs, and sometimes additional jobs at night, thereby having very little daytime contact with the child. Moreover, the nursery or school attendant, who may see the child far more often, is usually not available for questioning. A parent can usually assist with that part of the history regarding the child's home environment and household infectious contacts, but if the child is in a day care center or in a shared custody situation, such information may be only partially helpful.

If on examining a patient with suspected sinusitis, no cloudy discharge is found in the nose or throat to confirm the diagnosis, then the physician will have to rely almost entirely on the history from the older adolescent or adult as to what they blow out of their nostrils or clear out of their throats. Occasionally an adult patient will bring in a specimen, which can be very helpful. The child or parent, on the other hand, may encounter considerable difficulty in obtaining a specimen or in providing a reliable description as to the character of the discharge.

Observing your child, you may have noted a slight, often short-lasting cough, usually occurring after midnight and toward early morning when sleep is generally lighter. If this cough recurs each night, it frequently indicates a persistent sinusitis with an infected postnasal drip irritating the lower throat, larynx, trachea, or bronchi either directly from spillage or more likely by infected droplet contamination to the lower airway. The deeper or slow-wave sleep, known as non-rapid-eye-movement delta sleep, usually occurring earlier in the night, and especially in younger people, may tend to suppress a sinusitis-initiated cough, if it is fairly mild and not caused by a significant bronchitis. Bedtime cough medicines, some antihistamines, caffeine, alcohol, antidepressants, and sleep medications can, of course, affect the intensity as well as the time of onset of a nighttime cough. A persistent or chronic cough day and night is more likely the result of a true bronchial infection, which of course can be associated with a prolonged sinusitis, since any infection in one end of the respiratory tract seems eventually to involve the other.

The presence of a nasal tone in the voice of a child may sometimes be very helpful to you as well as to your doctor in determining the presence of a sinus blockage, which in many instances may also indicate the persistence of a sinus infection, as well as the need for further antibiotic treatment. In a few instances, this may be your only clue as to the existence of a sinus infection in your child, and even then a nasal allergy or enlarged adenoids may cause a similar problem and tend to confuse the picture. A nasal tone to the voice may also help identify sinus blockage in an adult, especially for a maxillary sinus, but usually not quite so pointedly as in the child, whose other resonance chambers are smaller and often more crowded.

You may have also noted a glob of infected discharge expelled from your child's nose into the swimming pool water, a not uncommon occurrence in a child who has purulent sinus discharge and a blocked nose. In an adult who has larger and usually less obstructed nasal passages, such discharge would be more likely to pass down the throat and be swallowed or expectorated.

A dry crusting around the nostrils of a child or infant, especially when it has a slightly discolored appearance, may be the only suggestion of an infected sinus drainage, and it would be helpful to the physician if you could recall such a finding, since it may have been wiped away before your visit to the doctor. This would of course be an unusual finding in the older adolescent or adult.

You may also have observed in your child an obvious increase in mouth breathing, possibly due to nasal congestion and especially noticeable when eating or sleeping. This is also important for the doctor to know, since it could indicate increased nasal obstruction and possibly a sinus infection in the child, whose smaller nasal passages tend to block up more easily.

In my experience, tenderness to finger pressure or to tapping with the finger over an infected sinus is not a common finding in the usual sinusitis patient but would certainly be more apparent to the discerning adolescent or adult than to a child. The exception to this would be an empyema, or fluid level, in an acutely infected frontal or maxillary sinus, which could be quite tender to palpation or to tapping over the sinus in both adults and older children.

Swelling around the eyes with an uncomplicated sinus infection is far more common in children than in adults. Children's tissues are more elastic, have a more active blood supply, and contain a greater amount of loose areolar tissue, making them more inclined to swell with inflammation or injury. Children are also more inclined to develop dark circles around their eyes, or shiners, as they are sometimes called, especially when a sinus infection has been present for a while.

If your child starts turning up the volume of the TV, indicating a hearing problem, it might also be indicative of an underlying sinus problem. Eustachian tube swelling and blockage can occur from an infected sinus discharge passing close to its opening in the nasopharynx just behind the nose. The drainage coming from the sinuses located in the front of the nose (the anterior ethmoids, frontals, and maxillary) passes just beneath the eustachian tube opening on that side, and the drainage from the sphenoid and posterior ethmoids in the back of the nose passes just above the eustachian tube opening. Of course, the diminished hearing may only be obvious if both eustachian tubes are blocked. You can test your child for one-sided eustachian tube blockage and hearing loss by closing one ear off with a fingertip and whispering softly in the other ear. A history of recurrent or prolonged ear infections, repeated episodes of fluid in the ears, or a history of having had ear tubes, especially in an infant or child, would make it necessary to rule out a persistent sinus infection as a major contributing factor. It was a revelation to me when I realized just how often chronic sinusitis and recurrent ear infections or ear fluid problems occurred together in children as well as the dire necessity of always treating both.

Sinus headaches, which were found in about 60 to 70 percent of the older adolescents and adults that I treated for sinus disease, were infrequently found in the child or early adolescent, even when a fairly extensive sinus infection was present. Some pediatricians and pediatric otolaryngologists, who probably see more children with sinus infections on a daily basis, have reported a slightly higher incidence of sinus headaches in children than I was aware of in my practice, but still not nearly so frequent as with the older adolescent or adult. In the older people, the type and location of the head pain, the time of onset and disappearance each day, whether it is exacerbated by bending over, lifting, straining, coughing, or shaking one's head, whether it is improved by heat or cold applications, whether oral decongestants or antihistamines tend to relieve it, or if a decongestant or steroid nasal spray alone provides any relief, and whether the discomfort is improved significantly by any particular pain medicine, such as aspirin or Tylenol, would all be extremely helpful to know in diagnosing sinusitis in the observant adolescent or adult. However, such information is seldom available from a child, and rarely from a parent. If a child, even if he or she has chronic sinusitis, complains of headaches, they could still be coming from some other source than the sinuses and could even be due to something more serious.

Children, with their still-developing immune systems, their usually very close daily contacts with one another, and their generally poor hygiene (they seldom wash their hands, rarely cover their mouths when they cough, cough in each other's faces, wipe their noses on their hands, and like to share their food or toys), naturally have more frequent colds and therefore more sinus infections than the correspondingly healthy adult. Children's respiratory infections and sinus flare-ups are more often complicated by associated ear, throat, and lung infections, which may tend to overshadow the more subtle sinus disease. This may make it very difficult to determine exactly when their sinusitis started and approximately how long it has been present, whereas the adult can usually tell just when it all began. This usually faulty information, plus a child's smaller nasal passages, smaller sinus openings, and greater tendency for membrane swelling, usually makes it necessary to prescribe antibiotics and decongestants for a much longer period in order to relieve sinus blockage and to cure the patient. It is also more difficult in the child to ascertain when the cloudy discharge has finally cleared or when it shows up again, since a child usually can't tell you and since an adequate fiber-optic exam of a child's nose is nearly impossible without a general anesthetic. Most of the time, when sinusitis is finally diagnosed in a child, the doctor has to assume that it has been present for considerably longer than the symptoms or the usually unreliable history would indicate, unless of course the infection can definitely be tied into a particular bout of head cold or flu or to the time of insertion of a foreign body into the nose.

After a course of treatment, the older adolescent or adult can usually tell if the sinonasal discharge has become clear and whether it has remained so, whereas the early adolescent, child, or infant may have to return to the doctor's office usually more than once to determine this. To confirm this, the doctor can usually shrink down and locally anesthetize the older adolescent's or adult's nose for an endoscopic exam. However, when dealing with an untrusting child and searching for evidence of a cloudy sinus discharge, the doctor must depend on a usually rather brief glimpse into the nasal passages with only a head light, and many times an equally brief view of the posterior throat and palate opening when the child gags.

The vertical reddish streaking occasionally seen in the back of the throat of people with sinusitis, consisting of minute clusters of inflamed lymphoid tissue, usually initiated by an infected postnasal drip, is often helpful in making the diagnosis of long-standing or recurrent prolonged bouts of sinusitis in a child. This streaking may, however, be entirely absent in the adult, even with chronic sinus disease, or it may sometimes be present in the adult as a holdover from prolonged sinus infections in childhood, even though no sinus infection may now exist. This membrane inflammation from a persistent infected postnasal drip may occasionally extend down into the esophagus to aggravate an already existing peptic esophagitis with an increase of heartburn, belching, and sometimes hoarseness. Gastroesophageal reflux (GER) of stomach acid backing up into the nose has been identified as a cause of chronic sinusitis, especially in children, and both conditions do sometimes coexist. However, from my own experience, this was an uncommon finding. For the infant who frequently regurgitates through the nose on a fairly continuous basis and the adolescent or adult who notices a bitter taste in the mouth followed by a burning in the nose, it is certainly a distinct possibility, but in both instances, the nasal membrane irritation would have to continue over a fairly extended period to cause a chronic sinusitis. This regurgitation of stomach contents may seldom reach as far as the nose or sinus openings, especially in the adolescent or adult, and is more likely to irritate the larynx or tracheobronchial tree to cause hoarseness or bronchitis. A chronic bronchitis from GER could, however, through reverse droplet infection of the nose, cause a rhinosinusitis. In the cleft palate child, however, daily repeated contamination of the nose by food and drink is of course frequently responsible for a chronic sinusitis.

Children are more inclined to run a fever or exhibit an elevated white blood count with a sinus infection, especially since other areas of their respiratory tracts, their adenoids, or their ears may also be involved at the same time and especially since children's respiratory tracts and their systemic response to infection seem generally more reactive than those of most adults.

Adults and occasionally older adolescents will usually admit to any systemic symptoms related to their sinus infection, such as being overly tired, feeling weak in the legs, and having a diminished appetite, difficulty concentrating, sometimes muscular aching, and difficulty sleeping, but in a child or early adolescent, these symptoms will usually go unrecognized or ignored.

Because of a child's very small nasal and sinus structures and the many difficulties encountered in trying to examine them adequately, the physician may be more inclined to order a CAT scan of a child's sinuses when a subacute or chronic problem is suspected, especially if the child doesn't respond to treatment, and it may sometimes be done even as a follow-up to prolonged treatment to determine whether residual sinus disease still exists. In the adult or adolescent, the less expensive plain sinus X rays, or even just a very thorough exam of the nose and sinus orifices with fiber-optic telescopes, may be all that is needed in many instances, and perhaps all that will be authorized. With the ever-increasing efforts to reduce the cost of medicine, physicians will have to rely more and more on their own diagnostic abilities and less on laboratory and X-ray studies.

The older adolescent or adult with sinusitis may complain of a post-nasal drip, usually more noticeable on arising in the morning, sometimes causing gagging or vomiting, especially in people who have very sensitive throats. Such a complaint or even an awareness of a postnasal drip is very unusual in a child. Some adults, however, who are chronic mouth breathers with very dry throats and who may have no sinus problems at all may sometimes experience similar gagging problems with their normal mucous drainage.

Adults and older adolescents with sinusitis will often have morning sore throats, which, like most early-morning sinus headaches, go away after you have been up and around for an hour or so, especially after drinking a cup of coffee or after having breakfast. The child, on the other hand, is either unaware of this or unconsciously accepts it, since many times he or she hasn't learned to discriminate between what is normal and what is abnormal or how he or she should feel or shouldn't feel. This may also in some instances account for a child's apparent lack of sinus headaches. Even adults who have had chronic sinus problems for a long time may begin to accept the way they feel as normal and many times don't realize how they should feel until they have been treated with antibiotics for a while and gained some relief.

Most discerning adults are aware of nasal blockage and will usually be able to say whether it is intermittent or constant, on which side it occurs, and even tell you when it is more or less obvious, for instance, during the night, in the early morning, after drinking an alcoholic beverage or ingesting a milk product, when lying down, lying on their side, sitting up, bending over, exercising, and so on. A child or early adolescent, on the other hand, may be totally oblivious to nasal blockage, even though it may be marked and even very evident to those around them.

Bad breath in association with a chronic sinus infection may occur in both adults and children, but it is not diagnostic of sinus disease, since it can also occur as a result of bad tonsils or adenoids, dental cavities, gum infection, a furrowed or coated tongue, esophageal regurgitation, chronic mouth breathing, and lung infections. When bad breath occurs in a child, it usually attracts more attention, since it is nearly always an unexpected finding and a rather shocking surprise to a parent. If there is a particularly foul odor to a child's breath, you should be concerned about the possibility of a foreign body in the nose producing a foul-smelling infected discharge. The greater tendency for children with chronic sinusitis to mouth breathe and its drying effect on a bacteria-laden sinus discharge in the back of their throats make them ideal subjects for bad breath, especially because bacteria are responsible for most of the offensive odors in our environment.

Although temporary bacterial contamination of the bloodstream (known as a bacteremia, or as a septicemia in its more severe form) may sometimes occur from an acutely obstructed sinus infection in both adults and children, it is more likely to develop in very young children, and is usually caused by a *Strep. pneumoniae* or an *H. influenzae* organism. These same bacteria, so commonly found in acute sinusitis, are, along with *Staph. aureus,* more often responsible for orbital cellulitis, an inflammation of the structures surrounding the eye that can sometimes cause blindness. Orbital cellulitis is usually due to an ethmoid sinus infection and is also more common in young children, especially under age six. The tendency for marked obstruction of their very small sinus drainage openings due to excessive swelling, the rich blood supply to their tissues, and their rather immature immune systems all seem to make young children more susceptible. Of course, the close proximity of the ethmoid sinuses to the orbits, with only a very thin, sometimes missing layer of bone separating them, is a major factor in developing orbital cellulitis at any age.

Children who have chronic sinus disease are also more often infected with one of these same organisms or possibly with *M. catarrhalis*, another form of bacteria commonly found in acute sinus infections. Adults with chronic sinusitis, when not experiencing an acute flare-up, will usually be infected with several different bacteria including *Staphylococcus,* sometimes *Pseudomonas,* and especially anaerobic bacteria that grow only in the absence of oxygen. If you consider chronic sinusitis in the adult, with its usually long-standing sinus obstruction enhancing the depletion of oxygen within the sinus cavity, its excessive scarring interfering with blood supply and oxygen transport to sinus membranes, and its diminished cilia sweep creating stagnation of mucous flow, it is not surprising that anaerobic bacteria, which cannot survive in the presence of oxygen, would tend to flourish there. However, for a doctor to demonstrate these anaerobic bacteria by culture requires a very careful technique and is not always successful.

The treatment of sinusitis, although primarily medical for both children and adults, may vary considerably between the two. As previously mentioned, children have smaller nasal passages and smaller sinus drainage openings, as well as a tendency for their nasal and sinus membranes to swell excessively with colds or sinusitis, and would therefore benefit even more from the use of oral and nasal decongestants. Because of this swelling with excessive sinus blockage and the fact that they may have had their sinus infection longer than a parent may realize, children will usually have to take an antibiotic for nearly twice as long as most adults with a similar infection. Because of this and the difficulties usually encountered in persuading children to take their medications, their sinus problems are more often undertreated. For the same reasons, children would be more inclined to produce antibiotic-resistant organisms and may therefore need a change of antibiotic more often. Children also seem to cultivate and pass on more virulent strains of bacteria and viruses—a fact that most adults who are exposed to them on a daily basis will adamantly confirm.

Because children have twice as many upper respiratory infections as adults each year and therefore often twice as many episodes of sinus involvement, their need for medical treatment in this regard may occur twice as often. The higher incidence of allergic rhinitis in association with chronic sinusitis in children usually means that they may have a greater need for allergy evaluations and treatments as well.

With regard to the surgical approach to sinus disease in the child versus that in the older adolescent or adult, we must realize that the cartilaginous and bony structures of a child's nose and sinuses are still developing and expanding, and that significant damage to these structures from injury or excessive surgical trauma could enhance or even limit their growth, not to mention the limiting effects on tissues and structural expansion sometimes caused by postsurgical or posttraumatic scarring. Scar tissue formations can literally close off or seal sinus cavities, thereby rendering them nonfunctional and unhealthy. In such instances, chronic sinus infection or sometimes even a cyst or mucocele will develop. Also, some patients unpredictably scar more than others. As to what effect this postsurgical scarring or limitation of sinonasal structural development early in life may have on sinonasal function later in life, doctors can only speculate.

Even though sinus surgeons may be somewhat hesitant to list subacute or chronic sinusitis as an indication for an adenoidectomy, and some insurance companies may be reluctant to approve the procedure, the rather simple removal of enlarged, chronically infected adenoids in the child who has persistent or recurring sinusitis can sometimes make a significant difference in his or her sinus problems. Adenoids, because of their deep folds and scarred pockets, usually lack any cilia activity to keep them clean, may tend to collect and harbor harmful bacteria, which either through direct spread or through moisture droplet contamination can sometimes prolong a rhinitis (and therefore a sinusitis) and even cause it to recur after a successful course of antibiotic treatment. Adults, on the other hand, whose adenoids are usually very small, would not be expected to benefit significantly from their removal insofar as their chronic sinus problems are concerned.

The long-standing practice of transilluminating a frontal or maxillary sinus by using a very small light in a darkened room to see if the sinus is cloudy and therefore possibly diseased may sometimes be helpful in older adolescents and adults. However, this technique is often of little or no value in young children, since even their major sinuses are still very small and their puffy cheeks may tend to defuse the light. Moreover, a darkened or cloudy frontal sinus on transillumination, as sometimes found in an adolescent or adult, doesn't necessarily mean an infected or badly scarred sinus. It could mean a very small or even absent frontal sinus and may require an X ray to determine this.

When it comes to endoscopic sinus surgery (ESS), you should remember that the very diminutive size of a child's nose and sinuses results in a much narrower working area for the sinus surgeon, usually poorer visibility, and often greater difficulty in identifying surgical landmarks. Because of this and the proximity of certain vital structures such as the eyes and the brain, the chances of surgical injury to one of these structures could be greater in the child. This, along with the likelihood of more postoperative swelling in younger tissues, as well as more adhesions, and with even greater difficulty in controlling any postoperative bleeding in a potentially uncooperative patient, would certainly make significant sinus surgery in the child a more formidable procedure. It may at times challenge all the experience and capabilities of the surgeon and should therefore be undertaken in most instances only after extensive prolonged conservative treatment fails. Parents should also realize that excessive sinus scarring in childhood, either from prolonged or repeated infections, from trauma, or in some instances from an extensive surgical procedure, may sometimes increase the chances of sinus problems developing later in life.

CHAPTER THREE

What Are the Signs and Symptoms of Sinusitis?

What Is a Sinus Headache, and How Can You Tell If You Have One, and What Can Be Done about It?

DIFFICULTIES IN DIAGNOSING SINUSITIS

One thing that is particularly disturbing to many people who have chronic sinusitis is that even though they feel miserable, there are often no impressive outward signs of disease; not to their family, their boss, their teachers, their friends, and sometimes not even to their doctor. In other words, they have nothing convincing to show for their illness, nor anything to make people realize just how badly they feel, or even that they are really sick at all. There is usually little or no fever, especially in the adult, unless there is an associated acute viral infection such as a very bad head cold or flu, or unless a more serious complication of the sinus infection has developed. I recall all too often being informed by sinusitis patients that they had been told they couldn't possibly have a sinus infection because they didn't have a fever.

If you have an uncomplicated sinus infection, the white blood count, often a good indicator of a bacterial infection elsewhere in your body, is usually normal or only slightly elevated. It may even be low if the sinusitis is part of a viral respiratory infection. The main indicator of a sinus infection, namely, pus or cloudy discharge coming from a sinus, may be missed by the examining physician, since depending on the degree of sinus blockage, pus may be discharged into the nose only intermittently or sometimes not at all. This infected drainage passing down your throat, known as a postnasal drip, may be particularly disturbing to you, especially in the morning, and may even cause you to gag and vomit. If you see your physician in the afternoon, the usual time for most office appointments, your infected postnasal drip may have disappeared, only to show up later. It should be emphasized, however, that all of us have a constant postnasal drip, normally amounting to a pint or more a day of perfectly clear mucus, and it is only when it becomes thickened from drying out or discolored from infection that we may become aware of it. A drying out of the throat from continuous mouth breathing as a result of strenuous exercise, excessive talking, singing, or nasal blockage can sometimes make you aware of your normal mucus flowing over these very dry membranes in the back of the throat, and it too can make you gag, especially if you have a very sensitive throat. Repeated efforts to clear this mucus from your throat can lead to the throat-clearing habit. Unfortunately, this habit is sometimes difficult to break, since the more you clear your throat, the more you irritate it, and the more you irritate it, the more you feel you have to clear it. Even so, the awareness of a postnasal drip—even one that makes you gag—is not indicative of sinusitis unless the mucous drainage is discolored or cloudy.

When your physician first peers into your throat to look for infected sinus drainage, he or she may not see any cloudy discharge because you may have already swallowed it, but the slight gagging sometimes caused by the tongue depressor can produce a squeezing down or milking action of your palate and cause the momentary appearance of a bubble or glob of cloudy infected mucus from behind the uvula. It may be gone in a second, but even when briefly noted, it is extremely helpful in the positive diagnosis of sinusitis. The persistence of a nasal tone to your voice after a cold can often be a good indicator of a blocked sinus and possibly a lingering sinusitis. Swollen, inflamed, somewhat reddish nasal membranes with associated symptoms of nasal blockage strongly suggest a sinus problem, but the absence of such findings doesn't rule out sinusitis. Swollen nasal membranes can also occur from allergic and nonallergic rhinitis but are more often pale to bluish-red in appearance unless there is a superimposed sinus infection, which would tend to make them more inflamed and usually a deeper red.

CAT SCAN, MRI, AND PLAIN SINUS X RAYS

For a doctor to put you through routine sinus X rays or CAT scans to confirm the diagnosis every time you have a sinus flare-up is not only unwise but economically unfeasible. Routine sinus X rays may often provide very little definitive information with regard to the ethmoid and sphenoid sinuses. If X rays do show some cloudiness, especially in the ethmoid sinuses, it could be due to scarring or subperiosteal thickening from an infection many years before. X rays may reveal a mass or air-fluid level in one of the larger sinuses but can be misleading when it comes to demonstrating a mass, active sinus membrane swelling, infection, and retained fluid or pus in the ethmoid or sphenoid sinuses. Here a CAT scan or sometimes an MRI may be much more revealing than plain sinus X rays but is not justified for most acute sinus flare-ups because of costs and the radiation exposure with a CAT scan, unless of course some complication or a chronic problem is suspected. A partial or very limited CAT scan is now being used and should provide most of the needed information at less expense and with less total radiation. MRI studies have the advantage of not exposing the patient to radiation but are generally not as helpful as a CAT scan in demonstrating sinus disease, where good bone definition is often needed. An MRI may sometimes be helpful if there is suspected fungal sinusitis, as well as in certain cases where further radiation exposure by a CAT scan might be considered unwise.

NASAL AND SINUS CULTURES

Nasal or sinus cultures with bacterial sensitivity studies for the various antibiotics are sometimes helpful in a diagnostic workup for a subacute or chronic problem but are only occasionally necessary if you have an acute sinus flare-up. Most culture reports are not available for three or four days, especially over a weekend, and most acute sinusitis patients may already demonstrate clinical improvement by then. Nasal cultures may tell your doctor only what kinds of bacteria happen to be present in the nose and not necessarily what exists in the sinus. In some instances, the findings may even represent contamination of the culture swab by bacteria clinging to the nasal hairs or to the skin of the nostrils. Bacterial sensitivity studies, on the other hand, can be helpful only if your doctor is fairly certain he or she has correctly identified and cultured the bacteria responsible for the sinus infection. Using a very small applicator and swabbing only the discharge from within a sinus opening should give fairly accurate results provided that your doctor doesn't touch the other nasal membranes, and the nasal hairs, or the nostril skin when introducing or withdrawing the culture swab. Small children will seldom permit a proper nasal culture. They will often jerk their heads or refuse to allow the introduction of a nasal speculum in order to avoid touching the nostril skin or hairs. Often the physician's best chance for a fairly reliable culture in a child is to obtain one through the mouth just behind the uvula when the child gags slightly.

To more accurately identify the infective organism, the doctor might culture the infected discharge from within the sinus cavity itself, which requires an invasive operative procedure, and even then may not be successful in obtaining a positive culture. I have obtained many cultures directly from obviously infected sinus cavities during surgery and requested that they also be tested for anaerobic bacteria that grow only in the absence of oxygen, and still had some of the cultures show no growth at all. This was especially true if the patient was already on an effective antibiotic or if the pus had been sealed off in the sinus cavity for a prolonged period, possibly allowing the buildup of nitric oxide in the sinus cavity as well as permitting the enzymes and antibodies in the retained mucous secretions to perform their works. Nitric oxide is produced by sinus membranes and is known for its antibacterial and antiviral capabilities as well as for its ability to improve cilia activity. In a diagnostic workup, cultures would still be considered worthwhile for any complicated sinus cases, very sick patients, those with subacute or chronic sinus disease, and any patients not responding to treatment.

SYMPTOMS OF SINUSITIS
CLOUDY NASAL DISCHARGE

It should now be apparent that possibly the best evidence and one of the most convincing signs of a sinus infection is your own observation of a cloudy discharge on blowing your nose or clearing your throat, realizing of course that infected matter cleared from the throat might sometimes have been coughed up from the lungs. You should be aware of this possibility, since you will often have to decide yourself whether the infected discharge was coughed up from your lungs or cleared from the back of your throat. Sometimes bringing to the physician's office a sputum sample either cleared from your throat or preferably blown from your nose will aid your doctor in identifying the presence of infection, although the sample will often be too contaminated and too old for a culture.

When cloudy sinus discharge is not found, your physician has to rely heavily on the history of the illness and whatever symptoms and signs you may have noted to make the diagnosis. In acute sinusitis, the patient or parent, most of the time, will recall a head cold or flulike episode at the start, since most viral respiratory infections are often followed by some degree of sinusitis. Viral head colds will often start with sneezing and a burning sensation in the nose, sometimes a soreness in the throat and above the palate, with associated nasal congestion and sinus blockage, occasionally a headache or face pain, sometimes a cough, and often with outpouring of nasal discharge, fairly clear at first and then usually by the third or fourth day frequently turning cloudy. Sometimes the discharge may be blood tinged from too strenuous blowing, from drying out of the nasal membranes, or from excessive use of nose sprays. If a sinus infection began as an episode of flu, it may start with a sore throat followed by hoarseness and cough, nonproductive at first and then usually productive of an infected, often greenish to brownish to yellowish mucus, or less often appearing whitish and opaque like milk. The flulike viral episode, usually involving the throat and lower respiratory tract in the beginning, may fairly often progress to the upper respiratory tract, nose, and sinuses, with symptoms rather similar to those previously described for a head cold. It too may be followed in three or four days by a bacterial sinusitis with a cloudy nasal discharge.

Some systemic symptoms are usually present in both instances but are usually much milder with the usual head cold than with flu. In both instances there may be a slight fever (more so with the flu), some generalized muscular aching occasionally involving the joints, loss of appetite often along with loss of taste and smell, and some tiredness or fatigue. As previously stated, the white blood count is usually within normal limits or slightly depressed with most viral infections, unless there is a complication such as early pneumonia or blockage of a bronchus from swelling or from an infected mucus plug. Either may cause an area of atelectasis, or airlessness, within a segment of the lung followed by fever and an elevation in the white count if the blockage is not rapidly relieved, usually by deep breathing and coughing. Some elevation of the white count and a fever are usually more evident in children with respiratory infections.

SINUS HEADACHE

With head colds and flu there may be a generalized headache and tenderness to pressure over your eyeballs, the latter usually being more apparent with the flu. Your eyes may ache some and water. A sensation of blockage in one or both ears from eustachian tube swelling may occur, especially in children. As the head cold progresses and your sinuses become more obstructed from nasal membrane swelling, the generalized headache or pressure feeling may shift to your face, cheeks, forehead, around your eyes, and sometimes to the top or back of your head, occasionally localizing to only one side depending on which sinuses are mostly involved.

Next to seeing a cloudy discharge from a sinus opening, the headache or face pain, when present, is the second most important symptom in identifying a sinus infection and in determining which sinuses are infected. Although every patient with a bacterial sinusitis should at some point have a cloudy discharge, in my own experience, only about 60 to 70 percent of the sinusitis patients 16 years of age and older that I examined complained of sinus headaches. Also in my experience, the elderly rarely complained of sinus headaches, and children even less often. The elderly also seemed to have fewer sinus problems, and that was generally true even for those who had suffered with sinusitis in their earlier years. Older individuals usually undergo a flattening of the surface membrane cells in their upper airways along with a decrease in mucus-secreting goblet cells. The former could result in some enlargement of the sinus drainage openings, and the latter in a thinner, freer, flowing mucus, both of which might contribute to the lessening of their sinus problems. Nevertheless, when the sinus headache is present, it is usually the most disturbing symptom of all and usually the one influencing you to seek early medical attention. It is usually characterized by a fairly deep dull pain of slight to moderate intensity and usually located in the brow area, between or behind the eyes, in the cheeks or in the back of the head depending on which sinuses are involved. Nausea is seldom associated with sinus headaches and when present may be related to medications or to alcohol intake the night before. Although sinus headaches can involve almost any part of the head, the brow and inner bony margin of the eye next to the nose are generally the most common locations for sinus pain. This is particularly true for the characteristic early-morning and late-afternoon ethmoid sinus headache or the midmorning to mid-afternoon frontal sinus headache. Since both frontal and ethmoid sinusitis often refer pain to the same brow area, the time of onset and departure of the headache is therefore very important in deciding which sinus is responsible. Moreover, the pain of frontal sinusitis is usually more intense than ethmoid pain.

MAXILLARY SINUS HEADACHE

Maxillary sinus pain usually centers around the involved cheek, frequently between the cheek and the nose, but may refer pain to your upper teeth and sometimes to your ear or the back of your head on the same side as the diseased sinus. Since ethmoid infection often accompanies maxillary sinusitis, there may be pain in the inner brow area as well. Although many people may have ethmoid sinusitis alone, whenever the other sinuses are diseased, either the anterior or posterior ethmoid sinuses will usually become infected also.

SPHENOID SINUS HEADACHE

Because of their location deep within the skull and their many surrounding nerves, your sphenoid sinuses, when infected, may refer pain to almost any part of your head, including the top of your head, behind your eyes, the back of your head, and even your temples. Sphenoid sinusitis may sometimes make the skin on top of your head very sensitive to combing or brushing your hair. Both sphenoid and maxillary sinus headaches are usually more disturbing during the late morning and afternoon. Since sinus headache is nearly always a daytime headache, the time of onset and departure during the day, the location of the pain, and the period of maximum discomfort will not only help in confirming that it is a sinus headache but will often help in identifying which sinuses are involved. Also realizing what makes your headache better or worse may further substantiate the diagnosis. When your headache is not severe, it will usually improve or even disappear with the use of nasal decongestants, taking an over-the-counter pain medicine, or sometimes after applying hot compresses and resting; whereas damp weather, air pressure changes, bending over, lifting, straining, shaking your head, coughing, breathing cold air, stress, and exercise will often make your sinus headaches worse. If your suspected sinus headache should persist throughout the entire night, which would be most unusual, it could be a headache due to some other cause or from a sinus infection that has extended beyond its bony confines to involve more vital structures. Asking sinusitis patients if their headaches are still present should they awaken in the middle of the night can be of considerable diagnostic help, especially since the alert observer will nearly always answer, "No, but it comes back again the very next day and at about the same time."

EMPYEMA FLUID LEVELS

If the headache or sinus pain should increase very significantly, especially in your frontal or cheek sinuses, then the possibility of complete sinus blockage with retained pus producing an empyema and showing an air-fluid level on X ray or CAT scan would be likely. Tenderness to finger tapping over the maxillary or frontal sinuses or discomfort on pressing upward beneath the upper bony orbital rim would help with this diagnosis, but these signs may still be absent in some cases. Also, an associated upper tooth discomfort is not an uncommon finding with empyema of the maxillary or cheek sinus. Empyema of a maxillary sinus may also produce the sensation of something moving or sloshing around in your cheek when you are walking down steps or stepping off of a curb.

The sphenoid sinuses, when totally obstructed, may develop a similar problem, but because of their location deep within the skull, they are properly named "the hidden sinuses" and are very difficult to evaluate for an empyema without a CAT scan. The ethmoids may also become totally blocked, but because of their very small size and their inflamed, swollen membranes often completely filling their small cavities, an air-fluid level may be absent or completely missed even with a CAT scan.

The headaches of acute sinusitis are usually more painful, but the daily annoying headaches experienced by many subacute and especially chronic sinus sufferers can be very discouraging, especially knowing that when they go away they will most likely return. Children and young adolescents, on the other hand, even with chronic sinusitis, are seldom bothered by sinus headaches, or so it seems. If your child complains of headaches, even though a sinus infection may be present, you may still have to look for another possible cause, especially if the head pain doesn't improve during treatment for the sinus infection.

Because sinus pain and headache, when present, can be the most disturbing and many times the most revealing of all the sinusitis symptoms, a more detailed discussion of this much neglected subject will be provided in the next section.

CHILDHOOD SINUSITIS

NASAL DISCHARGE

Since the medical history given by a child as to the character of a nasal discharge is usually not very reliable and sinus headaches are often absent, and since a parent may be working and therefore limited in his or her observations, the physician will often depend much less on the history and more on the findings in diagnosing sinusitis in a child. The most significant finding in childhood sinusitis is the same as with the adult, namely, the presence of a cloudy discharge in the nose or in the throat. When it can't be seen in the front of the nose, any dried crusting around the nostrils, especially if discolored, is often a clue that infected discharge has been there and is a fairly common finding in very small children with persistent sinusitis; however, it might have been wiped away by the parent before bringing the child to the doctor's office. As to finding infected discharge in the back of a child's throat, observing the palate area when a child gags slightly on a tongue depressor may, as previously mentioned, reveal a bubble of cloudy discharge squirting down from behind the palate or uvula and may sometimes be the only confirming evidence of the presence of a sinus infection in a child.

INFLAMED LATERAL BANDS

Finding reddish vertical streaks in the back of the throat, especially near the sides, often referred to by the physician as infected or inflamed lateral bands, may also be very helpful in diagnosing long-standing or chronic sinusitis, especially in children. These red streaks are due to very small clumps or clusters of inflamed lymphoid tissue, which sometimes give the appearance of the so-called cobblestone throat and which are usually a direct result of the continuous flow of infected drainage from the sinuses.

BAD BREATH

Bad breath may sometimes indicate an infected sinus discharge, but it isn't diagnostic, since other things such as chronically infected tonsils, diseased adenoids, dental cares, a coated tongue, esophageal reflux, gastrointestinal upset, chronic mouth breathing, a dry mouth, and even lung infections may cause bad breath as well. If bad breath does persist in a child and is getting worse, your doctor should also look for a possible foreign body in the nose, especially if there is also a persistent cloudy discharge from only one nostril. Although nasal foreign bodies are seldom present in adolescents or adults, the use of nasal feeding tubes, oxygen catheters, or plastic breathing tubes may cause a foreign body reaction in the nose resulting in rhinitis, sinusitis, and sometimes an odor. Internal anti-snoring devices or gadgets used to prop a nostril open at night for better breathing may also cause a foreign body reaction with mucous stasis, irritation of nasal membranes, and rhinosinusitis. These devices are rarely properly sterilized, are handled and inserted by contaminated fingers, interfere with sinonasal mucous flow, and can very easily introduce harmful bacteria into the nose.

NIGHTTIME COUGH

A slight nighttime cough, usually noted after midnight or during the early-morning hours and frequently for only a very short period, and many times not disturbing enough to awaken the child but possibly arousing a parent, is another likely finding in childhood sinusitis with a persistent infected postnasal drip. If your child coughs day and night because of a true bronchitis, you should still suspect an underlying and persistent sinusitis as a possible instigator, since any prolonged infection in one end of the respiratory tract may eventually involve the other.

MOUTH BREATHING

An increase in mouth breathing due to nasal blockage or a parent's awareness of a persistent nasal tone to a child's voice, often suggestive of maxillary sinus blockage, would both be very helpful for the physician to know.

NASAL TONE

A nasal tone may also be noted in the adult, especially when a maxillary sinus is blocked. Enlarged adenoids or allergic rhinitis may also create a nasal tone in a child, but when the larger sinuses are blocked, especially the maxillary, the nasal tone may sometimes sound a little more forward in the nose and slightly different from the hyponasality in the child created by enlarged adenoids, at least to the trained observer. Of course, both or all three may be present now that adenoids are seldom removed, and a persistent sinus infection may cause them to enlarge considerably. Although sinusitis may not directly affect a child's appetite, the problem of chewing and swallowing with an obstructed nasal airway may tend to limit a child's feeding interests as well as sometimes make a child fidgety and irritable.

DIMINISHED HEARING

If your child constantly turns the TV up loudly, you should suspect chronically blocked eustachian tubes and therefore the possibility of an underlying sinusitis, but you may become aware of a hearing problem only if both the child's ears are blocked. Diminished hearing from a swollen blocked eustachian tube on only one side may go unnoticed by a parent but may still be caused by a persistent sinus infection on that side. I have examined many adults with eustachian tube blockage problems, especially noticeable when flying or scuba diving, who also gave a very strong history of prolonged sinus infections in early life and long before ear tubes became popular.

PAIN IN TEETH

In older adolescents and adults, if a maxillary sinus is blocked or badly swollen from an infection, you may experience not only pain and tenderness in the cheek but also pain in the upper teeth on the same side, which occasionally may radiate along the nerves to the lower teeth on that side. This associated tooth discomfort occurs because the nerves to the upper teeth lie just beneath the floor of the maxillary sinuses, and any infection there may irritate these nerves to cause a toothache. Sometimes this referred tooth discomfort is so disturbing that you might have to consult a dentist to be certain that it is referred pain from a sinus infection and not primarily a diseased upper tooth that could even be infecting your sinus. Many times the tooth discomfort may be so acute that you will already have seen a dentist before consulting a sinus specialist. Moreover, whenever a maxillary sinus infection fails to clear up or continues to recur, an infected upper tooth or buried tooth root from a previous extraction should be suspected as a possible cause of the sinus problem and should be investigated, usually with a dental consultation and dental X rays.

TRANSILLUMINATION

If your doctor suspects a maxillary or frontal sinus infection, and X rays are not yet available, he or she will sometimes shine a light through your mouth in a darkened room or from each cheek through to your hard palate to transilluminate the maxillary sinuses or place it beneath the brow to transilluminate the frontal sinuses. This procedure may be worthwhile in older children and adults, since it may often tell your doctor whether that sinus is clear or cloudy. If the sinus is found to be cloudy, however, it could mean active sinus disease with membrane swelling and retained pus, or scarring from old disease without any activity now, or possibly a very small or absent sinus, especially with regard to the frontals. The doctor will then have to decide from the rest of the findings as to which it represents, and, of course, an X ray or CAT scan may sometimes be necessary in making this decision. This transillumination procedure has been used for more than a century but may have little diagnostic value in young children because of their puffy cheeks and very small sinuses. Transillumination of the sinuses, like plain sinus X rays, may give misleading information and sometimes make your doctor miss the diagnosis completely but when added to the other findings may still be helpful in coming up with the correct diagnosis.

EUSTACHIAN TUBE BLOCKAGE

Pain in an ear may result from a maxillary sinus infection by referring pain along nerve pathways to an ear or from inflammation and swelling of the eustachian tube itself due to infected sinus drainage passing close by the opening of the eustachian tube on its way to the throat. This eustachian tube swelling from infected sinus drainage, although usually far more common in a child, may sometimes cause ear problems in an adult with the accumulation of fluid in an ear, diminished hearing, ringing in an ear, occasional discomfort, and sometimes dizziness, and it may even progress to an ear infection.

SORE THROAT AND NASAL CONGESTION

When asked about the sore throat from an infected sinus drainage, many people will often point toward the palate and may also say they feel it in one or both ears. The sore throat typical of a sinus infection is usually a fairly mild morning sore throat and along with nasal congestion might be considered one of the more significant symptoms in making the diagnosis, especially in someone with a rather subtle sub-acute or chronic sinusitis or even with an acute sinusitis that has persisted for several weeks. This sore throat is usually the result of a nighttime accumulation of infected sinus discharge or pus in the back of the throat, and especially from bacterial toxins collecting there to cause inflammation and swelling. Nasal congestion with mouth breathing and drying out of the throat at night will usually exacerbate a sore throat. The throat pain is usually not severe, but like the early-morning ethmoid headache, it is usually there every morning when you awaken. It too usually goes away after you eat breakfast or drink a cup of hot coffee, which will stimulate your circulation, relieve swelling, and enhance the flow of mucus down your throat. A glass of water, hot cereal, and orange juice may work almost as well. This sore throat from infected sinus drainage may sometimes return during the day, usually in the evening, especially if the throat dries out from mouth breathing due to excessive talking, singing, or exercising.

HOW YOUR DOCTOR DIAGNOSES SINUSITIS

In making the diagnosis of sinusitis in the adolescent or adult, an accurate description of any postnasal drip or discharge from the nose is extremely important, particularly whether it is thick or thin, discolored or clear, and exactly what color, such as green, yellow, milky white, or blood streaked, and whether you think you coughed it up from your chest or cleared it from your throat. You may be asked to submit a specimen of the material blown out or coughed up on the next visit, especially if there is any uncertainty regarding the character of your sinonasal drainage, and especially if none can be seen by the physician during the examination. Frequently, people will describe sinus drainage as clear when it is really milky white, and cloudy when it is really foamy clear, with clear being normal and cloudy white indicating infection. It is important to remember that a sinus discharge doesn't have to be yellowish or greenish to be infected; a cloudy white discharge resembling milk or even skim milk is considered infected as well, but usually due to a different bacteria.

Often a sinus headache, especially in the very observant adult, may be diagnosed from a reliable history given over the phone or at least with a fairly brief examination. However, for your doctor to properly evaluate the more complicated case will require a meticulous history as to the time, location, and character of your head pain as well as what intensifies it and what relieves it, and especially if it disappears at night; whether it is helped by lying down, sitting up, sleeping elevated, or by the application of heat or cold and some say both, by taking Tylenol, aspirin, or other NSAIDs, by voluntarily induced gagging or vomiting, or by applying pressure to the area of pain. Your doctor will also want to know if you obtain any relief using a steroid, saline, or a decongestant nasal spray, by taking a decongestant pill or an antihistamine, or both, and whether the head pain is made worse by bending over, lifting, straining, coughing, sneezing, head shaking, walking down steps, diving, or flying. Knowledge of any accompanying visual disturbances, nausea, vomiting, dizziness, or discomfort in the eyes, ears, teeth, or neck will also be important to the examining physician.

Your physician may also inquire about possible allergies, nasal congestion (especially during the night and on which side), whether you are more comfortable sleeping elevated or on a particular side, and whether you have noticed any nasal burning, loss of taste or smell, sneezing, coughing, lack of concentration, lack of energy, tired eyes, or a feeling of weakness in the legs. Some people who have chronic sinusitis will say that their legs feel like jelly. A few may notice some increasing memory loss or forgetfulness, and some may also develop asthma with wheezing. Since children have small nasal passages to start with, and since their nasal membranes tend to swell excessively, sometimes blocking their posterior nasal drainage, you may have observed a cloudy discharge running out of the front of your child's nose and down the upper lip, often leaving a dried, slightly discolored crusting behind, and it is important for your doctor to know this. The examiner will also want to know how often a child sneezes and whether he or she frequently wipes a runny, itchy nose in an upward motion with the palm of the hand, an act often referred to as the "allergic salute," usually indicating a superimposed allergic rhinitis. If this palm wiping occurs very often, the child may develop an identifying skin crease across the bridge of the nose just above the nasal tip. You may also note dark circles under your child's eyes, or allergic shiners. Occasionally, while swimming, a child with sinusitis will expel a glob of cloudy infected discharge into the water from one or both nostrils, and this would be important evidence of a sinus infection.

Your doctor may also inquire about any neck injuries, especially related to neck fractures or surgery, and whether sinus blockage problems with nasal congestion and possibly increased nasal secretions began shortly thereafter. I have observed this development in some cases following neck injury and in a very few cases following neck surgery. It may be due to interference with the sympathetic nerve supply to the head, resulting in overactivity on the part of the counterbalancing parasympathetic nerve supply sometimes resulting in persistent nasal swelling and sinus congestion.

To confirm the diagnosis of sinusitis, the conscientious physician will first look for the telltale cloudy sinus discharge in your nose or draining down your throat. Your nose will also be inspected for any obstructive deformities such as enlarged turbinates, a deviated septum, a collapsed valve, growths or polyps, and to see if your nasal membranes are swollen and inflamed, especially around a sinus opening, where your doctor will also look for cloudy infected drainage as well. It is also important to determine whether your nasal membranes are pink, pale to bluish-red, or a deep red, with mildly pink being normal, pale to bluish-red suggesting allergy, and deep pink to deep red usually indicating varying degrees of infectious inflammation. In determining this, it is important to look with a bright white light with a narrow spot, since throat and nasal membranes will usually appear very reddish when examined with a weak or yellowish to orange light characteristic of most flashlights. I mention this because I have been called on numerous occasions, usually at night, by someone peering into a friend's or spouse's nose or throat with a dull flashlight and erroneously finding it very red and believing it to be infected.

Many times the medical examiner will shrink the inside of your nose with a topical decongestant for better visualization and apply a small amount of local anesthetic to painlessly examine your nose and nasopharynx with lighted magnified telescopes. The examiner will usually make two or three passes with the endoscope on each side, usually angling it upward to view the sinus drainage openings. This may reveal not only an infected discharge and redness around a specific sinus opening but also anything that might be obstructing the nose or a sinus such as a foreign body, polyp, cyst, tumor, septal deviation, enlarged or deformed turbinate, thickened erectile tissue, excessive scarring or adhesions, abnormal swelling, or even chronically infected adenoids behind the nose.

This type of examination is nearly impossible when the child is awake and if pursued may permanently endanger any future doctor-patient relationship. Occasionally a child will permit a cotton pledget with a decongestant on it to be placed just within the nostril on each side for a few minutes before examination. If so, it will open up the nose, and this can be a big help to the examiner. If the occasion should arise when a child with a persistent sinusitis may require a general anesthetic for some other reason, a thorough examination of the nose and sinus openings with the fiber-optic scopes at the same time, again using a topical decongestant, may prove very helpful in determining which sinuses are infected and whether there are any obstructive abnormalities such as a polyp, cyst, tumor, or enlarged turbinate. It would also provide a special opportunity to look for a nasal foreign body, which could be responsible for the sinus infection.

The examiner may tap on your frontal or maxillary sinuses with a finger or on any suspicious-looking upper teeth with a metallic probe to see if they are sensitive and therefore suggestive of disease. He or she may inspect your ears to see if they show evidence of eustachian tube blockage such as a retracted eardrum or the presence of fluid, which can result from an infected sinus drainage causing inflammation and blockage of a eustachian tube opening. Although dark circles around the eyes may sometimes occur with sinus infections or allergic rhinitis, especially in children, of a much more serious consequence would be the finding of swollen, inflamed eyelids, especially on only one side and possibly related to an orbital cellulitis, usually from an ethmoid sinus infection.

Orbital cellulitis may begin as a redness and slight swelling of the eyelids known as preseptal cellulitis, which is probably more often due to bacterial toxins from a nearby ethmoid sinus infection. In this early stage, intense antibiotic therapy for the sinusitis may be all that is needed, but if the infection should breach the sinus wall to produce an abscess beneath the periosteal lining of the bony orbit, or invade the orbital cavity itself, surgical drainage of the orbit or any suspected abscess along with surgical drainage of the guilty sinus is usually indicated. Since both the mild and serious types will usually produce redness and swelling of the eyelids, one of the best clues to identify the more serious kind is bulging or protrusion of the eyeball itself, known as proptosis, and here again a CAT scan may help to confirm the diagnosis.

Your physician may also question you about any family history of diabetes, cystic fibrosis, hypertension, immune disorders, chronic lung disease, anemia, and other conditions that might influence an infectious process in your sinuses. Your home, school, and working environments may also be scrutinized, along with your exercise routine, living and sleeping habits, hobbies, suspected allergies, and whether there are any chronic infectious problems, especially of the respiratory tract, lungs, or sinuses, in any other family members, close friends, carpoolers, playmates, or household pets.

When further confirmation is needed, especially as to the extent of the disease, whether there are any complications, and how much permanent damage exists, plain sinus X rays, or better still a CAT scan and in some instances an MRI, may be ordered, although the CAT scan is generally the most helpful. As previously mentioned, the overlapping densities and shadows created by most of the 22 bones of the skull as viewed on plain sinus X rays will often interfere with satisfactory visualization of the sphenoid and ethmoid sinuses. However, both the CAT scan and MRI are able to avoid these overlapping effects, and the use of an intravenous contrast media with a CAT scan or MRI may provide additional information. A sometimes limited follow-up CAT scan to determine the success of treatment and whether there is any residual sinus disease, especially in subacute or chronic cases, may have to be delayed for 4 to 6 weeks, since sinus swelling can easily last that long after an infection has cleared or even following surgery and could therefore confuse the issue.

If your case is more complicated, your physician may want to take a nasal culture and request bacterial sensitivity studies, including testing for anaerobic bacteria and occasionally for fungi, in order to identify the responsible organism and hopefully determine what antibiotic will be more effective against it.

In certain instances, allergic fungal sinusitis should be suspected and looked for in any young healthy adult who has nasal allergies, chronic sinusitis involving many sinuses on both sides, and multiple nasal or sinus polyps that keep recurring, especially when the sinusitis fails to respond to more than adequate treatment.

In a sinusitis workup, a careful history will often provide a clue as to whether an allergy evaluation is indicated. Sometimes a general medical workup including various laboratory studies may be necessary in difficult cases or in those not responding to adequate treatment.

WHAT IS A SINUS HEADACHE,
AND HOW CAN YOU TELL IF YOU HAVE ONE,
AND WHAT CAN BE DONE ABOUT IT?

Of all the sinusitis symptoms, the sinus headache can be the most complicated as well as the most difficult to explain, and yet a well-known textbook of medical physiology devotes only three short sentences to this subject. What is even more intriguing is that a review of six textbooks on otolaryngology revealed similar very limited discussions of sinus headaches, each less than five sentences. Although some did include a few diagrams showing the distribution of sinus pain, there was even some disagreement in that regard. Two of them did mention frontal sinus headaches as occurring after arising and then disappearing in the afternoon, but only one textbook noted the increase in frontal sinus pain toward the middle of the day. None of them mentioned that frontal sinus pain is often worse after you have been up for awhile whereas ethmoid pain usually gradually improves after you get up and move about. There was also no mention of characteristic early-morning onset of ethmoid sinus headache or its usual disappearance several hours later, especially after being up, nor its tendency to recur in the late afternoon. One book did mention maxillary sinus pain as being usually more apparent in the early afternoon. Amazingly enough, there was no mention of the absence of sinus pain at night, a very important fact that may be extremely helpful not only in diagnosing sinusitis but also in differentiating sinus headache from other types of head pain. Most of the textbooks described sinus headache as a deep, dull pain, but two disagreed as to whether it could also be throbbing in nature.

None offered any explanation for the regular daily occurrence and disappearance of sinus headaches or any information that might explain their absence during the night. If a sinus headache should persist throughout the night, a doctor has reason to be concerned about a possible extension beyond the bony confines of the sinus to the central nervous system resulting in a brain abscess, cavernous sinus thrombosis, or meningitis. In such instances, the headache may become more generalized and often more intense and may even shift to the back of the head. This extension from a sinus to the central nervous system or brain may sometimes proceed through infected clots, or thrombi, in very small vessels, often making it impossible to demonstrate early progression of the disease even with a CAT scan.

TIMING AND LOCATION OF SINUS PAIN

In most cases of sinusitis, it is the headache or face pain that so often influences you to seek medical attention, and at the same time, it is the rather unique daily disappearance of this head pain that is frequently responsible for delayed or canceled doctor's appointments. As soon as the headache disappears, you may mistakenly assume you are getting well, cancel your appointment with the doctor, and are often very surprised to see your sinus headache return the very next day. Except when it is part of a viral respiratory infection such as a head cold or flu, it is practically never a generalized headache but usually asserts itself in certain specific areas of the skull and many times on only one side. This can often be of considerable help in diagnosing that it is a sinus headache as well as in determining what particular sinus or group of sinuses is responsible. In addition to the head and face discomfort, a sinus infection may also cause pain in a tooth, the jaw, an ear, the mastoid, the temples, the eye, the back of the neck and in very rare instances even a shoulder. This very rare sinus pain in a shoulder, once known as Sluder's lower half headache, is more likely due to a neuralgia originating from a nerve ganglion in the back of the nose and, unlike the dull ache of sinusitis, usually causes a deep boring or burning pain in the cheek, nose, or the area around an eye. Posterior ethmoid or sphenoid sinusitis has been suspected of initiating this sphenopalatine ganglion response in some instances and is therefore blamed for the shoulder pain. However, since there is some overlap between the pain nerves in the head and the cervical nerves in the back of the neck, sinus pain itself may in this manner be sometimes referred to distant areas such as the back of the head, the neck, the jaw, and possibly in rare instances to a shoulder.

ETHMOID AND FRONTAL SINUS HEADACHES

If you develop a headache around an eye, between the eyes, or in the forehead, occurring in the early morning, usually on awakening, and if it then goes away in an hour or two after getting up, sometimes returning for several hours in the early evening, it is nearly always due to ethmoid sinus blockage. Some possible exceptions would include the early-morning hangover headache from too much to drink the night before, which is usually in the same location, very similar to the ethmoid sinus headache, and frequently due to ethmoid sinus block-age from membrane swelling due to alcohol. Then there is the early-morning headache sometimes caused by sleep apnea depriving the brain of adequate oxygen during the night. A third possibility is the early-morning headache caused by a slow carbon monoxide leak in the house or car, which of course could be deadly. Nausea, a common finding with carbon monoxide headaches, is usually absent with sinus headaches, unless of course you also had too much to drink the night before or should become aware of a postnasal drip and begin to vomit.

If, on the other hand, the morning headache is in the brow area but doesn't develop until midmorning, increases toward the middle of the day, and then gradually disappears toward the middle of the afternoon, it is nearly always due to a frontal sinus infection and is frequently accompanied by X-ray evidence of a frontal sinus air-fluid level or so-called empyema, which means pus within a cavity. When a frontal sinus is acutely infected and obstructed in this manner, there is often ethmoid and maxillary sinus involvement on the same side as well, since the drainage openings of all three sinuses are very close together and tend to infect each other. As a result, there could be an associated maxillary sinus pain in a cheek, especially noticeable in the early afternoon, as well as ethmoid pain in the brow area or around an eye, occurring each day several hours before the onset of the more intense midmorning headache of frontal sinus disease. All three sinus infections, when present, will have to be cleared up, or the usually more serious frontal sinus infection will very likely return (it may anyway if the obstruction to the frontal sinus drainage duct or opening is not permanently relieved).

Both frontal and ethmoid sinus headaches are usually located in the same area of the skull, namely, the forehead or brow region, especially when the anterior ethmoids are involved. The main differentiating factors between the two, however, are their times of onset and departure, as well as the tendency for frontal sinus pain to intensify toward the middle of the day, when ethmoid pain will have already departed. Ethmoid sinus headache may sometimes recur in the late afternoon, when frontal sinus pain will usually have disappeared.

Typically, ethmoid sinus headaches usually start between four and six o'clock in the morning, sometimes waking you up. Some people will say that the pain is always there in the morning when they open their eyes. However, after you are up, moving about, and have had breakfast, the headache will usually gradually disappear, occasionally, but not always, recurring between four and six o'clock in the evening. It will then disappear again around dinnertime or by early bedtime at the very latest, only to reappear at about the same time early the next morning.

In a very different way, frontal sinus headache, once referred to as sun pain because it becomes more intense as the sun reaches the middle of the heavens and then wanes as the sun descends, will usually develop midmorning, somewhere between nine and ten o'clock, often closer to ten, intensify toward the middle of the day, and usually disappear between three and four o'clock in the afternoon, varying of course with the change to daylight saving time. Wolff's classic neurological textbook on headaches mentions frontal sinus pain as commonly developing at about nine o'clock in the morning, gradually becoming worse, and then terminating toward evening or on retiring. Bedtime is actually very late for frontal sinus pain to disappear unless it is accompanied by an evening ethmoid sinus headache as well. If you have both frontal and ethmoid sinusitis, which is not uncommon, the headache may cover both time spans continuously from early morning to late evening; however, the much more intense and usually more serious frontal sinus pain during the middle of the day will nearly always dominate the picture.

SPHENOID AND MAXILLARY SINUS HEADACHES

Sphenoid and maxillary sinusitis both cause daytime headaches, and in my experience, both are usually more prominent toward the middle of the day or in the early afternoon. Sphenoid sinus pain has been reported as predominantly an early-morning headache, but this may be due to its frequent association with a posterior ethmoid sinusitis, especially since fewer than 3 percent of sinus infections are believed to involve the sphenoid sinuses alone. However, this incidence could increase with more frequent use of the CAT scan, which is particularly helpful in diagnosing sphenoid disease.

Maxillary pain usually occurs in a cheek or upper tooth but may also be felt beside the nose, in the jaw, or in the temporal area and is frequently associated with ethmoid sinusitis. This means that an early-morning headache above or around an eye may be present as well. Occasionally maxillary sinus pain may be felt in the back of the head on the same side as the involved sinus and may sometimes be referred to an ear on the same side as well.

Sphenoid sinus headaches, because of an extensive network of nerves and vascular structures adjacent to these sinuses, may refer pain or headache to a variety of areas including the top of the head or vertex, the back of the head, frequently behind an eye, occasionally the forehead, sometimes the temporal area, and, according to some observers, even a shoulder. The headache is often very intense and may sometimes require a narcotic for relief. In some instances, it may even make the top of the head very sensitive to the combing or brushing of your hair. Although sphenoid and maxillary sinusitis may both cause pain in the back of the head, often only on one side, when the headache is due to maxillary sinusitis, there may be associated cheek or upper tooth discomfort also on the same side. Bilateral temporal head pain may sometimes occur with bilateral sphenoid or maxillary sinusitis, but it is probably more often the result of muscular tension in the back of the neck and scalp. However, its location, signs of local tenderness, and time of onset and disappearance are rarely so defining as with sinus headaches. Because sphenoid sinus pain may be present in almost any area of the head, any unusual or inadequately explained headache, especially when located on only one side, deserves at least a limited CAT scan early in its diagnostic workup to rule out sphenoid sinus disease, since early diagnosis and treatment can be crucial.

SINUS HEADACHE PAIN AND ITS RELIEF

Sinus headache is usually a persistent dull aching pain, practically never sharp or knifelike, and many people describe it as more of a deep pressure feeling. A throbbing pain is seldom noted but when present sometimes indicates a more serious sinus problem. The sinus headache is usually exacerbated by shaking your head, bending over, coughing, sneezing, lifting, and straining and is usually improved to some extent by staying quiet and relaxing or lying down on the uninfected side or with your head elevated. The one exception is that getting up will often make the early-morning ethmoid sinus headache go away sooner. Applying warm, moist heat to your face and forehead is much more effective in providing lasting relief than applying a cold pack. However, some sinus headaches may require fairly intense medical treatment including antibiotics and even surgical drainage of the involved sinus before a sinus headache will go away and stay away.

Most people describe their sinus pain as a fairly deep, rather constant dull ache, known physiologically as slow pain. At times it can be quite severe, and yet a few who have had it on a daily basis for a long time may hardly be aware of the pain. When the headache is present, you may become irritable, short-tempered, and forgetful, and you may often find it difficult to concentrate. Any alcohol intake may tend to exacerbate it, especially on the following morning. Exercise, excitement, mental stress, and exposure to cold air can also make the pain worse. Many sinus-prone individuals who drink, especially if they consume more than 1 to 1.5 ounces of 80-proof whiskey or the equivalent amount of wine (5 ounces) or beer (12 ounces) in an evening, may often bring on a sinus blockage-type headache the next morning. This is especially true for someone with unhealthy, scarred, or partially obstructed sinuses. This headache is usually fairly typical of the early-morning ethmoid sinus headache, is mostly located above, in between, or around the eyes, is present on awakening, is usually bilateral, and in many instances is very likely due to ethmoid sinus blockage from membranous swelling caused by too much alcohol. The alcohol-induced toxic headache, however, even when partly related to ethmoid sinus blockage, is far more likely to cause nausea and is often more generalized. Alcohol in sufficient quantity dilates small blood vessels, causing tissue swelling throughout the body.

Tissue swelling seems to be less well tolerated by the ethmoid sinuses due to their relatively poor blood supply, and because any membranous swelling is confined to very small bony cavities. They would therefore register earlier discomfort from the increased pressure on nerve endings near their drainage openings or within their walls, especially if already inflamed, scarred, or partially obstructed. Since the anterior ethmoid sinuses generally have the smallest drainage openings of any of the sinuses, usually averaging between 1 and 2 millimeters in diameter, any membrane swelling from too much alcohol might be expected to block them first and result in a vacuum-type headache from air absorption within the sinus cavity. The other sinuses, being much larger by comparison, usually having larger drainage openings and containing a greater amount of compressible or expansible air, would generally be less affected by any temporary membrane swelling or early vacuum formation before producing a painful reaction.

Keeping your alcohol consumption level down throughout an evening is important not only to avoid sinus blockage headaches the next morning but also to discourage an acute sinus flare-up if you suffer from chronic sinusitis. Diluting alcohol intake with other liquids as well as food during the course of the evening can also be very helpful. If you are prone to sinusitis or ethmoid blockage headaches and you must drink, take your 1 to 1.5 ounces of 80-proof whiskey in a very tall glass, well diluted, and make it last all evening.

SLEEPING ELEVATED

As previously mentioned, sleeping with your upper body elevated or in a sitting position will usually minimize, delay, and sometimes even abort the early-morning ethmoid sinus headache, and some people with ethmoid sinusitis, as well as a few heavy drinkers prone to such headaches, often discover this on their own. However, if you must sleep fairly flat, you can still minimize your nasal and sinus blockage on the bad side by sleeping with the healthier, less troublesome sinuses down against the pillow. Having your bad sinus up will not only reduce swelling but also promote better drainage.

The milder types of sinus headache are often temporarily relieved by a decongestant pill such as pseudoephedrine or a decongestant nasal spray. Aspirin, Tylenol, or one of the nonsteroidal anti-inflammatory drugs, very similar to aspirin and known as NSAIDS, including Motrin, Advil, Daypro, Nuprin, Indocin, Naprosyn, Feldene, Ibuprofen, Ansaid, and Orudis, should also provide temporary relief for the mild to moderate sinus headache. If any of these medications should effectively relieve your sinus headaches, your physician should know about it, since it helps him to determine the intensity of your headache, and sometimes the seriousness of the sinus problem as well. Occasionally, a long-acting decongestant pill taken at bedtime will diminish or prevent the early-morning ethmoid sinus blockage headache, but it may also keep you awake. In such instances, the combination of a long-acting decongestant with one of the sedating antihistamines, both taken at bedtime, may avoid the insomnia and still thwart an ethmoid sinus headache early the next morning. Again, such information, especially if it works, would be helpful to your doctor in making a diagnosis. You should remember, however, that when you take a drowsiness-producing antihistamine, you should avoid the additional intake of alcohol, tranquilizers, sedatives, or sleeping pills. Moreover, the regular prolonged use of a first-generation antihistamine may also cause thickening of sinonasal mucous secretions. Trial of a decongestant nasal spray on awakening in the morning might add additional relief as well as useful information if the spray is successful in relieving the head pain, especially if it works very quickly, since it might then suggest a nasal airway abnormality aggravated by nighttime swelling from the lying-down position as a possible cause.

TURBINATE HEADACHE (CONCHA BULLOSA)

A rapid relief of head pain with a decongestant nasal spray could also mean that the headache or eye or cheek pain could be due to middle turbinate swelling or enlargement, causing the so-called middle turbinate headache syndrome. In such instances, pressure against nerve endings in the nasal septum or in the lateral wall of the nose from middle turbinate swelling can sometimes cause rather intense pain, especially since the area of the sinus openings just under the middle turbinate is generally considered to be the most sensitive part of the nose. In fact, it is generally believed that sinus pain or headache may often originate from an inflamed sinus drainage opening as well as from the inflamed and swollen turbinate overlying and protecting it. Sometimes a middle turbinate may become distended by a large hollow space or sinus cavity within its bony core known as a concha bullosa. Any additional nasal swelling, such as initiated by a head cold or allergy, or from breathing a primary irritant, as well as from lying down (especially on that side), may cause pressure pain or headache originating within the turbinate, the lateral nasal wall, the septum, or the sinus cavity itself. Since this hollow space within the turbinate is lined with a ciliated mucus-secreting membrane like the other sinus cavities, it may, by obstruction of its drainage opening or by developing a polyp or mucocele, cause an expanding pressure-like feeling within the nose and headache or pain in the cheek, nose, eye, or brow.

Occasionally pressure pains may also develop from surface enlargement or swelling of an inferior or superior turbinate. A CAT scan and sometimes applying a topical anesthetic very locally to the turbinate to see if it relieves the head or face pains may help to confirm the diagnosis of pain due to turbinate enlargement. Treatment, of course, would be to reduce the size of the turbinate, either medically or more permanently by surgery, or sometimes by a freezing technique known as cryosurgery if the enlargement involves only the soft tissue covering. If the nasal septum is deviated and also pushing against a turbinate, this too may cause head or face pain and may have to be corrected at the same time. Whenever two opposing membranous surfaces within the nose swell and press against each other, cilia activity and mucous flow will cease in that area, and if this stasis continues, a localized persistent inflammation with infection, ulceration, scarring, and adhesions may occur.

TIMING OF SINUS HEADACHES

With an ethmoid sinus headache, it is sometimes difficult to determine the exact time of onset because some people are heavy or late sleepers, and some may have had several drinks the evening before, which can influence the intensity and time of onset or awareness of early-morning ethmoid pain. This early-morning ethmoid blockage headache can usually be blamed on peak sinonasal membrane swelling, mostly from the lowered position of the head during sleep, especially since it can often be diminished and sometimes obviated by sleeping elevated or in a semi-sitting position. The pain is usually relieved in an hour or two with the reduction in head and sinonasal swelling from the head-up position of getting up and moving about. This increased reduction in sinonasal swelling after arising is aided not only by the gravitational flow of blood from the head due to the upright position but also by the change from the resting state of heart and lung activity during sleep to one of increased cardiopulmonary activity from being awake and up and about, and the corresponding increase in circulation, heart rate, and blood pressure. The usual result is an improvement in venous congestion with a more effective mobilization of fluid throughout the entire body as well as in the swollen membranes of the head, nose, and sinuses. However, none of this sufficiently explains why ethmoid pain or headache sometimes returns in the late afternoon, usually between four and six o'clock, apparently unassociated with cocktail time, only to disappear again an hour or two later that evening.

The very precise timing of frontal sinus pain, with its midmorning onset becoming more intense toward the middle of the day and disappearing usually between three and four o'clock in the afternoon, often associated with a fluid level on X ray, has been observed by numerous patients and even experienced by myself on a number of occasions years ago. This kind of pain nearly always indicates a rather serious sinus problem and may even require drainage on an emergency basis. It is therefore important that you are very much attuned to the nature of frontal sinus pain and that you alert your doctor should it develop. Unlike the ethmoid headache, frontal sinus pain doesn't seem to be delayed or minimized by sleeping elevated, getting up early, or even sleeping late. In fact, it is often increased by most forms of activity. Like sinus pain in other areas, when present, frontal sinus pain is particularly exacerbated by shaking your head, bending over, lifting, and straining, and the frontal area may also be tender to palpation or to tapping with a finger directly over the sinus cavity or brow area. In such cases, pinching the inner brow area between the thumb and forefinger and with the thumb just beneath the upper bony rim of the orbit will usually elicit pain.

VACUUM HEADACHES, BAROMETRIC PRESSURE, AND YOUR BIOLOGICAL CLOCK

Not only will a positive pressure buildup in an infected sinus cavity from inflammatory swelling and the accumulation of infected discharge often cause a sinus headache, but a vacuum-type sinus headache may occur from the absorption of air trapped within a completely obstructed, but not necessarily infected, sinus cavity. Although a positive pressure buildup in a sinus cavity from inflammatory swelling might be slowed some by the air absorption of the sinus membranes, this air absorption might also be diminished significantly by the presence of an acute inflammatory process. In my practice, I measured pressure levels in more than a dozen totally obstructed and acutely infected frontal sinuses showing air-fluid levels on X ray, and all revealed a slight to moderate positive pressure buildup. This is in rather marked contrast to the obstructed but uninfected middle ear, which has been shown to absorb air rather rapidly, usually developing a partial vacuum in 20 to 30 minutes after persistent eustachian tube blockage occurs. During and after plane flights, it is mostly the negative pressure or vacuum effect in an obstructed and usually uninfected sinus that causes most of the head and face discomfort.

Early in my career, I was emphatically reminded by some of my patients that while flushing out their maxillary sinuses, drawing back on the syringe and creating a vacuum was much more painful than pushing on the plunger and increasing the positive pressure within the sinus cavity. This effect was also impressively demonstrated to me when suction was applied to my own frontal sinus through an incision in the brow and I experienced an excruciating pain. Here a vacuum or suction might cause stretching or tugging on pain nerves within the periosteum, or bony covering of the sinus cavity, and could be responsible for much of this discomfort, especially since the soft membranous linings of sinuses are considered to be fairly insensitive to pain. In children, especially, the periosteum covering their bony structures, which include the inside bony walls of their sinuses, is thicker and more vascular, contains more soft tissue, and is more loosely connected to the underlying bone by numerous elastic fibers. All of these factors serve to cushion any pressure effect or a vacuum pull on nerve endings there and could even be a factor in the infrequency of sinus pain and headache in children, who seem to have much more elasticity, or give, in all of their tissues.

In most instances that I have had to surgically drain an acute frontal sinusitis showing an air-fluid level and have temporarily inserted a hollow tube for subsequent irrigations, thus releasing any further pressure buildup within the sinus cavity itself, I have noticed that the timely onset and persistence of frontal sinus pain, although often diminished, would continue to occur in most cases at the same time of day until the infectious inflammation and swelling had subsided some. This would suggest that the inflammatory responses within the sinus walls, especially near their very sensitive drainage openings, might have a more significant effect in initiating or sustaining a frontal sinus headache than the buildup of a positive pressure within the sinus cavity itself.

For the present, however, we can only speculate as to whether the somewhat rhythmic coming and going of sinus headache and the almost complete absence of pain at night is in some way tied into our biological clocks, or to some kind of "clock gene," as recently found in mice, to hormone release or a nighttime reduction thereof, to the analgesia system, to endorphins and their opiate receptors in the brain, to the body's complicated inflammatory response, to an increased release of serotonin or certain prostaglandins, to nitric oxide accumulation in a blocked sinus cavity, to cyclic membrane swelling, to nervous system fatigue, or to some combination thereof.

One might also wonder if the very minimal drop in atmospheric pressure known as the solar tide, occurring during the day from

10:00 A.M. until about 4:00 P.M., might be a factor. This is almost the exact duration of frontal sinus pain and also represents the period when most of the discomfort occurs from the other two larger sinuses as well. These normally very slight highs and lows in barometric pressure are based on local time, since this is a worldwide phenomenon moving constantly around the globe, more obvious in the tropics but slightly distorted in the middle latitudes by the jet stream and other atmospheric phenomena. This of course would not explain the pain noted in the much smaller ethmoid sinuses, usually occurring for several hours before or after the solar tide, nor would it explain the complete absence of sinus pain during the same period of atmospheric pressure drop from 10:00 P.M. to 4:00 A.M. during the night but also during a period when solar energy is absent. We do know, however, that a very minimal drop in atmospheric pressure from an approaching storm can cause sinus pain and headache in certain individuals who have obstructive sinus disease. Unfortunately, we really don't know just how much solar energy, gravity, electromagnetic waves, and the atmosphere around us interrelate with our biological clocks and our biological functions.

It would appear that to arrive at a reasonable explanation for the rather bizarre daily onset and disappearance of sinus headaches in general, we would also have to find a plausible explanation for the usually complete absence of sinus headaches during most of the night. So far, no one has.

CHAPTER FOUR

Why Is Sinusitis Such a Complex Common Disease?

SINCE MOST HEAD colds and many of the 40 million flu cases occurring each year are either accompanied or followed by some degree of sinus involvement, that alone makes sinusitis one of our most common diseases. When you also consider the frequency with which it is found in combination with allergic and nonallergic rhinitis, with rhinitis of pregnancy, with chronic lung diseases, and with 70 percent or more of late-stage AIDS patients, sinusitis becomes a major health and socio-economic problem as well.

The actual incidence figures for sinusitis are impossible to obtain, since most of the acute cases are either self-treated or clear up on their own. However, people who seek medical attention because of a sinus infection, and can therefore be counted, are estimated at close to 50 million cases a year. Many of these people, of course, suffer from chronic sinusitis, which the U.S. Department of Health and Human Resources has estimated at more than 30 million cases in the United States alone, thus making it the nation's most prevalent chronic disease. The rapid advances in special equipment for diagnosing sinus disease should make this figure even higher, since many subacute and chronic cases have been overlooked in the past.

Conservative estimates indicate that sinus infections caused 73 million limited-activity days in 1992, and 13 million antibiotic prescriptions were written for sinusitis during that same period, which is more than twice the number recorded in 1985. Medical costs for the diagnosis and treatment of sinus infections in 1992 were estimated at between 2 and 3 billion dollars, and that doesn't include any special exams such as CAT scans and MRI or even endoscopic sinus surgeries (ESS), which are now estimated at close to 300,000 a year and performed mostly for chronic disease. It would be impossible to even estimate the amount of money spent on over-the-counter medications that are consumed each year to alleviate various sinusitis symptoms.

Worldwide estimates of sinus infections would undoubtedly run into astronomical figures, especially since head colds and flu, the usual forerunners of acute and subacute sinus infections, are so very common in almost every populated area today, thanks to the burgeoning of international travel and the influx of tourism into nearly every corner of the world. The global spread of respiratory viruses from plane cabin contacts has no doubt contributed its share as well.

Sinusitis can also be a very complex disease and may become even more so when it is neglected or ignored. At times, it can be so insignificant that you are completely unaware that you even have it, and it may even go away entirely by itself without your ever knowing. On the other hand, sinusitis can be so complex that if it goes untreated or inadequately treated, it may cause a chronic lung infection, chronic cough, asthma, and difficulty breathing, as well as a persistent sore throat, laryngitis, esophagitis, gagging, vomiting, bad breath, tearing, diminished taste, loss of sense of smell, insomnia, headache, chronic fatigue, a feeling of weakness in the legs, loss of appetite, irritability, lack of concentration, forgetfulness, toothache, ear infection, diminished hearing, dizziness, and sometimes even blurred vision, double vision, and blindness. On very rare occasions, it may cause a brain abscess or meningitis with convulsions, coma, and death. Sinusitis can also play a role in infections in other parts of the body far removed from the sinuses such as a heart valve infection, chronic prostatitis, and kidney or bladder infections. If this sinus relationship should go unrecognized and therefore untreated, the remote problem may often persist or continue to recur. A sinus infection can even be passed on to other family members, pets, and close companions, as well as from them to you, and unfortunately can even last a lifetime.

Although most people are aware of the symptoms of acute sinusitis, many may pay little attention to the often milder symptoms of subacute and chronic disease, especially in the beginning, even though both of these conditions in the long run may have far more serious consequences. It is also a disease for which the diagnosis can be completely missed, even with a careful examination by a competent physician. Even the severity of a chronic sinus infection may sometimes show a complete lack of correlation between the CAT scan findings and the microscopic exam of diseased tissue obtained at surgery. The usual clues of an acute bacterial infection, such as fever and an elevated white blood count, are also mostly absent in bacterial sinusitis, whereas the very same infection with the same virulent bacteria in another part of the body—such as an arm or leg—not confined to a bony cavity might very well produce a high fever, chills, and a markedly elevated white count. Even though the infection in both instances may respond to antibiotic treatment, the sinus infection will not clear up completely until adequate sinus drainage and sinonasal air exchange have been reestablished, which can sometimes take a very long time and may even require very prolonged antibiotic therapy. This makes relieving the sinus blockage just as important as treating the sinus infection, and for a complete cure, both should proceed together.

The presence of a sinus infection may be completely overshadowed by an accompanying ear, eye, nose, throat, or lung infection, and yet it may be largely responsible for their existence. Many times if sinusitis goes untreated or ignored, it will become chronic, and so may the associated disease. If you are afflicted with it, especially in the subacute or chronic forms, you may have nothing to show for nearly always feeling bad, often missing work or school, and yet rarely gaining any sympathy from the boss, a teacher, friends, and family. Moreover, since you seldom feel good, it may show up in your work, in your studies, and even in your disposition.

Even though a headache is often the most disturbing symptom noted by the majority of sinusitis patients, and usually the one that brings you to the doctor, 30 percent of my adult sinusitis patients did not complain of sinus headaches. To further complicate the picture, those that do have sinus headaches will usually experience them at various times during the day depending on what sinuses are involved, but practically never at night, even with the worst kind of sinus infection. Furthermore, children and the elderly rarely admitted to sinus pain or hurting even after careful questioning, again revealing the very complex nature of the disease. Some sinusitis patients will also gag and vomit from their postnasal drip, whereas others with the same kind of sinusitis and the same kind of infected drip may be totally unaware of it.

An episode of sinusitis may be influenced or even initiated by any one of a hundred or more different contacts or exposures in your working, schooling, traveling, and living environments, including the many things you breathe, touch, and swallow every day. It is, therefore, a disease whose onset, persistence, and prognosis can be drastically affected by your choice of a particular job, a certain working environment, an office building, a type of home and its location, air-conditioning and the kind of heat you have, as well as the location of the vents; by a particular climate, a school or college environment, the clothes you wear, your recreational activities, personal habits, hobbies, pleasures, allergic history, social activities, modes of transportation, human and animal contacts, weather, humidity, temperature variations, and pollution exposure; as well as by your general health and medical care, and sometimes even by the medicines you take, the air you breathe, and the food you eat. Just as too little humidity can make sinusitis worse, so can too much humidity.

Many people can throw off even the most virulent sinus infection on their own with little or no treatment, whereas others with much milder infections may have to be treated with prolonged intense antibiotic therapy and sometimes even with surgery to get well and stay well. Some acute sinus flare-ups respond to almost any antibiotic on one occasion, and the next time respond to almost none. It always disturbs me greatly to hear an authoritative person say that antibiotics should not be used for something as simple as a sinus infection for fear of causing bacteria-resistant organisms. Such people should take a moment to realize just how unpleasant and complicated inadequately treated sinusitis can become and that much more antibiotic treatment may be required later if certain acute or subacute sinus infections are either ignored or treated in too simple a manner.

In many instances, you may be given entirely different opinions by different doctors, including sinus specialists, as to how your sinus problem should be treated, and understandably, this may cause you great consternation. Often a doctor will fall back on his or her own past experience in the treatment of similar cases, which may account for some of this. A sinus doctor may also change his or her mind as to what is the better course of treatment, especially for a subacute or chronic sinus problem, after seeing you for a second or third time.

The medical treatment for some cases of subacute and chronic sinusitis may also present complexities other than the proper choice of a steroid spray, a decongestant, or an effective antibiotic that may be safely tolerated, possibly for a prolonged period. Proper treatment may also require a thorough investigation and treatment of any contributing factors such as allergic rhinitis, immune deficiency, diabetes, hypothyroidism, and other systemic disorders. The identification, avoidance, and control of certain environmental factors that could be contributing to a persistent sinus problem might also have to be diligently pursued, further adding to the complexities of the disease.

Even though some degree of sinusitis may accompany most head colds and many episodes of flu, normally healthy sinuses, thanks to their own built-in self-cleaning capabilities and provided they do not become persistently obstructed, can usually cleanse themselves of any retained infectious organisms, pus, and other contaminants and quickly revert to their original healthy state principally on their own. They are able to accomplish this through a very complex system of local immune response, mucous secretions containing bacteria-destroying enzymes and antiviral agents, the production of bacterio-static nitric oxide, rapid cilia regeneration, and a very effective sinonasal sweeping process.

The diagnosis of sinusitis can sometimes become very complex if the patient or doctor is unable to identify a cloudy, infected discharge within the nose or coming from a sinus. This of course may be missed if a sinus is completely blocked, if the doctor should happen to inspect the nose and sinuses at the wrong time, or if the patient is a child or very unobservant adult. The history, which is usually so helpful in making the diagnosis of sinusitis, may be unreliable or even totally lacking when taken from a child's working parent or in a divided-custody situation. Routine sinus X rays, which may often reveal retained pus with an air-fluid level, membrane thickening and scarring, as well as polyps, cysts, or other growths within the larger sinus cavities, will usually tell very little about the ethmoid or sphenoid sinuses. Even a CAT scan cannot always tell you if what you see is the result of an old or a recent sinus infection. Transillumination, or shining a light through a maxillary or frontal sinus, may also give a faulty impression as to the presence of disease. An endoscopic exam under local anesthesia with two or three passes of the scope on each side may be very helpful in identifying a blocked sinus, nasal polyps, inflammation, or an infected discharge but requires a trained specialist and cannot be done in a child without a general anesthesia. Endoscopy is not always accurate in identifying a sinus infection, especially if a sinus is completely obstructed or if you have been on antibiotic therapy for a while. Even a positive culture from the nose doesn't necessarily identify what kind of infection exists within the sinus cavity itself.

Some persistent cases of sinusitis may be so complicated as to require the opinions of a half-dozen or more consultants other than the ear, nose, and throat specialist (otolaryngologist), possibly including an allergist, a radiologist, a family practitioner, a pediatrician or internist, a hematologist, an endocrinologist, a pulmonary specialist, a dental surgeon, a neurologist, sometimes a neurosurgeon, and in rare instances even a psychiatrist.

More than a score of different operations on the sinuses and a dozen or more on the nose have been devised and are still performed in the treatment of sinusitis, and many people may have submitted to more than just a few before they were cured and some not even then. I underwent 11 such operations, all on one side, before finally obtaining complete relief, but unfortunately there is no guarantee that even a dozen surgical procedures will afford a complete cure.

There are also some very good reasons why endoscopic sinus surgery, as well as sinus surgery in general, can be so complex at times. To begin with, not only is the X-ray anatomy of the sinuses consistently different in everyone, but there are often bony anomalies present that could expose certain nearby vital structures to surgical injury, and this possibility is not always predictable from a preoperative CAT scan. Also, a number of individuals with chronic sinusitis will have had previous sinus surgery followed by significant postsurgical scarring, and often with loss or displacement of the usual landmarks so helpful in guiding a subsequent surgical procedure. Finally, the very narrow approach through the nose to the operative field, where visibility may be further diminished by bleeding as well as by swollen or polypoid tissues, will sometimes present a very complex challenge to even the ablest of endoscopic sinus surgeons.

As will be further demonstrated later, the symptoms, diagnosis, and especially the treatment of this very complex common disease may vary not only from patient to patient but also significantly from infancy to childhood to adolescence to adulthood, and people who have prolonged sinus infections in early life could very well have them come back to haunt them later.

CHAPTER FIVE

Is Sinusitis Contagious?

CONTRARY TO WHAT many people think, if you have sinusitis with a persistent cloudy sinonasal discharge due to a bacterial infection, you may over a period of time infect someone with whom you are in close, fairly continuous contact, often breathing the same air, as for example, husbands and wives, brothers and sisters, parents and children. Infection is even more likely to occur if the exposed individual is rendered more susceptible because of a reduced sinonasal cleansing action of his or her own, perhaps due to a recent viral respiratory infection, an allergic or nonallergic rhinitis, or excessive sinus scarring from previous sinus infections. This does not mean that those so exposed will necessarily develop chronic sinus disease, but this too can happen, especially if the cross-contamination is permitted to exist over a fairly long period and goes untreated. Again, the transmission of the disease depends on the closeness of the relationship, the length and frequency of the exposure, the virulence of the bacteria, the degree of contamination, your own immunity or resistance, and especially the efficiency of your own sinonasal mucus-cleansing action in being able to eliminate infection before it can become firmly entrenched. I have found chronic sinusitis in many children whose parents or grandparents gave a history of chronic sinus disease, often starting long before the child was born, many times dating back to their own childhood, and frequently with a history suggesting that they may have contracted it from one of their parents or siblings. Even a classmate or playmate with a bacterial sinusitis and a constantly dripping nose, or one who is coughing and sneezing, can be a potential hazard to others, especially during the closed-in winter months, when children are usually crowded together in carpools or confined to small playrooms with all breathing the same air or handling the same things.

Grade school teachers, who are almost continuously exposed to all kinds of respiratory infections during the winter months, are especially susceptible, and I often found it difficult to keep them free of sinus infections. Other factors in the schoolroom, day nursery, and home environment that can lower your resistance, encourage the transmission of respiratory infections, and exacerbate sinus problems include exposure to dry and drafty heat; sitting, sleeping, or studying near a heat or air-conditioning vent; breathing irritating cigarette or cigar smoke; breathing all kinds of sprays, perfumes, and powders, including detergent powders; sleeping or working in or near a freshly painted room, even with the windows open; sleeping, sitting, or playing directly in front of a closed window in cold weather; exposing yourself to wood dust, plaster dust, or excessive house dust; and even riding to school in a car or bus seated next to the heater or air-conditioning vent. Any of these conditions may dry out or irritate the membranes of the nose and cause rhinitis with inflammation, swelling, and sinus blockage. This in turn may reduce the effectiveness of the sinonasal mucus-cleansing action, thus making you more susceptible to any bacteria and viruses in the immediate environment as well as to developing a sinus infection.

If you have a woodworking shop in your home, you should make certain that it is well ventilated with window or tank exhausts and vacuumed frequently but never swept, since sweeping will stir up the very fine dust particles and circulate them in the air. Heat and air-conditioning ducts may then pick the dust up and transmit it throughout the house almost indefinitely. Dust from salt-treated wood and even from old-time favorites such as mahogany, walnut, cherry, fir, and redwood can be especially irritating to nasal membranes and to the lungs. Glues, paints, solvents, sealants, and wood-finishing products can contaminate the entire house if their tops are not on tightly. All of this can make you, your child, and your spouse more susceptible to a sinus infection and encourage the spread of respiratory infections within the home. A chronic sinusitis in one member of your household might even exacerbate or prolong a chronic bronchitis in one of the other occupants.

Hand-to-hand followed by hand-to-mouth, hand-to-nose, or hand-to-eye contact between siblings, parents, and playmates can be a major factor in spreading the infection. Simple acts such as pushing open a door, turning a knob, flicking a light switch, pressing the button on the water fountain, flushing a toilet, shaking hands, and even exchanging food, candy, toys, and bikes at home, in school, or at kindergarten can result in cross-contamination, especially if a child is dripping pus and wiping his nose on his hand or sleeve. Since these are fairly routine daily performances that can't be avoided, frequent hand washing with a fairly mild antibacterial soap can make a difference and is an excellent habit to cultivate. A recent study in Michigan found that children who washed their hands at least four times a day had 24 percent fewer sick days due to colds or flu. Fortunately, microorganisms won't survive on most objects for more than a few hours unless moisture is present, and then they may last for several days. An exception, of course, is the tuberculosis germ, which can survive for a very long period even in a perfectly dry area. Handkerchiefs are rarely used anymore because they contaminate hands, pockets, and purses and often remain contaminated for days. By the same token, you should use hand or facial tissues only once and never store them in a pocket or purse after usage, especially if you have obvious pus or cloudy discharge from your nose or are coughing it up from the lungs.

In some instances, an infected sinonasal discharge from a pet dog or cat can infect other members of your household. Infected drippings from pets may be transmitted from hand to mouth or simply by breathing the dust stirred up from rugs or floors. These contaminated dust particles in rugs are propelled into the air by sweeping, brushing, vacuuming, and even walking. I have seen particle counts where sitting down on a chair cushion or just walking on a rug ejected clouds of invisible dust particles into the air, and these may be contaminated by dust mites and bacteria as well. Dust from litter boxes or birdcages can be similarly contaminating, as noted in cases of psittacosis, a lung disease contracted from parrots. Most of the cases I saw with cross-contamination of the sinuses from pets to humans involved the *Staphylococcus* bacteria, and in most instances, the patient would temporarily clear up on an appropriate antibiotic but refused to remain well until the source of the contamination, namely the pet, could be tracked down and treated. Cultures from both pets and humans would usually show similar organisms with similar antibiotic sensitivity studies, but it was not always possible to tell who had infected whom. Since each represented a source of reinfection to the other, however, both had to be treated and cleared up at the same time.

Whenever a sinus infection keeps recurring in a child or adult, it may be necessary to examine and often culture his or her frequent contacts, be it a parent, spouse, sibling, companion, or playmate, and if a sinus or respiratory infection is found, it too should be treated. In addition to frequent hand washing with a mild antibacterial soap, some control over the spread of respiratory infections in a household may be maintained by having your own drinking glass and toothpaste, using paper towels or separate towels and washcloths, temporarily sleeping in separate beds when acutely infected with a head cold or flu, using tissues once and then discarding them, and never sharing nose sprays or drops. With most cross-contamination, a lot depends on how contaminated, moistened, or oily your hands were when the organisms were seeded, and how soon the subsequent contact with them was made. There is more evidence now to show that the amount or degree of the contamination, especially for viruses, is an important factor in contracting an infection.

Dampened towels and washcloths are always a good source of contamination. This has especially been noted in the spread of viral conjunctivitis within the household and should be remembered, since it could apply to viral head colds and flu as well. Fortunately, in such instances, viruses, unlike bacteria, can't multiply on moist surfaces alone but have to enter a living cell to reproduce.

CAN SINUSITIS BE INHERITED?

Parents frequently ask this question after being informed that their child has chronic sinusitis, especially if a parent or grandparent has had a similar problem. The child could very well have gotten it from a parent, or even from a grandparent, but through prolonged contact—not through the genes.

Although there is no known genetic passage of sinus disease itself, a person's predisposition for allergic rhinitis, or for allergies in general, known as atopy, which usually runs in families and seems to be genetically passed on, may provide all the impetus needed to develop a chronic rhinitis and therefore a chronic sinusitis. Inheriting certain body characteristics or systemic abnormalities can also lead to sinus problems in an offspring. A nose of a particular shape, possibly inherited from a parent, especially a very small or very narrow nose that may not tolerate swelling without sustained blockage and sinus obstruction, could make you prone to sinus infections.

CLEFT PALATE

Another condition that appears to follow genetically determined predisposing factors in many instances, and that is frequently associated with sinusitis almost from birth, is cleft palate. This occurs in about 1 in 800 births in the United States and appears to show up in the embryo near the end of the second month. From the very first day of life, the cleft palate child has a major feeding problem, which may in turn cause very significant sinus problems. The main purpose of the palate is to separate the delicate tissues of the nose and nasopharynx from the usually very contaminated mouth, and to close off this area during the process of drinking and swallowing so that food and drink go down the esophagus into the stomach and not up into the nasopharynx or nose. A person with a cleft or divided palate, or sometimes even a badly scarred, paralyzed, or improperly functioning one, may experience contamination of the nose and therefore the sinuses almost every time he or she eats or drinks. Repeated contamination of the nose by food and drink will produce a foreign body reaction in the nose resulting in irritation, inflammation, and swelling of the delicate nasal membranes, followed by infection. Nasal inflammation and swelling, or rhinitis, may then cause sinus blockage, often resulting in a persistent sinus infection.

Since this contamination is a daily occurrence in the cleft palate child, by the time the palate is surgically closed, sometimes as early as 4 to 6 months and usually by age two, the beginnings of chronic sinus disease may have already started. Further interference with proper sinonasal function in the cleft palate patient due to other nasal and septal deformities, scarring from repeated nasal or palatal surgeries, or further nasal contamination by food due to an unsuccessful palate closure or fistula formation may all tend to enhance a sinus problem. This does not mean that chronic sinusitis in the cleft palate child cannot be prevented, treated, and even reversed once it has developed, but it does require diligence and cooperation on the part of the parent and the physician to be successful.

After examining hundreds of cleft palate patients from five eastern states over a 35-year period, I found better than two- thirds of them afflicted with some degree of chronic sinusitis. Most of those spared had been given frequent antibiotics for various infections including sinusitis, ear infections, bronchitis, and wound infections following surgery during their early years, especially before palate closure. Even some of those in whom chronic sinus infection was averted by early antibiotic therapy would later succumb to chronic disease because of the many nasal and septal deformities associated with this condition. The cleft palate child has so many obvious problems, including dental, audiological, speech, nutritional, psychological, cosmetic, and socioeconomic, to name just a few, that something as common as a sinus infection usually takes a backseat, not only in the eyes of the parents but often with the family doctor. Since most of these youngsters have, by the time they are young adults, submitted to numerous surgical procedures related to their palate problem, they usually don't want any additional surgery related to a sinus problem. It is my sincere hope that the cleft palate child will be given vigorous treatment for sinusitis in early life, every time a sustained sinus infection is noted, and thus possibly avoid chronic sinusitis and extensive sinus surgery later.

CYSTIC FIBROSIS

There are other conditions or systemic diseases that are inherited and carry a predisposition to sinusitis. Perhaps the most familiar is cystic fibrosis (CF), often referred to in the past as the most common genetically transmitted lethal disease affecting people of Caucasian ancestry. Cystic fibrosis is also found in other races, but not nearly so often. It is mainly an abnormality of the secreting glands of the body, including those in the pancreas, intestines, gallbladder, and liver, as well as those in the membranous walls of the respiratory tract and sinuses. It is in the respiratory tract and sinuses where most of the serious, very disturbing, and sometimes fatal symptoms develop, especially early in the disease. The very sticky secretions produced by CF result in plugging of the secretory ducts, the sinuses, and the smaller bronchial tubes, thus creating stagnation of mucus, with blockage of drainage followed by infection. The cilia sweeping action is sometimes so markedly hindered by this very sticky mucus that some have described it like pulling taffy. The earlier name applied to this disease was mucoviscidosis because of the very thick and viscid mucus it produced. Eventually cyst formation and scarring, or fibrosis, may pervade the glandular ductile system, thus accounting for the disease's present common name.

Cystic fibrosis also causes a collection of excess salt or sodium chloride in the surface membranes and skin, which has given rise to the sweat test for cystic fibrosis, a diagnostic patch test applied to the skin that reveals the presence of any excessive amount of salt secreted by the sweat glands. Because of this excessive salt secretion, some people with cystic fibrosis may experience body salt depletion in hot weather, a condition called hyponatremia. However, the most notable and constant symptoms are usually those related to chronic infections of the lungs, nose, and sinuses. About one-fourth of them will develop nasal and sinus polyps, and because of this, any child or young teenager found to have nasal polyps should in most instances be tested for cystic fibrosis, especially since the test is painless and simple. Questionable test results may in some instances have to be confirmed by DNA testing. With advanced disease, liver, heart, and lung complications are not uncommon. Pancreatic and intestinal problems are also noted. People with cystic fibrosis usually require oral and intravenous antibiotics repeatedly throughout their lives, and having them available has been a major blessing in prolonging life, since most of these people, before antibiotics, would die in childhood, and usually from lung infections. Genetic treatment may someday offer the best chance of prevention as well as a cure.

OTHER DISEASES LEADING TO SINUSITIS

Several other inherited diseases of lesser renown also affect cilia motility and the flow of mucus in the respiratory tract and sinuses. One such disease is called Kartagener's syndrome, a subgroup of immotile cilia syndrome or dyskinesia, a Greek derivative indicating bad or difficult movement of cilia. Fortunately, Kartagener's syndrome is a rare disease and is only mentioned here because of its unusual characteristics and its devastating effect on the mucous flow of the respiratory tract and sinuses resulting in chronic infection. In this condition, the cilia throughout the body are defective, all the way from those lining the respiratory tract and sinuses to the ciliated propulsion hair on the tail of the sperm. All of these cilia are immobile and cause mucous stagnation or stasis, resulting not only in chronic lung infection and chronic sinusitis but also in sterility. If a patient has chronic sinusitis, chronic lung infections, and suspected sterility, then a chest X ray may confirm the diagnosis of Kartagener's syndrome, since close to 50 percent of these patients have a condition called situs inversus. "Situs" means site, position, or location and when coupled with "inversus" under these circumstances means that the locations of the body organs are inverted, transposed, or turned about. The liver, gallbladder, and appendix may lie in the left side of the abdomen instead of the right, the stomach and intestines may be turned around, and the spleen and heart may occupy the right side of the body instead of the left. This transposition of organs may be partial or complete. A simple chest X ray may reveal the heart on the wrong side and help in making the diagnosis early. However, since only about half of the cases will have this, a negative chest X ray will not rule it out. Some people with this condition may also develop nasal polyps.

There are other systemic diseases with inheritance factors that can make infections more difficult to control and therefore sometimes play a role in the development of chronic sinusitis. These include diabetes, certain anemias, including sickle-cell, as well as some forms of low thyroid function or hypothyroidism. Both hypothyroidism and ane-mia can impair cellular metabolism, which is important for healthy sinus membranes, efficient ciliary activity, and adequate glandular secretions. Low thyroid function may also render you more susceptible to viral respiratory diseases such as colds or flu and therefore more open to sinus infections.

There are also some noninherited systemic diseases that deplete the body's ability to control infections in general as well as within the sinuses. These include other types of anemias, leukemias, malignan-cies of the lymph tissues called lymphomas, acquired hypothyroidism, and notably the acquired immune deficiency syndrome (AIDS). Other conditions of impaired immune response following chemotherapy, extensive radiation for cancer, or immunosuppressive therapy for peo-ple receiving transplants as well as those with a deficiency in the body's immune globulin (hypogammaglobulinemia, often noted in infants during the first year or so of life) would likewise make you more sus-ceptible to sinus infections. People with severe burns, certain chronic kidney diseases, and GI protein-loss disorders, usually with a corre-sponding loss of T cells, may also develop troublesome sinus infec-tions. A more severe deficiency in immune globulin, called agammaglobulinemia, which may be inherited or acquired and also usually accompanied by diminished T cell or antibody formation, will often lead to very obstinate sinus problems.

Your doctor may have to consider all of these possible contributing factors when diagnosing and treating a chronic sinus infection.

PART TWO

Prevention and Treatment of Sinusitis

CHAPTER SIX

If You Have a Chronic Sinus Problem, What Questions Should You Ask Your Doctor,

and What Questions Should You Ask Yourself?

IF YOU ALREADY have chronic sinusitis or appear to be heading in that direction, it should now be apparent that there are certain things you need to know about yourself, your living and working conditions, your environment, your general health, your nose, and your sinuses to evaluate the problem properly and, with the aid of your doctor, hopefully reverse it. Unfortunately, your doctor may not be able to provide you with all the answers, since as you have already learned, chronic sinusitis can be a very complex disease, and your doctor can't pick your sinuses apart bit by bit to examine them. However, doctors do have certain diagnostic aids such as CAT scans, MRI, bone scans, special allergy tests, and magnified lighted telescopes that can systematically investigate your sinus problems and provide you with most of the answers.

With this in mind, this chapter provides you with questions for a careful self-appraisal along with certain pertinent questions that your sinus doctor may be able to help you with. The answers to these questions should not only tell you if you are doing the right things but, along with your other findings, should provide you and your physician with some idea as to the extent of your sinus disease, how long it has been around, which sinuses are involved, the adequacy of their drainage and air exchange, whether they are constantly infected or just intermittently so, how badly damaged they are, whether you have a subacute or chronic problem, if you need sinus surgery or whether medical treatment may suffice, what local or systemic factors are contributing, the part that your living and working environments might play, whether allergy is a factor, and most importantly what measures should be undertaken to clear your sinusitis up permanently and what your chances are of accomplishing this.

QUESTIONS TO ASK YOURSELF

Is the discharge from my nose always cloudy or only cloudy part of the time; and if it is a part-time thing, what seems to bring it on, and what tends to make it go away?

Do I always have a cloudy sinonasal discharge following a cold or flu, usually lasting for more than 10 days, and does it nearly always require an antibiotic to clear it up? If so, for how long do I usually have to take an antibiotic to accomplish this, and how long does my sinonasal discharge usually remain clear after completing the antibiotic?

Is there anyone among my close associates such as my spouse, my children, other household occupants, working partners, carpoolers, household cleaners, babysitters, and household pets who may be carrying a chronic respiratory infection or sinusitis and thereby infecting me or other members of my family?

Am I drinking adequate fluids every day, avoiding low-humidity environments and drafts, and adding humidity when needed and practical to keep my respiratory membranes moist and my sinonasal mucous secretions flowing freely?

Am I doing what I can to avoid excessive exposure to membrane-irritating sprays, cheap newspaper print, firsthand and secondhand smoke, paint odors, solvents, soap powders, sprays, chemicals, dusts, molds, perfumes, scented tissues, and scented soaps and lotions; and when it is obvious that I may be hypersensitive or allergic to any of them, am I avoiding them altogether?

If I have year-round allergic rhinitis with an associated sinusitis or asthma, am I doing all I can to control dust, molds, animal danders, cockroaches, and dust mites at home and at work, as well as limiting my exposure to their allergens?

Am I avoiding humidity and temperature extremes inside and outside the house as well as inside and outside air pollution, including excessive pollen exposure, as much as possible?

Do I avoid sitting or sleeping in front of, beneath, or next to heating or air-conditioning vents at home, at school, and at work, and do I also try to keep exposure to such drafts at a minimum when riding in a car or bus?

Do I limit my alcohol intake and avoid the kinds of alcoholic beverages that may tend to make my sinuses worse?

Do I pay close attention to my diet and try to avoid foods that might tend to thicken the mucus in my respiratory tract or bother my nose and sinuses, and do I pay attention to suspected food allergies and try to eliminate them from my diet altogether?

Do I insist on keeping house pets when I know that I am allergic to them; and if I must keep them, do I ban them from the bedroom and bathe them weekly?

While exercising, do I avoid jogging on very cold or smoggy days as well as getting overheated and then cooling off too quickly, and do I refrain from swimming in heavily chlorinated or contaminated water? Do I avoid swimming altogether during the winter months when viruses are so prevalent, as well as diving or swimming underwater without a nose clip? Do I wear a hat when I go outside even if only for a few seconds from early fall to late spring?

If I am pollen sensitive, do I avoid exercising outdoors and even going outside, if I can avoid it, when the pollen count is high? Do I use pollen filters in my house and car, try to eliminate pollen from my hair, shoes, and clothing, keep my windows and doors closed, change my air-conditioning filters frequently in pollen season, and avoid breathing it when brushing my hair as well as that of my pets?

Do I take sensible precautions when someone in my home or at work comes down with a contagious respiratory virus not only to protect myself but also to prevent it from making the rounds of other members of my household? Do I wash my hands frequently with a mild antibacterial soap and encourage my family to do the same?

Do I use good judgment in my everyday living to dress warmly, to avoid sleeping or sitting in a draft or next to an open window or even directly in front of a closed window in cold weather, and especially to avoid sleeping in too cold a room, to refrain from painting in a closed room or sleeping in a freshly painted room, and to wear a truly effective mask when sawing wood, spraying shrubs, spreading dirt or fertilizer, sanding, raking leaves, pitching hay, or cutting grass? Do I avoid going outside or to bed with a damp or wet head, and do I keep my feet warm and dry, avoid public hot tubs, steam baths, and saunas, drink at least seven or eight glasses of liquid a day, eat nourishing foods, obtain enough sleep, and never fly with a cold, sinusitis, or flu if it can possibly be avoided?

If I awaken with sinus blockage, a headache, or a congested nose every morning, have I tried sleeping on a 7-inch sleeping wedge with a pillow on top of that to see if it helps; and if so, have I informed my sinus doctor about it?

Do I always make certain my colds or sinus flare-ups have completely cleared and that there is no lingering cloudy discharge?

Did I make a wise choice as to the location of my house or apartment, the kind of heat I have, or the climate in which I chose to settle, and did I also choose a healthy climate when selecting a college for myself or for a family member?

And last but not least, do I seek responsible medical advise promptly when it becomes obvious that things are not going as they should and that my own efforts to treat my sinuses are not working?

QUESTIONS TO ASK YOUR DOCTOR

Do my sinuses seem to drain adequately even when my nose is irritated and swollen from allergy or from breathing certain irritating inhalants encountered in my daily living and working environments? If not, what medications, avoidances, or treatments should I undertake to improve my sinus drainage?

Does the sinonasal cleansing action for my nose and sinuses seem to be efficient enough to prevent stagnation or pooling of their mucous secretions, and if not, which sinuses are not functioning properly, and what can or should be done about it?

Is there any evidence of excessive scarring in my nose or sinuses, from either previous surgery, injury, or earlier prolonged infections as far back as childhood, that might have impaired my sinonasal circulation, mucous secretions, cellular metabolism, cilia sweep, local enzyme and antibody activity, or the free flow of mucus and air through my sinus openings?

Are there one or two sinuses that are always obstructed and therefore always infected and, as a result, tend to infect my other sinuses?

Are there any benign tumors, cysts, polyps, cancers, mucoceles, bony growths, fistulas, foreign bodies, infected tooth roots, bone fragments, or congenital anomalies in my sinuses that might interfere with their normal function and cause a chronic sinus problem to develop?

Do I have any nasal abnormalities such as a deviated nasal septum, benign growths, foreign bodies, polyps, cancers, cysts, enlarged or abnormal turbinates, chronic swelling, excessive scarring, adhesions, mucoceles, fistulas, nasal valvular collapse, allergic or nonallergic rhinitis, or any congenital anomalies that might impair breathing, misdirect normal airflow, depress cilia activity, induce drying out or pooling of mucous secretions, or cause blockage of sinus drainage openings; and are there any of these things that can and should be corrected?

Do I have gastroesophageal regurgitation of stomach acid or food into the back of my nose on a fairly frequent basis, causing a persistent rhinosinusitis? If so, what can I do about it?

Is my body's immune response adequate to fight and control sinus infections and not impaired by any disease, blood disorders, chemical imbalances, medications, or deficiencies?

Do I have any other chronic infectious problems such as an infected upper tooth or retained tooth root, infected adenoids, or infected bronchi or lungs that might be contributing to a persistent infection in my sinuses; and conversely, could my sinus infection be contributing to infectious problems in other parts of my body?

Am I taking any medications that might tend to dry up, thicken, or otherwise interfere with my sinonasal mucous flow, inhibit its cleansing action, or in any way diminish the mucous blanket protecting my sinuses and respiratory tract?

Am I taking any medications, breathing any irritants, or using anything locally in my nose that might depress or inhibit the cilia sweeping action or that might cause burning, swelling, irritation, or inflammation of my nasal membranes or sinus openings?

Do I have any significant allergy problems that might keep my nose, sinuses, and their drainage openings inflamed and swollen, and if so, what should I do about it?

Is there any evidence of a fungus infection in my nose, throat, or sinuses, and are there any darkened specks or light brownish putty-like matter in my sinonasal secretions or sinus washings that might suggest it?

Do I have any circulatory, metabolic, organ, or hormonal deficiencies that might cause a low-grade chronic swelling of the tissues in my nose, with blockage of my sinuses, or that might impair the ability of either to resist infections?

Do any of my living, working, playing, eating, drinking, and sleeping habits encourage head colds, bronchitis, or sinusitis?

Some of this may sound too restrictive for your day-to-day living when, in truth, it is mostly good common sense. If you are a sinus sufferer or find yourself heading in that direction, if you have frequent colds or frequent sinus flare-ups that tend to persist, or if you have ever been told that you have a chronic sinus problem, asking these questions, making necessary changes, and following your doctor's advice can make a great difference in your quality of life.

CHAPTER SEVEN

What Can Be Done to Prevent a Head Cold or Flu From Going to the Sinuses?

UNFORTUNATELY, VERY LITTLE can be done to prevent a head cold or flu from going to your sinuses, but there are things you can do to lessen the chances of contracting a head cold or flu as well as to minimize the often associated sinus infection and hopefully prevent any permanent sinus scarring.

When a head cold virus attacks your nose or upper respiratory passage, there is nearly always some associated sinus involvement. Most of the time, the involvement is very minimal, usually producing some mild inflammation with sinus membrane swelling, an increase in mucous secretions within the sinus cavities, and occasionally a tightness or sinus pressure-like feeling in the cheeks or face. This membrane swelling with blockage and pooling of mucus within the sinus cavities has been demonstrated by CAT scans and MRIs taken of normally healthy sinuses early in the course of a head cold. The generalized headache, systemic symptoms, and sometimes significant fever noted many times in the beginning of a viral respiratory infection, especially with an attack of flu, are usually due to a generalized invasion of the body by the virus and seldom due to any sinusitis that may accompany it. Although there is no sure way to prevent sinus involvement by a viral respiratory infection such as a head cold or flu, if the sinuses remain open and continue to drain well, they will usually clear up in the same 5 to 10 day period it normally takes you to recover from a cold.

The sinonasal discharge will usually turn cloudy by the third or fourth day of a cold due to the body's cellular response and in some instances due to the destruction of cilia followed by stasis or stagnation of mucous flow resulting in bacterial overgrowth. Studies have suggested that the rhinoviruses that are responsible for almost half of the head colds in adults and even more in children are not nearly so damaging to nasal cilia in the first week of a cold as some of the other cold viruses and especially the flu virus. Sinuses that are normally healthy, however, will usually recover rather quickly and begin to sweep themselves clean of infected discharge in just a few days. If a sinus cavity should become significantly blocked due to swelling from a viral infection, then a bacterial sinusitis may follow and may occasionally require antibiotic treatment.

So far there is no conclusive scientific evidence that large doses of vitamin C, zinc lozenges, or herbal extracts will prevent a cold, shorten its duration, or even minimize its symptoms. We do know that too much zinc can cause a sore throat or upset stomach and that vitamin C or ascorbic acid, even in normal dosage, may sometimes cause a gastrointestinal upset with diarrhea or esophagitis with heartburn.

Vaccines and antiviral agents may minimize some flu attacks, and decongestants will help reduce any associated bronchial or sinonasal swelling, thereby improving drainage; but final resolution of the infection will usually depend on the rapid recovery of both the bronchial and sinonasal sweeping action along with the body's immune response and in some instances may also depend on proper and responsible medical care.

Head colds, like flu, are due to respiratory viruses, and more than 200 different kinds of viruses have been identified as being responsible for head colds. That is why it has been so difficult to manufacture a vaccine for head colds. Because there are usually only three or four dominant flu viruses expected to occur in a particular season, on the other hand, manufacturing a vaccine for flu is far more practical. One drawback, however, is that the viral cultures for the flu vaccines have to be grown and then manufactured well in advance of the flu season. Since the decision as to which flu types should be included in the vaccine is predicated on the previous year's flu epidemics, there can sometimes be a surprise or two for the vaccine dispensers when the flu season finally arrives. However, if the vaccine does provide complete coverage and the shot is administered at least 4 to 6 weeks before exposure, it will greatly reduce your chances of contracting flu. If you should develop the flu, the vaccine will usually minimize your symptoms and frequently diminish any complications. To avoid any late-winter or early-spring epidemics of flu, however, you may sometimes require another shot later in the season, since they are mostly effective over a 3 to 4 month period.

A nasal spray vaccine is also being promoted for protection against both A and B strains of the flu virus. It is made from weakened strains of live influenza viruses, rather than from the dead viruses used in regular flu shots. So far, a vaccine for the very prevalent respiratory syncytial virus (RSV), which often behaves like a form of flu, has been unsuccessful, although a serum of pooled antibodies against RSV has been selectively tried. Like flu, RSV can be more serious in the elderly, and even more so in small children, since the virus may involve the very small bronchioles of their lungs as well as cause asthmatic-like wheezing, especially during the first two years of life. Like flu and the adenovirus, RSV is often temporarily destructive to cilia and may cause a rhinosinusitis flare-up as well. Rhinoviruses and coronaviruses, which together cause most of our colds and upper respiratory infections, are not as damaging to cilia but still initiate most of our sinus infections.

Respiratory viruses are mostly airborne and usually enter the body through the nose, mouth, and lungs. The eyes are another invasive route where a virus moving along with contaminated tears may pass rather quickly through the nasolacrimal ducts into the nose, thereby ending up in the respiratory tract as well. This transmission and invasion of your body by respiratory viruses may be helped along the way by sneezing, coughing, spitting, drooling, and blowing your nose, as well as through hand-to-hand, hand-to-mouth, finger-to-nose, and hand-to-eye contact. Viruses are more often spread by fairly direct contact but may catch a ride on moisture droplets or even fine dust particles in the air and infect you on a bus, plane, train, or boat, in a car, across a room, or even down a hallway if the air currents are flowing in your direction. Under certain circumstances, viruses may be transported in food and drink and even transmitted by means of shared toys, drinking glasses, tableware, paper money, coins, doorknobs, doorplates, light switches, telephone handpieces, gas pump handles, salad bar utensils, keyboards, copiers, steering wheels, faucet and toilet handles, hand railings, shopping carts, stamps and envelopes, playing cards, poker chips, billiard cues, throwing darts, bowling balls, and credit cards—and especially the loaner pen used in signing them, which may already have been used by a hundred different people that same day. Viruses may also be transmitted by damp towels and washcloths, facial tissues, handkerchiefs or shared cloth napkins, and anything else someone has handled and left an infected moistened handprint or finger smudge behind, and especially through a handshake, a kiss, or other intimacies.

Just using your paper towel to open the door of a public restroom when you leave can make a difference in the spread of germs. Having your own napkin ring with an identifying mark or sometimes even with your initials, a common practice years ago, is one answer to limiting the spread of germs within the home. Using someone else's nose drops or spray, a very easy way of transmitting an infection, should never be permitted, and they too should be tagged with the owner's name. Smoking, breathing other irritating pollutants, being overly tired, depressed, or stressed out, excessively dieting, having PMS, a suppressed immune system, lack of sleep, or hypothyroidism, getting your feet wet, or being exposed to drafts or to the elements have all been blamed for an increased susceptibility to head colds, but the virus must still be present in the respiratory tract, probably in significant numbers, for you to contract one. A virus or bacteria can live on your hands for hours, on a damp washcloth, and even on some hard surfaces for several days, but a virus must eventually enter a body cell and its nucleus in order to survive and reproduce or replicate. Therefore, an understanding and awareness of possible transmission routes and frequent hand washing with a good antibacterial soap may offer you the best chance of completely avoiding a viral respiratory infection.

At a party, you should, whenever possible, avoid eating with the same fingers with which you shake hands, and you should wash your hands with a mild antibiotic soap as soon as you return home, especially during the flu season and especially if you are prone to sinus or lung problems. Never floss without thoroughly washing your hands first, and by all means keep your fingers out of your nose and mouth. Biting your nails and sucking your thumb can lead to all kinds of infections. Remember that if you have a cold or flu virus, you are infectious usually from the day before any symptoms develop until three to five days after onset. During this period, as a matter of consideration, you should avoid exposing others as much as possible, especially those prone to sinusitis or those with chronic lung disease, for whom a respiratory virus infection could even prove fatal. If you have a fresh cold or flu, be a good Samaritan and avoid others, sneeze or cough into tissues whenever possible, and don't infect whoever does the laundry by blowing your nose on a cloth handkerchief.

Several antiviral medications are recommended for flu caused by the influenza A virus, particularly in high-risk patients and especially if they were unable to take the vaccine well ahead of time either because of putting it off or having a known sensitivity to it. Two in particular are known by the generic names of amantadine and rimantadine. They have no effect on an infection with influenza B strains, however. These medications should be taken with caution if you have a history of seizures. Their concentrations in the blood may be reduced some by taking aspirin or Tylenol. Doctors will be especially cautious in prescribing amantadine for anyone taking a medication that affects the central nervous system, and there have been reports of suicide in a few patients taking them. Pregnant and nursing mothers should avoid these medications. They should be started as early as possible in the disease, preferably within 24 to 48 hours of onset of the flu, and continued for approximately 7 to 10 days or preferably for 24 to 48 hours after the symptoms disappear. A resistant influenza A virus may develop from prolonged prophylactic use of these drugs, and taking either medication should therefore be kept to a minimum, especially since these resistant strains could be transmissible to others. The dosage will be reduced considerably if you have impaired kidney or liver function or congestive heart failure, and if you are over age 65.

These medications, however, will not totally prevent an influenza A infection and may not completely relieve the symptoms but will often minimize them. They are generally considered safe and are occasionally prescribed for small children as well. They do not interfere with the effectiveness of the flu vaccine and when necessary may be given along with a late flu shot administered for protection later in the flu season. However, you should not look on these medications as a substitute for an influenza vaccination or as an excuse to avoid one. They can be very useful in the high-risk person who is unable to take a flu shot because of a hypersensitivity to the egg culture media or to some of the vaccine's components. They can also be important to the sinusprone individual, since a bad case of flu can be followed by a persistent bronchitis and a sinusitis as well.

Once your body's outer defenses, and especially its mucus-coated membranes, are breached by a flu virus and it enters the bloodstream, the virus may travel throughout the body, unless of course it can be stopped and quickly neutralized by antibodies, destroyed by T cells and enzymes, or gobbled up by phagocytes, the body's own Pac-Man.

If the virus survives, one may notice a generalized systemic response in the form of a fever and sometimes chills, fatigue, loss of appetite, and generalized aching along with a sore throat, hoarseness, generalized headache, chest congestion, and cough.

Flu, or influenza, is potentially a far more serious disease than a head cold and is responsible for more than 20,000 deaths in the United States each year. Flu can be especially dangerous for the elderly, for people who have chronic heart or lung disease, and for the generally debilitated patient as well. Uncomplicated colds rarely produce a significant fever, but with a flu infection your body temperature may rise as high as 102° F to 104° F, and sometimes higher, especially with ear or lung complications. A head cold usually completely disappears within 7 to 10 days, but the weakness, fatigue, and cough following an episode of flu may last for 3 to 6 weeks and sometimes longer.

An invading cold virus, being predisposed to the upper respiratory tract, will tend to concentrate itself in that area, and its major symptoms will therefore involve the nose, throat, sinuses, and sometimes the ears, although you may subsequently develop a cough and bronchitis. Since the flu virus usually prefers the lower respiratory tract, at least to start with, and even though it may often begin with a sore throat, hoarseness, and chest symptoms, it could end up in your nose and sinuses later. Hoarseness may be the only clue to steer you away from someone at a midwinter party, business meeting, or community gathering who may be coming down with a flulike virus—and who is very likely contagious, since this symptom may appear even before a sore throat, cough, or nasal congestion, and many times before the person even realizes that he or she has a contagious viral infection.

After reaching the larynx, the flu virus will usually proceed to the trachea, bronchi, and lungs, causing a dry cough initially, but frequently followed in 1 to 3 days by a wet, productive one. In some cases, flu may cause a viral pneumonia, and this should be suspected, especially in the elderly, whenever there is cough with associated chest discomfort, and usually a persistent high fever. With the flu, the material you cough up after the first day or two is often a pale greenish color but can be a tanish brown and occasionally may have the consistency of a fairly thick paste, thicker if you are dehydrated. Later it may change to yellowish or a milky white color, often depending on which of the subsequent bacterial invaders are dominant. In some instances, the flu virus may attack the nose or upper respiratory tract early, causing nasal congestion, sinusitis, headache, runny nose, nasal burning, and face or eye discomfort.

Sneezing, a fairly common symptom in the beginning of a head cold, is seldom noted with the flu, whereas frequent repeated sneezing could also be caused by an allergic rhinitis attack. At times, an infection with the flu virus may begin with a slight soreness in the back of the nose or upper throat and with discomfort occasionally referred to one or both ears. At other times, the virus seems to ignore the nose, ears, and sinuses almost completely, and although the attack may begin with a sore throat and laryngitis, it may then remain fairly well confined to the lower respiratory tract and lungs.

The entire respiratory tract offers the largest area of directly exposed tissue for possible invasion by an airborne virus. In addition, it is covered by an extensive, very delicate membrane, greatly increasing the chances for a break in its wall, through which infectious organisms may then enter the body. Unlike the body's other membrane surfaces that are covered with a protective mucous coating, the delicate respiratory tract is exposed to a tremendous variety of irritating pollution particles almost too numerous to count as well as to many drying elements in the environment, thus making the respiratory tract even more susceptible to irritation, swelling, drying out, and tissue damage as well as to the breakdown of its protective mucous barrier. The GI tract also offers a large area for membrane invasion by inhaled and swallowed organisms, but its approach is usually well guarded by a pool of hydrochloric acid within the stomach and by numerous digestive enzymes throughout, all of which can be very discouraging to invading bacteria and viruses.

As with any invasion, the success of the viral attack will often depend on their numbers and concentration, how successful they have been in breaching the body's defenses, how quickly they were able to spread out once inside, how virulent or destructive they are, how prepared the body's immune system is to meet the challenge, whether you have antibodies left over from a previous similar infection or from a vaccine shot, and finally whether your body is in good shape, healthwise, and has stored enough reserve supplies to withstand a heavy and possibly sustained onslaught.

There is no doubt that many unsuccessful incursions by potential viral invaders are going on in our bodies much of the time, but the body manages successfully to repulse them mostly unbeknownst to us. All of us have experienced the feeling that we are about to catch a cold or viral sore throat and have been very surprised the next day that it hadn't materialized and was totally gone, which may on occasions represent a repulsed attack. Also, it is generally known that when a virus, especially an airborne one, infects a member of a household, other occupants in fairly close contact with him or her will usually have the same virus in their nose or throat and still may not contract the disease. Before the polio vaccine was discovered, the polio virus was frequently found in nose and throat samples from the other family members of a polio victim but many times without their ever developing the disease. This is also true of the rhinoviruses, which are mostly responsible for the common cold, and which are often present without our knowing it, many times without causing any head cold symptoms. Although young children, with their immature immune systems and their often frequent exposures to respiratory infections, may average six to eight head colds a year, adults rarely have more than two or three, and usually fewer as they grow older, even though there are more than 200 different head cold viruses.

With so many people from different areas now traveling throughout the world, especially in confined plane cabins, as well as on buses, boats, and trains, exposure to the many different cold viruses must certainly occur on a frequent basis. It is highly possible that some kind of cross-immunity does exist to prevent us from succumbing to so many different head cold viruses every year. If you do have more than three or four head colds a year, you might be including one or two episodes of flu, an episode of respiratory syncytial virus (which may infect a large number of small children as well as an occasional adult), and also possibly some recurrent acute flare-ups of sinusitis, which may occur rather frequently in some patients and may resemble a cold. Even flare-ups of allergic rhinitis may be misinterpreted as a head cold by some. I and some of my colleagues who were frequently exposed to our patients' many respiratory viruses found that we would usually stay free of colds or flu until after returning from a vacation. Then we would often contract the first respiratory virus we encountered. We noted this even when we hadn't flown on a plane, which of course would have made us more susceptible. This would certainly suggest that small but frequent and often unnoticed viral incursions into our bodies may stimulate the immune system just enough to provide some short-term protection or immunity, which in a sense is the same principle employed now for using a weakened live flu vaccine in a nasal spray.

Extensive work with the AIDS virus has shown us that exposure to

larger viral concentrations can greatly increase the chances of contracting a viral infection, and we have also noted that some strains of
a particular virus may be far more vicious or virulent than others and
likewise more resistant to treatment. Bacteria may sometimes behave
in a similar way, as recently demonstrated by the so-called flesh-eating
group *A beta Streptococcus,* an extremely virulent strain of the strep
throat and scarlet fever variety. Fortunately, scarlet fever has taken on
a milder form known as scarlatina, although it is still caused by the
same strep organism, but apparently of a weaker strain.

I am also reminded of numerous cases I treated in which an adult
was generally a lot sicker with a respiratory virus if he or she contracted it from a child rather than from another adult. It is just possible that a child, with his or her increased heart rate, faster breathing,
better tissue oxygenation, more active glandular secretions, and a
more vigorous cellular metabolism in young, healthy tissues, may very
well revitalize and strengthen a sluggish, somewhat dormant virus,
thus making it more active or virulent. By the time these viruses have
passed through several other young, vigorous bodies crowded together
in carpools, nursery schools, or kindergartens, they may conceivably
take on an even stronger and more resistant status, thus rendering the
unsuspecting parents or doting grandparents even more vulnerable.
All adults should take note of this and follow extra hand-washing precautions when around a child who has an upper respiratory infection
or flu.

When you contract a respiratory virus from someone else and it
attacks your nasal membranes, it is not surprising that the sinus cavities, which are often less than a millimeter away, may likewise become
involved. Both the nose and sinuses are connected by common openings as well as by a continuous layer of cells, lymphatics, and blood
vessels. Since viruses or bacteria invading nasal membranes can spread
by continuity from cell to cell as in cellulitis, as well as through lymphatic or blood vessel flow, or by cellular subdivision as in the case of
a virus, it would be very unnatural for an infection to travel along
these common tissue planes and vascular channels from the nose to
the edge of a sinus drainage opening or duct and then to stop, especially since this same nasal membrane, with its extracellular fluids and
extensive vascular network, continues through this opening and into
the sinus cavity itself. The same situation would arise with a middle-
ear infection, where infectious organisms would hardly be expected to
stop at the opening between the middle ear and the mastoid cavity, and

yet any outward clinical evidence of mastoiditis is rarely noted with middle-ear infections.

Any symptoms of sinus involvement at the beginning of a cold would often tend to be masked and completely overshadowed by the very acute cold symptoms as well. Later in the cold, any cloudy discharge that squeezes through a partially blocked sinus opening may appear one minute and be gone the next, possibly not to reappear again until that night or the next day. This is one reason why the diagnosis of a suppurative sinus infection is so often missed, since the examining physician may observe a sinus opening for only a very short period, and the incriminating evidence of a cloudy sinus discharge may already have been swept away and down the throat, not to appear again until sometime later.

Even if a sinus opening is completely blocked by a mucous plug or nasal membrane swelling from a cold, this would not obstruct the passage of the cold virus or secondary bacterial invaders into the sinus cavity, since as previously mentioned, they can still travel from cell to cell or along submucosal tissue planes through an obstructed sinus opening to involve the lining membranes of the sinus cavity. Although there is some degree of sinus involvement with almost every head cold, it doesn't mean that a cold has to be treated any differently, since for most people, especially those with normally healthy sinuses, the body's immune response and continuous flow of sinonasal mucous secretions in taking care of the cold will usually resolve the sinus problem as well.

The exception to this is the individual with generally unhealthy sinuses, usually with a history of persistent sinus trouble in the past, especially following colds, often with sinus-obstructing scar formation or chronic sinusitis, and who may develop a head cold. If you are sinus prone, your doctor will most likely start you early on decongestant pills, sprays, or drops. After the third or fourth day of your cold, when the viral infection is waning, the dominant nasal bacterial invaders are beginning to take over, and the earlier clear nasal discharge has turned to a cloudy yellowish, greenish, or milky white color, an appropriate antibiotic might have to be prescribed in certain cases if you wish to avoid any protracted sinus problems. When you start taking an antibiotic at the beginning of a cold, however, the dominant bacteria that subsequently emerge to cause the rhinosinusitis will usually be resistant to any antibiotic you are already taking, and you may therefore require a different antibiotic for a cure. Of course, in many instances, thanks to your body's own immunity and an effective sinonasal cleansing action, you may still get well even while taking an apparently ineffective antibiotic. If the cold is complicated by an ear infection, or a high fever and chest pain suggesting early pneumonia or pneumonitis, you may have to start taking an antibiotic right away without the 3- or 4-day delay and then continue taking it for some weeks thereafter.

If an oral decongestant is well tolerated, doesn't cause nervousness or insomnia, and if you do not have a medical condition or are not taking a medication that would contraindicate its use, then much may be gained in the treatment of a sinus infection if you can continue taking the oral decongestant for the entire duration of the infectious process. Taking a decongestant by mouth, as compared to using a nasal decongestant spray, may work a little slower. However, it does have the advantage of reducing membrane swelling within the lower airways as well as the nose and sinus cavity, often with further relief of sinus blockage, shortening not only the course of the disease but also the duration of any antibiotic treatment, which is likewise very important. Helping an infected sinus to drain with the use of decongestants involves the same principle as incising an abscess elsewhere in the body, since in both instances the continued release of retained pus is usually necessary for a rapid and successful cure.

If you use a decongestant nose drop or spray instead of an oral decongestant for a cold or sinusitis, then you should use it as directed (directions are on the label) for no more than 3 to 5 days and discontinue using it if you experience rebound swelling, bleeding, or increased membrane irritation in the nose or throat. Sometimes you may develop a very troublesome and persistent sore throat with the continued use of a decongestant nasal spray. Changing to a nasal decongestant pill if any of these problems should occur or when the rather brief course of the decongestant spray is completed is often worthwhile. In children, with their very small drainage openings, narrow nasal passages, and their tendency to excessive membrane swelling, the oral decongestant will usually have to be continued for a longer period, provided it is well tolerated. Although I have certainly tried it, using a steroid nasal spray for an acute viral respiratory infection would seem to me to be a poor choice unless your doctor suspects an allergic rhinitis. Corticosteroids are immunosuppressive, and although it is difficult to prove, a steroid spray could interfere with the body's normal immune response to a viral attack both locally and systemically.

If your doctor prescribes an antibiotic for a bacterial sinusitis following a head cold, it should be continued for a minimum of 10 days to 2 weeks, and often longer for a child. A fairly safe rule, especially in a child, is to keep taking the antibiotic until the discharge is perfectly clear and then continue it for 5 to 7 days after that. This is the safest approach, since an infected cloudy discharge can sometimes remain trapped in a swollen sinus cavity and reinfect the sinus as well as other nearby sinuses if the antibiotic has been withdrawn too soon.

Other supportive therapy for the acute phase of the cold or rhinosinusitis might include getting adequate rest; drinking plenty of fluids; avoiding alcohol; not breathing cigarette smoke, perfumes, or other irritating pollutants; staying warm and avoiding drafts from fans, air-conditioning, and heat ducts; sleeping somewhat elevated; applying hot compresses to the face followed by a dry towel; using a mucus liquefier or cough suppressant when necessary; limiting antihistamines; possibly taking Tylenol or a similar analgesic for pain; and running a steam vaporizer or using a manufactured saline nasal spray for added moisture. Using a medication or spray to dry up the sinonasal secretions could be a definite mistake and will frequently prolong the infectious process.

If the cloudy discharge should return within 2 or 3 weeks after antibiotic treatment for sinusitis following a head cold, possibly along with some nasal congestion, headache, cloudy postnasal drip, cough, or morning sore throats, it usually means that the sinus infection never completely cleared, rather than indicating the onset of a new infection. Another 10- to 14-day course of the same—or preferably a different—antibiotic would again be indicated. Before you start the antibiotic again, a culture with bacterial sensitivity studies at this stage may sometimes be helpful but is not always necessary, although occasionally a resistant organism will develop, and a culture with sensitivity studies may occasionally reveal it. If you have chronic sinus disease, this regimen of therapy may have to be repeated a number of times before the discharge finally remains clear and may also have to be repeated again in the ensuing months should you have another flare-up of sinusitis following a head cold or flu. Most sinus-prone people usually have a history of having had to take antibiotics for a fairly long period after a head cold in order to get well and stay well. If you follow this approach carefully, however, it could mean the difference between having reasonably healthy sinuses, with only an occasional persistent sinusitis following a cold, and developing chronic sinus disease, often with numerous infectious flare-ups, possibly for the rest of your life.

CHAPTER EIGHT

What Complications Could Develop From a Sinus Infection?

COMPLICATIONS FROM A sinus infection may be confined to the sinus cavity itself to include its membranous lining, its mucus-secreting glands, its drainage opening, or its bony walls; or they could extend beyond the sinus cavity to involve other sinuses as well as important nearby structures such as the eyes, the brain, the pituitary gland, certain major vessels, important cranial nerves, and even the upper teeth. Either directly through infected drainage or indirectly by way of the bloodstream, a sinus infection may cause complications in some of the more distant organs or body structures including the lungs, the eustachian tubes and ears, the nasopharynx and adenoids, the heart valves, the prostate, the urinary tract, the pharynx, the esophagus, the larynx, the trachea, and the bronchial tubes.

Several complications of sinus infection are illustrated at the end of this chapter. Refer to the illustrations beginning on page 145 for more information.

CHRONIC SINUSITIS

Of all the infectious complications that might involve the sinus cavity itself, one of the most common—and one that many times could be avoided—is the conversion of an acute sinusitis to a subacute infection and thence to chronic disease. This occurs more often than you realize, usually following a head cold or flu. After 10 to 14 days, the acute symptoms of the viral infection and its associated sinusitis will have mostly disappeared, but there may still be a lingering low-grade subacute sinusitis with a persistent cloudy discharge, which you may only occasionally be aware of when blowing your nose or clearing your throat. If allowed to go untreated for weeks or months, this persistent infection may cause significant scarring with more permanent blockage of a sinus drainage opening resulting in chronic sinus disease. You may further recognize the gradual development of this rather subtle complication in yourself or in another adult by the presence of a mild nasal congestion that comes and goes, occasionally involving only one side of the nose, noted especially when lying down, and sometimes causing you to snore. Often there is a fairly mild early-morning headache, especially around the eyes, and sometimes a diminishing sense of taste and smell. An occasional awareness of a cloudy post-nasal drip, possibly a slight cough, and sometimes a rather mild morning sore throat may also be present. In a child, nasal blockage with a persistent nasal tone to the voice, sometimes accumulation of dried mucus around the nostrils, red streaking on the back of the throat, a slight nighttime cough, persistent ear blockage symptoms with signs of diminished hearing, increased mouth breathing, and sometimes an associated feeding problem may be the only indications of a subacute or early chronic sinusitis, especially when you can't see a cloudy sinus discharge in your child's nose or throat. Many times, however, only two or three of these findings may be present.

EMPYEMA

An infected sinus may sometimes develop a sustained total blockage with pooling of mucus and pus within the cavity, usually under pressure, known as an empyema of the sinus. With this complication, there is usually an increase in pain or headache. Sometimes there may be facial swelling and tenderness to finger pressure or tapping over the involved frontal or cheek sinus as well. Sinus X rays or a CAT scan will usually reveal an air-fluid level within the sinus, except in very delayed instances where the air may have been completely absorbed by the body and only the fluid or pus remains. Then the sinus may show up as densely cloudy on X ray due to its swollen, inflamed membranes and fluid content.

If the empyema or pus under pressure involves the frontal sinus, the pressure pain or dull headache will nearly always develop midmorning, intensify toward the middle of the day, and depart usually by midafternoon, only to return at almost the very same time the next day. This frontal pain will usually increase when you bend over, lift, strain, cough, or sneeze and is often rather severe.

If the empyema should involve a maxillary sinus, the cheek, the upper teeth, and on rare occasions even the lower teeth on that side may be painful, very closely resembling a typical toothache. This head pain is usually around the eye, beside the nose, or sometimes in the back of the head on that side. It occurs during the day and may get worse as the day wears on, often disappearing by late afternoon. The pain in the cheek and teeth will also increase when you bend over, lift, strain, or do anything else that increases the venous pressure in the head such as coughing or sneezing. The cheek may also become tender to deep pressure or to tapping with the finger. Sometimes the pain may be referred to an ear on the same side as well. You may also experience a jarring sensation in the cheek when walking down steps or stepping off of a curb.

The ethmoid and sphenoid sinuses may likewise develop an empyema with an air-fluid level. Because the ethmoids are so very small, however, and because they (like the sphenoid sinuses) are located fairly deep within the skull where other bony structures tend to hide them, the ethmoids are not so easily diagnosed with ordinary sinus X rays and may require a CAT scan for confirmation. Ethmoid headache is usually located around the eyes, between the eyes, or above the eyes. It usually develops between four and six o'clock in the morning or when you awaken and goes away by midmorning, sometimes to return in the late afternoon.

Sphenoid sinus pain is often worse during the middle of the day or early afternoon and may occur in almost any part of the head, but more often in the top, the back or the forehead, or sometimes the temple area or behind an eye. You should remember that headaches due to sinus infections are nearly always daytime headaches, and any impressive increase in sinus pain should make you suspicious of a totally blocked sinus with pus under pressure. Empyema of a sinus may require early surgical drainage to relieve the pain as well as to promote a rapid recovery, and especially to prevent any permanent scarring with blockage of a sinus drainage opening or duct that might cause more trouble in the future.

POLYPS

A complication may also develop involving the membranous wall of a sinus cavity, since the membranous lining may sometimes continue to swell due to an infection, allergy, aspirin intolerance, cystic fibrosis, or from some unknown cause and then protrude through the sinus opening into the nose to form a nasal polyp, an occurrence more often arising from the very small ethmoid sinuses. In some instances, a polyp may appear to develop as a result of a sinus infection, and at other times it might appear to develop first, block the sinus drainage opening, and then cause the sinus infection.

The presence of a polyp in your nose or sinus will usually have to be diagnosed by your physician, but you may suspect it if you are aware of something moving back and forth in a nasal passage when you breathe through the nose, or if you notice a gradual, progressive obstruction to breathing, especially on one side. Although the symptoms of polyps in the nose may be more obvious on one side at first, they could involve both sides. A sinus polyp that doesn't protrude into the nose or nasal airway but remains confined to a sinus cavity may produce no symptoms, at least not until the sinus drainage opening becomes obstructed by the mass, and may only then be discovered on routine sinus X rays or a CAT scan. Polyps not only obstruct breathing and sinus drainage but may cause loss of the sense of smell and with it the appreciation of taste. If allowed to continue growing, they may in rare instances even destroy surrounding bone and cartilage.

CYSTS AND MUCOCELES

Another complication of sinus disease also arising directly from within the sinus cavity, but this time involving the mucus-secreting glands, is the development of a simple mucous cyst or its more formidable cousin, the mucocele. Both arise when the mucous secretions of a sinus are totally obstructed, usually by scarring, and the mucous glands continue to secrete under their usual rather significant pressure. The so-called simple mucous cyst usually encountered in a sinus is a smooth, rounded sac containing a clear serous fluid, usually developing from obstruction to the drainage duct of a seromucinous gland, or from a small area of mucus-secreting membrane containing numerous glands being pinched off and blocked by scar tissue. In both instances, the formation of the cyst would be like blowing up a balloon with water.

The more formidable mucocele is usually a thicker-walled cyst often containing a much thicker fluid and more often developing from total and permanent blockage of a part or all of a sinus cavity. The mucocele is usually the result of infectious or postsurgical scarring, with complete obstruction of the sinus drainage opening and with gradual expansion of the cavity by retained mucous secretions under pressure, even to the point of eroding the bony walls of the sinus, the orbit, the nose, the brain, and the walls of any surrounding sinuses as well. When a mucocele becomes infected and fills up with pus, it is called a mucopyocele. As previously stated, mucoceles are more commonly found in the frontal and ethmoid sinuses, fairly often in association with cystic fibrosis. The anterior ethmoid sinuses are the most common source of mucoceles, mainly because they are a grouping of the smallest sinus cavities with the smallest drainage openings, which makes them more vulnerable to complete and permanent blockage with mucocele formation.

As they expand, both the simple mucous cyst and the mucocele are capable of obstructing sinus drainage openings and may then direct your or your physician's attention to them through the persistence of a sinus infection. Since sinus cysts are seldom visualized within the nose, the diagnosis would usually be made with sinus X rays or, better still, with a CAT scan. Either or both may sometimes develop following sinus surgery where postsurgical scarring may have sealed off an area of mucus-secreting membrane or even an entire sinus cavity and yet may not show up as a cyst or mucocele until some years later.

Although sinus surgery may have made mucoceles a more common occurrence, their treatment, thanks to endoscopic sinus surgery, has been greatly simplified, since in most instances surgeons no longer feel it necessary to radically excise them but merely to thoroughly drain them and thereby incorporate them into the drainage structure of the sinuses themselves. A sealed-off mucocele may develop, expand, and even destroy bone over a period of many years before finally making itself known. As a mucocele gradually enlarges, it may cause drainage obstruction of other nearby sinuses, an infected nasal discharge, sinus headaches, and sometimes numbness in a cheek when it involves a maxillary sinus. Occasionally the first symptoms noted may be visual disturbances from erosion of the orbit or from compression of the optic nerve behind the eye by a mucocele arising in the sphenoid or posterior ethmoid sinuses. Occasionally they may mimic a tumor invading the orbit and pushing the eyeball upward, forward, or to one side, often causing double vision. A frontal sinus mucocele may also extend behind the eye, invade the orbit, or compress the brain. Of course, if they do expand into the nose, nasal obstruction may be noted, mainly on one side. Since mucoceles, as well as polyps, are rare in the nose and sinuses of children, finding either of them in a child makes it necessary to rule out cystic fibrosis with a sweat test, or a

DNA analysis if the results of the sweat testing are questionable.

PERIOSTITIS AND OSTEITIS

Another complication also arising directly from an infected sinus cavity and one that can sometimes be very serious is an infection of the bony sinus wall. All bone has a protective covering known as the periosteum, and this may become involved with infection, to varying degrees, resulting in a periostitis. This is often fairly self-limited and usually clears up along with the sinus infection, sometimes leaving subperiosteal scarring that may show up on subsequent X rays as a cloudy sinus. If the bone involvement should progress further, it may result in an osteitis, a more significant complication, since it usually indicates a more protracted and prolonged sinus infection that is now beginning to involve not just the bony covering but the bone itself. Osteitis usually requires more prolonged antibiotic therapy and sometimes surgery. It can lead to a far more serious bony complication, fortunately one that is rarely seen now, thanks to antibiotics, namely, osteomyelitis of the sinus wall and surrounding bone. This can be a very destructive necrotizing disease involving the main body of the bone rather than just the surface and one in which the blood supply to the bone is usually compromised by the infection and the bone dies. It will sometimes show up on X ray and especially with a CAT scan or bone scan. At operation, the infected bone may be soft or mushy or sometimes may even present itself as an isolated island of dead bone known as a sequestrum. This type of bone infection will not respond to prolonged antibiotic therapy alone and nearly always requires surgical excision of the diseased bone with very prolonged antibiotic therapy to clear up the chronic sinusitis and to prevent further progression of the disease to the surrounding healthy bone.

There may be no early warning that bone disease has developed, and the findings may be only the usual cloudy sinus discharge from the nose or throat with the usual local symptoms of chronic sinusitis. Systemic symptoms of lethargy, a feeling of weakness in the legs, sometimes a mild temperature elevation, and occasionally an elevated white blood count, especially when there is significant bone disease, may be noted. A CAT scan and bone scan will usually make the diagnosis. Complications from involvement of any of the immediately surrounding structures such as the orbits and brain may also occur once the very confining and protective bony sinus walls break down.

In the days before antibiotic therapy, an individual with osteomyelitis of the frontal bone arising from a frontal sinus infection would sometimes develop a puffy swelling of the forehead due to bone erosion with pus collecting beneath the skin, known as Pott's puffy tumor. This was described by Sir Percival Pott a year before the American Revolution, but thanks to antibiotics, it is seldom seen now, especially in this country.

OTHER SERIOUS COMPLICATIONS

If you consider the complications of sinusitis that might occur when infection extends through and directly beyond the sinuses' bony walls, certainly the more serious ones would involve the brain or the eyes as well as some of the vascular structures and nerves connected to them. Although these vital structures are fairly adjacent to many of the sinus cavities, their intervening bony walls and periosteal coverings usually serve as formidable barriers to the spread of a sinus infection to the optic nerve and eyes as well as to the dura or other membranes covering the brain. Sometimes, however, the common bony walls separating them may be deficient due to invasion by benign or malignant tumors, by bone-destroying bacteria or fungi, as well as from congenital malformations, old or recent fractures, or even surgical procedures on the sinuses, thus allowing the spread of a sinus infection to these adjacent structures.

If a large defect in the bony wall separating a sinus from the orbit should occur with sinus surgery, it is important that your doctor avoid too tight a nasal or sinus packing, which could cause pressure on the eye and damage the vision. In some cases, a complicated sinus infection may bypass or breach its bony wall and by means of infected thrombi or clots in emissary veins or nearby vessels reach the optic nerve, the eye, the cavernous venous sinus, the intracranial cavity, and the brain. The veins connecting the orbits with the surrounding sinuses have no check valves, thus providing easier access for blood-borne infections in either direction.

ORBITAL CELLULITIS The warning signs to you or your physician of a bacterial invasion of the orbit, called orbital cellulitis, are redness and swelling of the skin around an eye, a swollen protruding eyelid, sometimes with bulging and limited motion of the eye, usually eye pain and headache, occasionally double vision, fever, elevated white blood count, blurred vision, and even blindness should the optic nerve or eyeball itself become involved. In the beginning, it may have a more benign appearance with fairly superficial redness and swelling of the eyelids mostly due to bacterial toxins from an adjacent sinus infection and known as periorbital or preseptal cellulitis. It may remain this way if you start intensive antibiotic treatment of the sinus infection immediately, or it may progress to actual bacterial invasion of the orbit causing a bacterial cellulitis and sometimes an abscess formation, often requiring surgical drainage. In the latter case, protrusion or bulging of the eyeball itself is usually indicative of a more serious bacterial invasion of the orbit with a possible abscess formation and should be regarded as a major warning sign. A CAT scan using an intravenous contrast substance will usually confirm the diagnosis. Orbital cellulitis is the most common serious complication of sinusitis and is most frequently associated with ethmoiditis. It occurs more frequently in children, especially under age six, and most of these cases respond well to intravenous antibiotics. Before antibiotics, almost one-fifth of adults and children with this disease died of meningitis.

MENINGITIS AND BRAIN ABSCESSES Brain or central nervous system involvement, including meningitis, may also occur when a sinus infection breaks through or extends beyond the confines of the sinuses' bony walls. In these serious infections, you may experience various neurological symptoms including a generalized, rather intense headache, sometimes photophobia (sensitivity to bright lights), stiffness of the neck, chills, sometimes a very high fever, marked elevation in the white blood count, and even delirium, convulsions, coma, and death. Meningitis more often occurs from ethmoid or sphenoid sinusitis, and brain abscesses more frequently develop from frontal sinusitis.

The two sphenoid sinuses lie behind the nose, just below and in front of the pituitary gland at the base of the brain, an area rich in major vascular structures and important nerves; and any infections involving either of these sinuses must be taken very seriously. Acute sphenoid sinusitis is considered to be the most common cause of meningitis arising from the sinuses. The two internal carotid arteries, each a major supplier of blood and oxygen to the eyes and brain, pass along the walls of the sphenoid sinuses, sometimes separated from them by only a very thin membrane.

CAVERNOUS SINUS THROMBOSIS Two very large venous blood lakes, or reservoirs, called the cavernous venous sinuses, lie on each side of the sphenoid sinuses and contain portions of five major nerves to the brain. Infectious involvement of these venous lakes may occur directly from a sphenoid sinus infection or indirectly by way of an orbital cellulitis. Fortunately, however, this is not a common occurrence, since almost one-fourth of those who develop such an infection may die (before antibiotics, this figure would often approach the 100 percent mark). When this complication occurs, you have very much the same signs as an advanced orbital cellulitis or orbital abscess with a very swollen inflamed droopy upper eyelid and a bulging eye as well as fairly intense eye and face pains, headache, double vision, and usually a rather significant fever. You will nearly always appear to be very ill, and if both eyes are involved, your doctor's diagnosis will usually be firm, since the infection can progress to the opposite side (especially if treatment is delayed), which orbital cellulitis alone usually won't do. A CAT scan may again confirm the diagnosis.

Fortunately, the bony walls of the sphenoid sinuses are normally very sturdy and, unless they are defective, rarely allow a breakout of infection to involve any of these very important surrounding structures. When it does happen, though, it can be extremely serious. Therefore, it is important to diagnose sphenoid sinusitis before complications develop, treat it vigorously with antibiotics, and if a sphenoid sinus is not draining or if it shows an air-fluid level on X ray or CAT scan, it should be opened up and drained as soon as possible.

Incidentally, the same condition of an infected cavernous sinus thrombosis with the same serious consequences can occur from the simple act of squeezing a pimple on the nose or cheeks in the so-called butterfly area of the face. These are usually staph infections that may travel along thrombosed ophthalmic or emissary veins at the inner angle of the eye to the cavernous venous sinus in back of the eye at the base of the brain, infect it, and cause it to thrombose or clot. Remember, when you are tempted to squeeze a pimple or blackhead on your nose or cheek, or even when you inadvertently or deliberately extract a hair from inside or outside your nose, you could be courting disaster.

PITUITARY GLAND The pituitary gland is situated just above and behind the sphenoid sinuses and is an important part of the hormonal system. It secretes hormones that regulate growth, fat mobilization, menstruation, reproduction, and lactation (milk production). Because the pituitary may stimulate the hormonal secretions of other endocrine glands scattered throughout the body such as the thyroids, the adrenals, the testes, and the ovaries, it was once called the master gland, or maestro. In rare instances, a complicated sphenoid sinus infection could spread to this gland, and although such a complication was very rare in the past, it could occur more frequently in the future with the increase in surgical instrumentation in and around the sphenoid sinuses.

Fortunately, even with long-standing chronic sinus disease involving all the sinuses, and even when infected with the most virulent kinds of bacteria, as long as you are generally healthy and the main tissue planes and bony sinus walls remain intact, uninterrupted by old or recent fractures, by invasive tumors, by congenital malformations, or by extensive sinus surgery, a sinus infection will rarely spread beyond its bony confines to involve these rather vital structures. Immuno-comprimised patients with invasive fungus disease, including those with late-stage HIV infections, appear to be especially vulnerable to such complications, however.

DENTAL COMPLICATIONS The upper teeth may sometimes become involved as a complication of a maxillary sinus infection if there is a defect or breakdown in the bony sinus floor covering their roots or the nerves supplying them. More often, however, an infection of an upper tooth or an infected tooth root left behind from a previous extraction will involve a maxillary sinus. In rare instances, a root canal on an upper tooth or a foreign-body reaction to misplaced filling material can cause a maxillary sinusitis. An upper tooth extraction that breaks through the floor of the sinus may cause maxillary sinusitis as well as a fistulous opening between the mouth and sinus requiring surgical closure. A dental cyst arising from the root of an upper tooth may invade the maxillary sinus located just above the tooth and cause blockage and pooling of the sinus secretions with subsequent sinus infection. However, when the dental cyst is excised from the sinus to relieve the blockage, the tooth must also be extracted, or the cyst will recur and the sinus problem will begin again. Diagnosing these dental complications of sinus disease may frequently involve your dentist and require dental X rays in addition to sinus X rays or a CAT scan.

DISTANT COMPLICATIONS

Complications occurring away from a diseased sinus include the transmission of infection to an undiseased sinus cavity whose drainage opening happens to lie close to that of the infected sinus, or it may extend to the adenoids, which lie behind the nose and are vulnerable to the flow of an infected sinus discharge. A diseased sinus may also infect a eustachian tube and ultimately a middle ear from infected sinus discharge passing close to a eustachian tube opening. As it passes down the throat, infected drainage from a sinus can also inflame your pharynx or larynx and, traveling even further down, may inflame the esophagus, possibly aggravating an already existing peptic esophagitis, or heartburn, caused by a hiatal hernia with stomach acid regurgitation.

THE LUNGS AND ASTHMA Droplet-borne bacteria caught up in the inhaled airflow over an infected sinonasal discharge can involve the trachea, the bronchi, and the lungs, causing acute or chronic infection, and even aggravate an asthmatic condition. Asthmatic wheezing might also result from rhinosinusitis by initiating a sinobronchial or nasobronchial reflex spasm of the bronchial walls. In all such instances, you should become suspicious of a possible underlying contributing sinusitis, especially if any of these problems began with a viral respiratory infection such as a cold or flu but failed to clear up or to remain clear after seemingly adequate treatment, and especially in such instances as an ear infection that keeps recurring, middle-ear fluid formation that persists, hoarseness that comes and goes, daily morning sore throats that won't go away, a lingering cough, an exacerbation of esophagitis, or asthma that seems resistant to treatment. Asthma may be triggered by a number of things, and sinusitis is one of them. Other common causes would include viral respiratory infections such as colds or flu, the inhalation of polluting irritants in the air, and the breathing or swallowing of protein substances to which you may be allergic. A family history of asthma may increase your chances of developing it, and if both parents have it, there is a 75 percent chance that a child will also develop it. When asthma and chronic sinusitis occur together, clearing up the obstructive sinus disease may improve and sometimes even relieve the asthma.

BACTEREMIA AND SEPTICEMIA Distant complications of a sinus infection may also occur from blood-borne bacteria, known as a bacteremia, or from the more severe kind called septicemia, and even from blood-transmitted bacterial toxins. This complication may involve any organ of the body, but blood-transported bacteria from a sinus infection seem more often to settle on a damaged heart valve, in a diseased or malfunctioning urinary tract, or in a prostate gland previously scarred by recurrent infections. I also recall a few patients with flare-ups of phlebitis in the legs in association with their episodes of sinusitis. This relationship was repeatedly demonstrated to me by a patient who experienced many episodes of phlebitis in his right leg occurring within just a few hours of a flare-up of his sinuses. In such cases, you or your physician might become suspicious of an existing sinusitis as a possible underlying cause after observing several time-related flare-ups of both, especially when some distant infectious problem fails to clear up with the usual treatment, or if it should continue to recur.

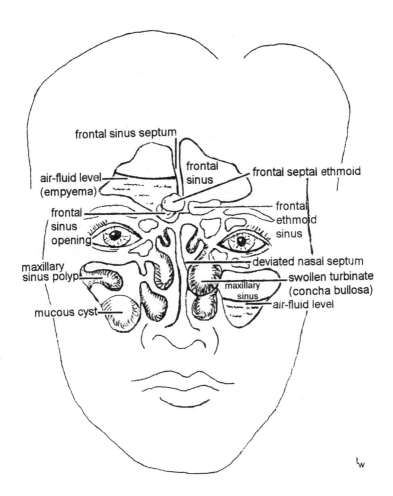

FIGURE 3. Blockage of the right frontal and maxillary sinuses with air-fluid levels present. The right frontal blockage appears to be caused by a misplaced and enlarged frontal ethmoid sinus arising from the septum between the two frontal sinuses. The drainage of the left maxillary sinus is obstructed by an enlarged middle turbinate, or concha bullosa, which also seems to be pressing against a deviated nasal septum. Another badly located frontal ethmoid sinus is partially obstructing the left frontal sinus drainage opening. A polyp and a rounded cyst-like structure are both noted in the right maxillary (or cheek) sinus but so far are not obstructing its drainage.

(Compare this figure with the healthy sinuses shown on page 12.)

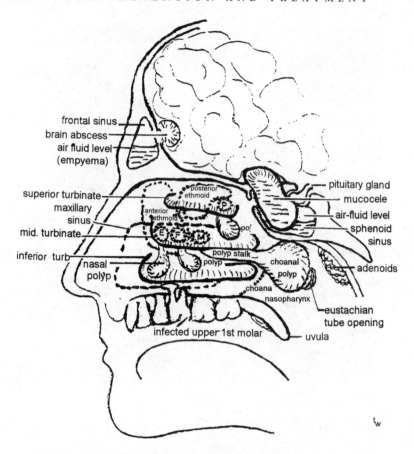

FIGURE 4. A side view of the nose and sinuses. The frontal sinus is partially filled with pus (known as an empyema), and the infection has ruptured the sinus's posterior wall to cause a brain abscess. A thick-walled mucocele is noted within the sphenoid sinus and has not only blocked the drainage opening, causing retention of mucous secretions, but also eroded the pituitary area and the base of the skull and brain. Nasal polyps can be seen arising from the anterior ethmoid (E), frontal (F), and posterior ethmoid (E) drainage openings. Another polyp on a very long stalk (known as a choanal polyp) extends through the maxillary sinus opening (M) and back into the nasopharynx, where it is partially blocking the air passage as well as the eustachian tube. Infection around a root of an upper first molar can be seen extending into the floor of the right maxillary sinus.

(Compare this figure with the healthy sinuses shown on page 13.)

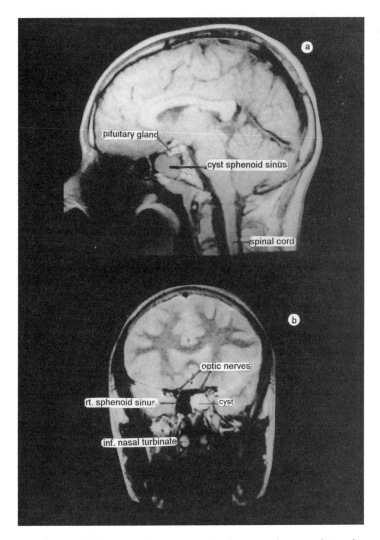

FIGURE 5. MRI views of a large cyst (and potential mucocele) in the sphenoid sinus as seen from the side (a) and front (b). These views reveal the cyst's closeness to the optic nerves and the pituitary gland.

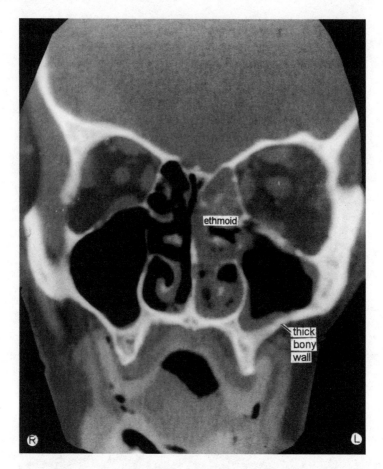

FIGURE 6. This CAT (CT) scan reveals chronic sinusitis involving the left ethmoid and maxillary sinuses, with impressive thickening of the bony walls and periosteal lining of the left maxillary sinus.

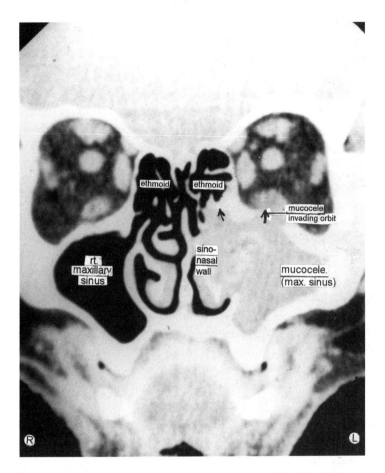

FIGURE 7. This CAT (CT) scan reveals a mucocele filling the left maxillary sinus and invading the left orbit through the maxillary sinus roof. It has partially destroyed the sinonasal wall between the nose and the left maxillary sinus and appears to have broken through into the left ethmoid sinuses. Inflammatory thickening of the bony left maxillary sinus wall is also visible.

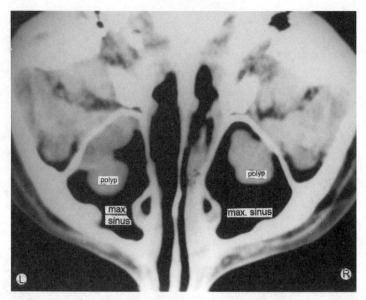

FIGURE 8. This CAT (CT) scan shows pedunculated polyps in both maxillary sinuses, but none are visible in the nasal passages in this view.

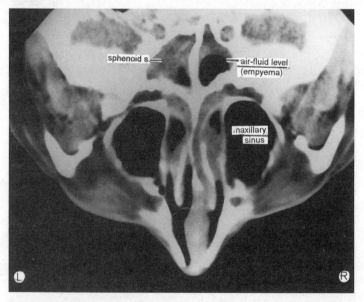

FIGURE 9. This CAT (CT) scan shows infection in both sphenoid sinuses The air-fluid level (empyema) on the right and the concave crescent shape of the fluid suggest pus under pressure.

CHAPTER NINE

What Is Proper and Responsible Treatment for a Sinus Infection?

And What Can Be Done to Prevent Acute Sinusitis From Becoming Chronic?

DETERMINING THE NATURE AND EXTENT OF THE SINUS INFECTION

Once a positive diagnosis of sinusitis has been made, often from the history and the finding of a cloudy infected drainage in your nose or throat, the physician, before recommending definitive treatment, will try to determine which sinuses are involved, how extensive the disease is, whether any complications exist, what local and systemic factors there are, whether your living and working environments play a role, if there is an associated allergy, lung, or ear problem, and how long your infection may have been present. It is also important to find out not only the duration of your present infection but, when possible, how long ago or at what age you first began to have sinus problems, how often your attacks have occurred each year since then, approximately how long each episode lasted, whether antibiotics were required, and, if so, for how long you had to take them to get well and stay well.

Your answers to these questions will often tell your physician whether he or she is treating a subacute or chronic problem that might require prolonged medical therapy with decongestants and antibiotics, allergy treatments, anti-inflammatory drugs, and possibly nasal or sinus surgery for you to completely recover, or if he or she is treating an infection of short duration in relatively undamaged and normally rather healthy sinuses that may even recover on their own or with the aid of a decongestant, or perhaps one that may require a short course of antibiotic therapy, usually over a 10- to 14-day period. The questions usually facing the physician when treating a more prolonged infection in generally unhealthy sinuses are what kinds of medical treatment should be tried first and for how long, whether surgery should be recommended early to establish better drainage and shorten medical treatment or later if medical treatment should fail, whether allergy investigation and possible treatment should be recommended early or later, and finally whether your working or living conditions could be contributing factors, and if so, what long-term corrective or preventative measures you might undertake to improve them.

Obviously most of these questions can't be answered immediately. With sinus disease, because it is more often a drainage blockage problem, the longer the infection has been present, the more persistent the swelling and blockage will be, and therefore the longer the course of antibiotics required to get well and stay well. It is therefore very important for the physician to know if he or she is treating a primary acute, a subacute, a recurrent acute, or a chronic sinus infection, since the duration of antibiotic therapy for each may vary considerably, and this is another reason your accurate history is so important.

Regular sinus X rays or sometimes a CAT scan may be necessary to confirm which of your sinuses are involved, whether there is any permanent damage to them from excessive scarring or bone involvement, whether there is an air-fluid level in a sinus cavity, or whether there are any obstructive masses such as polyps, cysts, or tumors that might require surgery to reestablish sinus drainage and provide you with a permanent cure. If, as sometimes happens, a small polyp should suddenly appear within your nose as part of an acute sinus infection and is obstructing a diseased sinus opening, it may require surgical removal early in the course of your medical treatment to facilitate drainage, clear up the infection, and prevent reinfection after you stop taking the antibiotic. In the more complicated long-standing subacute, recurrent acute, and chronic cases in people who have generally unhealthy sinuses, it may be necessary and for the same reasons surgically to correct any nasal abnormalities that might be contributing to the sinus blockage. Nasal surgery alone in some instances may also prevent a subacute sinus problem from becoming chronic.

If your physician suspects that a systemic disease might be influencing the persistence of a sinus infection, as in the case of diabetes, hypothyroidism, chronic lung disease, anemia, leukemia, chronic debilitating diseases, and immunodeficiency diseases such as AIDS, it may be necessary to obtain a general medical workup including various laboratory studies to confirm it so that appropriate treatment may be given. Nasal cultures and bacterial sensitivity studies may have to be obtained, especially in the subacute and chronic cases, as well as in acute cases with complications, frequent recurrences, or failure to respond to treatment. To culture every case of acute uncomplicated sinusitis is not economically feasible when you consider the limited information sometimes gained and that many acute cases may be well on their way to recovery by the time the culture report and sensitivity studies are received. Some nasal or sinus cultures may come back negative or even report a normal bacterial flora when it is very obvious that a sinus infection exists. Some of these culture-negative cases, especially those with chronic disease, may be infected with anaerobic bacteria, which grow only in the absence of oxygen and therefore require careful handling and special culture techniques for a positive result.

Of course, in most instances your doctor is culturing the nose and not the sinus directly, since the latter would usually require an invasive procedure. In those instances where your doctor can visualize infected discharge in a sinus drainage opening and can take a culture directly from this opening without touching the nostril skin or nasal hairs, there is a very good chance that it will be representative of the infection within the sinus cavity itself. If your physician has already put you on an antibiotic by phone, several days before coming to the office, or if you had already started on some leftover antibiotic several days before a culture was obtained, then the culture report may very well come back negative or with no growth. Of course, if you have a very prolonged sinus infection or one that has continuously failed to respond to adequate treatment, a culture and sensitivity studies including testing for anaerobic bacteria should be obtained, preferably before starting any further antibiotic treatment. This is especially true for someone with chronic sinus disease who may have to stay on an expensive antibiotic for a very long time and would certainly like some assurances that it is effective.

Initial nasal cultures and antibiotic sensitivity studies should also be obtained from sinusitis patients with diabetes, cystic fibrosis, immunosuppressed or debilitated conditions, as well as from those with significant complications such as a sinus air-fluid level, orbital cellulitis, brain abscess, meningitis, or a troublesome ear or lung infection. Since nasal or throat cultures, including bacterial sensitivity studies, are not always reliable in determining what bacteria are responsible for the sinus infection or whether you are taking the correct antibiotic, your doctor may have to depend more on your clinical improvement during the first week or so of treatment to determine if an antibiotic is working. If after 8 or 10 days of antibiotic therapy your thick cloudy sinonasal discharge has not become thinner or even slightly clearer, and your morning sore throats and headaches have not improved, then it might be wise to consider a stronger antibiotic, perhaps one that is bacteriocidal rather than just bacteriostatic or possibly one that is more effective against a different spectrum of bacteria.

To make the proper antibiotic selection even more difficult, some organisms such as *Staph* have learned to produce a penicillin-neutralizing enzyme known as penicillinase, and another very common ear, nose, and sinus bacteria called *H. Influenzae* have succeeded in developing an enzyme known as beta-lactamase that protects them not only from penicillin but also from some of the other beta-lactam antibiotics. If you should have long-standing subacute or chronic sinus disease, it may take as long as 10 days to 2 weeks, even when taking a very effective antibiotic, before you realize any improvement in symptoms, and sometimes at least 5 to 7 days before acute cases may notice any improvement. Unfortunately, some people expect immediate improvement and may want a different antibiotic when this doesn't happen. Nevertheless, if during that period of no improvement, or any time during the entire course of treatment, you should notice an impressive increase in your symptoms, especially for pain, you should notify your doctor, since more intensive treatment, including surgical drainage, and sometimes even hospitalization with intravenous antibiotics may be necessary.

If routine sinus X rays or a CAT scan should reveal an air-fluid level in one of your larger sinuses, such as the maxillary, frontal, or sphenoid, it nearly always means that your sinus is totally blocked and that purulent or infected material, often called pus, is trapped within your sinus cavity along with air, usually under pressure. This is often referred to as an empyema of a sinus. In such cases, it is preferable to drain your sinus early, not only to relieve the rather marked discomfort you may be experiencing and hopefully avoid any other immediate complications, but also to clear up your infection as soon as possible, thereby lessening the chances of sinus membrane ulceration with excessive scarring, particularly in the region of a sinus drainage opening or duct, and hopefully reducing the chances of more sinus obstructive problems later. This could be especially true for the 20 to

40 percent of frontal sinuses with fairly long or tortuous drainage ducts, which may rather easily become permanently scarred and permanently obstructed from a prolonged infection.

Although certain very virulent organisms may cause more damage to a sinus or its drainage opening than others, anytime a sinus infection is allowed to go on for as long as 6 weeks or more, especially if untreated, some permanent damage, usually with scarring of the sinus membranous linings, their mucus-secreting glands and ciliated cells, or even the drainage openings themselves, will very likely occur. As to whether the damage will be sufficient to convert an acute or subacute sinusitis to chronic disease, only time will tell. This often depends not only on the extent of scar formation but also on the location and whether it represents more scarring on top of existing scar tissue from previous infections. This emphasizes the importance of treating all sinus infections early and adequately, since any scar formation is always permanent and therefore accumulative. Fortunately for all of us, our sinuses do have the ability to recover and resume normal function even after a rather severe and prolonged infection and even with a certain amount of permanent scarring, if given a reasonable chance.

PREVENTION

Any discussion of sinusitis treatment would not be complete without some thought being given to preventative care. That should include any sensible changes in your living and working environments that might lessen your attacks, possibly prevent an acute or subacute condition from becoming chronic, or at least improve your daily enjoyment of life should an irreversible chronic problem exist. Your doctor will thoroughly quiz you about possible inhalant allergies, pollution exposure, and food allergies; your use of scented lotions, tissues, and powders; drug snorting; any effects from breathing newsprint; smoking and drinking habits; excessive caffeine intake; sports activities, including swimming and diving, especially in heavily chlorinated water or in excessively contaminated waters; any secondhand smoke exposures; possible contacts with other household members harboring a chronic respiratory infection, including pets, as well as any close friends, fellow carpoolers, students and teachers, nursery or school companions; types of hobbies; kinds of working environment; heat or air-conditioning draft exposures at home and at work; bathing habits such as taking a hot shower and then going directly outside in cold weather; washing your hair at night and going to sleep with a damp head; sleeping in front of an open or poorly insulated window or in too hot or too cold a room; exercising outdoors on too cold a morning or when the ozone or pollen count is high; breathing irritating vapors, liquids, and powders at work or in the home; any exposure to household sprays without good ventilation, or to the outside spraying of trees, grape arbors, shrubs, and insects without adequate protection; cleaning an attic or basement; sleeping in a freshly painted room; sanding, plastering, and restoring or cleaning of old houses.

Any of these may contribute significantly to your nose or sinus problems, and in each instance, wise judgment with a few precautions can make a big difference in your quality of life as well as prevent an acute or subacute sinusitis from becoming chronic. In each of these instances, with help from your doctor, you should try carefully to trace any possible source of nose or sinus contributing factors and try very hard to either eliminate, correct, or neutralize them.

CIGARETTES

Cigarette smoking should be conscientiously avoided, and second-hand smoke curtailed at home, in the car, and in the workplace whenever possible, since it is irritating to respiratory membranes and impairs cilia sweeping action. Cigar smoking, if you don't inhale, may not be as great a lung cancer risk, but it can be very irritating to respiratory membranes (and even more so than cigarettes for most people with rhinosinusitis) as well as a very definite cancer threat to your mouth, throat, and esophagus. Like cigarette smoke, cigar smoke will also reduce cilia activity, and since cilia similar to those in the nose, sinuses, and lungs are also found in the middle ears as well as within the eustachian tubes, their proper sweeping action is essential to clearing serous fluid, mucus, dead cells, or infected discharge from the middle ear cavity and thereby eradicating an ear infection. Children prone to ear, sinonasal, or bronchial problems should therefore avoid secondhand smoke in carpools, at home, or in school, since normal respiratory cilia activity is essential to good health.

ALCOHOL

Excessive alcohol intake can aggravate an existing sinusitis and may even precipitate an acute sinus flare-up if you have chronic sinusitis. Alcohol causes sinonasal membranes to swell, which may further obstruct an already partially blocked sinus opening. If you are prone to sinusitis and must drink, you should limit your intake to 1.5 ounces of whiskey, preferably vodka, or its equivalent in wine or beer over a

24-hour period. Excessive alcohol intake, like too much caffeine, will also increase your urine output, which may tend to dehydrate the body and cause a drying out or thickening of sinonasal secretions.

FLU SHOTS

Taking an influenza shot each year is also good preventative treatment if you are sinus prone, since some degree of sinusitis fairly often accompanies the flu. This would also be good advice if you live or work with sinus-prone individuals, as well as for the elderly, the debilitated person, the immunosuppressed, health care workers, those living or working in institutional settings, and those prone to lung diseases such as asthma, bronchitis, and emphysema. A single-shot vaccine for pneumococcal pneumonia, with a repeat in 5 years, would also be recommended if you are over age 60 or 65, since those who survive a prolonged episode of pneumonia could still end up with a bad case of sinusitis initiated by a persistent lung infection, which in turn could keep a lung infection or bronchitis going.

Some doctors feel that pregnant women whose third trimester may arrive during the influenza season, and especially women prone to complications of flu, should also be vaccinated. This might also apply to some pregnant women particularly prone to sinus infections, since it is often very difficult to control sinusitis during pregnancy, and a bad case of flu could bring it on. Prescribing antibiotics and decongestants for a sinusitis attack during pregnancy should be avoided whenever possible. Some preventative treatment here could therefore be important, provided of course your OB doctor agrees. Although it is true that some pregnant women with rhinosinusitis may clear up almost miraculously very soon after delivery, some untreated cases may develop excessive sinus scarring and end up with chronic disease. You would therefore be ill-advised to ignore sinusitis during pregnancy or to assume that it will go away of its own accord after delivery.

ALLERGIES AND POLLUTION

Nasal smears for an eosinophilic cell count, skin testing, elimination diets, food challenges, and special blood studies may be necessary to confirm suspected allergies in a sinusitis-prone individual. When positive results are found, you may hopefully be able to avoid those allergens, or you may have to be treated with steroid nasal sprays, decongestants, antihistamines, and sometimes allergy desensitization shots, better known as immunotherapy. Even if you require surgery, correcting or controlling any allergic rhinitis problems ahead of time will usually increase the chances of surgical success, and the same might be said for pollution exposures as well.

Filters and exhaust fans may be necessary to prevent glue vapors, paint odors, solvents, dust, and irritating powders originating from a basement workshop from getting into the air-conditioning or heat duct system and thereby traveling throughout the home. You should be reminded that some plastic resin glues contain formaldehydes, which can slow cilia activity as well as irritate and inflame the nose, causing a flare-up of sinusitis. Many glues also contain solvents or volatile organic compounds (VOCs) that evaporate into the air when the glue is mixed or applied and can be harmful to your health, especially to your liver, kidneys, and blood-forming organs, as well as the central nervous system. Breathing the fumes from some of these may also inflame your nose and sinuses. When the label says to use the product with adequate ventilation, you should bring in outside air and exhaust the room air, or better still, do the work outside while standing upwind and wearing an appropriate mask, or at least holding your breath. If the wind isn't blowing, you should practice the technique of holding your breath and walking away when a mask with a proper filter isn't available. When you anticipate prolonged exposure to an irritating vapor or dust inhalant, using an electric fan outside on a windless day to blow it away may prevent a sinus flare-up later. If you have a lot of gluing to do, use a proper filter mask. A good filter mask for vapors as well as for fine-particle dusts is a very worthwhile investment, not only for the sinus-prone person, but for anyone prone to respiratory problems or who may want to avoid future problems. Artists should also be reminded that their paints, felt markers, aerosol sprays, and cleanup solvents can cause skin rashes, eye problems, nasal irritation, and even sinusitis.

FAMILY MEMBERS AND PETS

When treating a very stubborn case of sinusitis or one that keeps recurring, your doctor may also have to take cultures from the nasal passages and throats of certain family members, as well as from any infected sputum they may cough up, especially if they are suspected of harboring a sinus or lung infection. Even though the cultures may be negative, if any family members have an obvious infection, they too will have to be treated to prevent them from reinfecting you or other members of the household. This also applies to any pets in the household should they reveal a cloudy nasal discharge.

COLD AND HEAT

Protecting the head and feet from excessive heat loss by wearing a hat whenever you are outside, even for very short periods from mid-September to mid-April in the temperate zone, or wearing socks and sometimes a ski hat to bed, especially if you sleep in a cold or drafty room, can make a significant difference to the sinus-prone individual. Painting inside can be especially hard on your sinuses and even more so in the wintertime when exhaust fans and open windows are not practical. Using a so-called odorless paint is just as bad, and sleeping in or near a freshly painted room any time of year within 10 days to 2 weeks after painting can be devastating to anyone prone to sinus infections. I have even seen this initiate serious sinus problems in some individuals not prone to sinusitis.

If you are prone to sinusitis, you should also avoid sleeping or sitting next to or beneath a heat or air-conditioning vent, since they both will tend to dry out the nasal membranes and thicken nasal secretions by continuously blowing the moisture cloud away from the face and body. If the bed or easy chair can't be moved, or the airstream can't be diverted by louvers or by placing a chest or dresser in front of it, then you should close it off completely and substitute another kind of heat, preferably of the radiant type without a fan, since you should not sleep in too cold a room, either. A bed next to an open window is bad any time of year, but especially in the wintertime, even if the window is closed and double insulated. Not only does cold air tend to congest the nose, but thermal conduction through the frame, glass, and sill will cause convection currents within the room next to a glass window or a glass door with cold air falling and warm air rising, and this is usually sufficient to create a fairly continuous draft over the bed and your head. If you sleep next to an open window, even in the summer, you may be exposed to the fallout pollution of the cooler night air, especially near industrialized cities or valleys, and this has been observed to aggravate lung or sinus problems on many occasions.

If you are prone to sinusitis, you should avoid being chilled, dress warmly, and protect your head and the back of your neck from drafts. When riding in a car, bus, or train, you should try to avoid any draft from a heater or air-conditioning unit. When traveling in the wintertime, it is better to dress warmly and keep the car heater fan on low, which will also reduce the amount of dust stirred up from the floor. Parents should check with the school bus driver as well as the teacher at school to be certain that their sinusitis-prone child is not seated directly in front of, next to, or beneath an air-conditioning or heat vent. If so, it is doubtful that any amount of antibiotic will completely eliminate the child's sinus infection.

Cold, pollution, and dampness, especially, may cause major problems for sinus-prone individuals, and you should protect yourself from all three as much as possible. You should not live or sleep in damp, cold basements or sleep in too dry a room. A good 10- to 12-hour vaporizer, preferably of the self-sterilizing hot steam type, can make a significant difference to your health in cold weather, when the relative humidity in most homes is usually very low, often in the twenties or low thirties (the ideal relative humidity for the proper functioning of the respiratory tract and sinuses should be in the 45 to 65 percent range). Unfortunately, whenever the relative humidity is allowed to fall below 30 percent, mucociliary flow in the nose may be significantly reduced.

If you are prone to sinus infections and have to be outside on a cold day or cold night, on returning home or to the office, you should go directly to the sink and apply a hot washcloth, hot towel, or even a pack of folded paper towels passed under the hot water spigot to your face and nose for 2 or 3 minutes. This has to be done carefully by very gingerly applying the hot towel or cloth to the skin of the face, cheeks, and nose to be certain that it is not too hot and then holding it there until it begins to cool. You should repeat this several times and then dry your face thoroughly. This should improve the circulation in your nasal membranes and sinuses. It will also lessen nasal congestion, add moisture to your nasal membranes, enhance mucociliary flow, and help to reduce any vascular spasm in your face, nose, or sinuses that may have been caused by exposure to the cold temperature. Many people are convinced that this procedure may frequently prevent a sinus flare-up and sometimes might even abort a head cold after being in close contact with someone who has one. Following this same procedure, but continuing it for 4 or 5 minutes each time and then repeating it three or four times a day, may also be very helpful in the treatment of an existing cold or sinusitis. Here again it is very important to dry your face thoroughly immediately after completing your hot applications and also to lie down with your head slightly elevated for a few minutes with a dry towel over your face to prevent it from cooling off too rapidly. Sometimes the use of a decongestant nose spray just before such treatments can be very useful in helping the sinuses to open up and drain.

PROMOTING SINUS DRAINAGE

Another way you might encourage sinus drainage, especially at night, is to sleep elevated on a 7-inch sleeping wedge with a pillow on top of that and when possible to sleep on your side with the noninfected sinus or sinuses down toward the pillow. This will lessen the nighttime swelling of the nasal passage and sinuses on the upper side and should encourage them to drain better. Many people who awaken every morning with a chronic ethmoid sinus headache may benefit by sleeping this way also.

NASAL DECONGESTANTS AND SALINE SPRAYS A nasal decongestant spray before retiring or once during the night can facilitate this drainage, but you shouldn't use it too often or for more than just a few days at a time. Some decongestant sprays may be used every 4 to 6 hours, and some are meant to be used only at 8-, 12-, or 24-hour intervals, so you should always make certain which kind you have. They should also be used only when the head is elevated and never when you are lying flat or in the head-down position, since in those positions, the spray will erupt in a stream instead of a mist. It is not necessary to inhale vigorously when you spray your nose, as that could immediately deposit too much of the spray in the back of your throat and lungs. A slight sniffing with each spray may create more turbulence within your nose and allow for a wider dispersion and distribution over your nasal membranes, which can be helpful. Inhaling it deep into your lungs or swallowing excessive amounts of a decongestant nasal spray could irritate your throat, larynx, and trachea and keep you awake as well as make you nervous and irritable, since these are nervous system stimulants that can be absorbed by the GI tract and lungs as well as by the nasal membranes.

The proper use of a nasal decongestant is to spray each nostril once, wait a minute or two and spray each side again, then repeat it once on each side for a third time, again with a minute or two in between. This permits your nose to open up a little further with each spray and allows for deeper penetration into the nasal passages. Saline sprays are used strictly to add moisture to the nasal membranes and to dilute or thin out infected discharge, causing it to flow more freely, and would therefore require no special spraying technique. One or two sprays of sterile saline solution every few hours will not harm your nose, but excessive use can make your nasal membranes spongy, which is also true of prolonged respiratory membrane exposure to steam inhalations, steam rooms, or inhalation saunas, which may often do more harm than good. For this reason, steam inhalations for people who have rhinosinusitis or bronchitis should not be used for more than a few minutes at a time and no more than two or three times a day. Steam, of course, is distilled water, which could harm respiratory membrane cells and their cilia were it not for the protective mucous blanket, which may sometimes be partly lacking, especially during a viral respiratory infection or for a short time thereafter.

The use of manufactured saline nasal sprays or salt solutions will not only help to keep nasal membranes moist in cold, dry weather but also speed recovery of damaged cilia, thin out infected nasal discharge so that it flows more freely, and often diminish the chances of nasal bleeding from infection, dryness, strong decongestant sprays, or from too vigorous blowing of the nose. Unlike homemade salt solutions, properly prepared saline sprays or solutions are specifically formulated so as not to irritate or harm delicate nasal membranes. Some people have even used them to dilute a bottle of adult decongestant nasal spray to half strength for less irritating effects on nasal membranes. For those prone to sinus infections, especially in cold weather, the timely use of a saline nasal spray may therefore play a preventative role as well. However, excessive continuous daily usage, the use of an old, previously contaminated spray or out-of-date sprays, or the use of someone else's spray could be counterproductive and even harmful. Also, when you use a saline spray, a nasal saline irrigation, or a salt-water gargle, especially if you mix your own, you may be adding extra salt to your body, and this could be important if you are on a restricted salt diet or prone to fluid retention.

STEAM ROOMS, HOT TUBS, AND SAUNAS

Steam rooms, hot tubs in poorly ventilated areas, and sauna baths, by offering too much humidity, may encourage the nasal membranes to remain swollen and even to swell more, since they can no longer release their own moisture. None of these is a healthy choice for the chronic lung patient, either, since the increased moisture in the air diminishes its oxygen content. The use of a hot tub for too long a period at a time, especially in a small, enclosed room, could be very counterproductive if you have sinus or lung problems, since excessive moisture can also cause the colonization and growth of molds and fungi, as well as a very treatment-resistant bacteria know as *Pseudomonas*. This strain of bacteria has been cultured from hot tubs, and I have also found *Pseudomonas* in the upper and lower respiratory tracts of patients in whom too much moisture had been introduced for too long a period. Fortunately, when *Pseudomonas* is found in someone with sinusitis, it is more often a secondary organism and frequently the result of inadequate sinus drainage and aeration. Many times it will disappear with treatment of the primary sinus invader, especially when the swelling subsides and good sinonasal air exchange with good drainage is reestablished. It can, however, be especially serious in premature infants as well as in people with immunodeficiency, who seem to be more prone to *Pseudomonas* infections as well as to various fungi and molds.

Unfortunately, there are very few antibiotics even moderately effective against the *Pseudomonas* organism. This is partially due to its very tough double-layered cell wall, and interestingly enough, it is this same characteristic that shields it from damaging sun rays and makes it very useful, in the dead form, as a carrier or transfer agent for the very sunlight-sensitive *Bacillus thuringiensis,* known to most farmers as B.t., a natural pesticide with few environmental side effects. Another strain of B.t., also when encased and protected by the *Pseudomonas* bacteria's double-layered wall, has been devastating to mosquito larvae as well as black flies and is being used extensively in large areas of Africa, Asia, and South America to prevent malaria and onchocerciasis, or river blindness. Of great interest to skiers is that a protein extracted from dead *Pseudomonas* bacteria permits snow makers to crystallize water molecules at warmer temperatures for ski resorts throughout the world.

To the physician, it is disheartening that a dead bacteria with so many good and useful qualities can at times in its live form be so devastating to the human body and responsible for so many deaths. Another previously mentioned very harmful bacteria is the *Legionella* bacterium, which lives on vapor droplets, is sometimes found in hot tubs as well as in central air-conditioning reservoirs, and can attack the lower respiratory tract as well as the sinuses in rare instances. It is responsible for Legionnaire's pneumonia, another sometimes fatal disease.

ALLERGIES AND ANTIHISTAMINES
The combination of sinusitis and allergy can create a difficult problem for the physician as well as for the sinusitis patient where treatment and preventative care are concerned. An allergy can cause your nose

to swell, and a swollen nose can block your sinuses. Blocked sinuses will usually become infected rather quickly and often remain infected as long as the swelling and blockage persists. Furthermore, completely controlling the allergy can be expensive, time-consuming, and at times unsuccessful. Some individuals may have their allergies year-round and, unlike those with seasonal allergies, can't predict when the nasal swelling, congestion, and resultant sinus blockage will occur.

Being able to take an allergy-blocking medication well before exposure and before nasal swelling develops is especially helpful not only if you have allergies but also if you are sinus prone with nasal allergies. People with seasonal allergy like to start their allergy-preventative medications a week or more in advance of the expected nasal swelling, and they can also estimate fairly accurately when they may discontinue treatment, usually with the first frost. This gives them a decided advantage. If, however, you are subject to year-round allergies, then you have no way of knowing for certain, when you leave home or the workplace, where or when you will encounter an allergen; and by the time you take your medication and it finally begins to work, significant nasal swelling and sinus blockage may already have developed.

It is far easier to prevent allergic nasal swelling than to reverse it once it has occurred. A decongestant spray to rapidly reduce the allergic nasal swelling followed by a steroid nasal spray on a regular daily basis should help considerably, but steroid sprays usually take a few days to even begin to work and most of the time should not be used more than once or twice a day depending on the type and the directions on the label. Whenever possible, you should start using a steroid spray a few days to a week or more before an anticipated allergic rhinitis episode. It is important for you to remember that antihistamines will often relieve or at least diminish most allergic symptoms but will not reduce nasal or sinus swelling. It usually takes a decongestant or a corticosteroid spray or pill to do that. However, antihistamines can limit allergic swelling in your nose or sinuses if started early enough.

STEROIDS
Since the word "steroid" is a shortened version of "corticosteroid" and is fast becoming a common word in our vocabulary, and since this same word is often used to designate two entirely different medications, each produced in its natural form by two pairs of entirely different glands within the body and each producing entirely different

effects, it would appear that some clarification is needed.

ANABOLIC STEROIDS First of all, we should dispense with the steroids that have nothing to do with the treatment of allergies and sinusitis. They are known as an anabolic steroids, or AS, and represent synthetic derivatives of testosterone, the male sex hormone secreted primarily by the testes. Some athletes use them as muscle strengtheners and bulk builders as well as physique enhancers. Some nonathletes use anabolic steroids because, as they say, they make them look good. When given by shot, they will promote, among other things, the buildup of complex proteins within the body. Although they are prescribed medically for specific hormone deficiencies in both sexes and for a few rare diseases, improper usage has given anabolic steroids a bad name, and we usually hear a lot about them each time the Olympics roll around. In some, they may cause mood changes and have been blamed at times for irrational behavior known as the steroid rage. The latter is not a certain entity and may sometimes be used as an excuse for very bizarre conduct.

CORTICOSTEROIDS The other steroid group consists of a number of slightly different synthetic hormones called corticosteroids or glucocorticosteroids, the better known and more potent of which is hydrocortisone. They are called corticosteroids because they are similar to the hormone secreted by the adrenal cortex, which forms the outer layer of the two adrenal glands that lie on each side of the body just above the kidneys. This essential hormone plays an important role in body tissue metabolism, growth, and development, as well as in the body's response to stress and injury. When prescribed as a medication, they are capable of exerting an anti-inflammatory effect on body tissues, thereby reducing swelling. This capability for reducing membrane inflammation and swelling makes corticosteroids useful for certain sinus and allergy problems, especially in the sinus-prone individual with allergic rhinitis. Even though they have been around for a very long time, the exact mechanism for their anti-inflammatory action is still unknown. They may also cause salt retention within the body, loss of calcium, fluid retention, weight gain, elevation of blood pressure, and excessive loss of potassium, and since they may play a role in liver sugar metabolism, prescribing them for a diabetic could cause some problems. They may also ignite an old dormant tuberculosis infection.

They are known by many different names such as prednisone,

prednisolone, hydrocortisone, cortisone, gluco-corticoids, gluco-corticosteroids, flunisolide, beclomethasone, fluticasone, and others. They are administered in many different ways, some intravenously and intramuscularly, some by mouth, others through eye or ear drops, vaginal applicators and suppositories, skin creams, rectal supposito-ries, as well as by lung inhalation or nebulizers, and of course by nasal sprays. Corticosteroids have saved many lives, prolonged life, saved vision, spared hearing, calmed hemorrhoids, promoted transplants, and enhanced the quality of life for millions of people. They are prob-ably second only to antibiotics in their many vital contributions to human and animal health, and probably even first as far as variety of uses is concerned.

However, they all have to be used with caution, since they are pow-erful medications and, when prescribed in significant amounts and for any length of time, tend to reduce the body's own production of this essential adrenal hormone. Therefore, after extended continuous usage, they can't be discontinued suddenly, since to prevent a crisis, the body must be given the opportunity to reestablish its own corti-costeroid hormonal production for use in times of stress by having you gradually reduce the dosage. Withdrawal of corticosteroids may some-times produce symptoms of joint or muscular pains, weariness, and mental depression. Some undesirable effects as far as infections such as sinusitis are concerned are related to the corticosteroids' immunity-suppressing characteristics, which may be even more significant in someone already immunodeficient. As such, the corticosteroids may tend to depress the body's natural response to infection and may also encourage fungal or yeast infections not only in the mouth and sinuses but in other parts of the body.

Children or adults taking large doses of immunity-suppressing cor-ticosteroids might encounter serious and even fatal consequences when contracting measles or chicken pox. In such instances, you should immediately notify your physician of a known exposure, since you may require antiviral medications or immune globulin shots as soon as possible. As far as sinus surgery is concerned, corticosteroids may tend to delay postoperative healing, and if you have been taking them and need to undergo surgery, you will usually need booster doses to prevent a surgical or postsurgical crisis. For the sinus patient, how-ever, these drawbacks are fairly often outweighed by the ability of cor-ticosteroids to counteract the effects of allergy, reduce inflammatory swelling in the nose, and sometimes minimize scarring; but when they are used in the presence of an infection, antibiotic coverage may be necessary to aid the body's suppressed defenses against further spread of the disease. Should the body lose all of its adrenal cortical hormone productivity for whatever reason, a condition called Addison's disease may result. This disease was made famous by one of its victims, President John F. Kennedy, who suffered from it for much of his life.

Corticosteroidal drugs by shot, pill, or spray can be very useful not only in preventing or relieving allergic swelling in the nose and sinuses but also in reducing any inflammatory swelling of respiratory membranes from breathing irritating inhalants, as well as that caused by fire or chemical burns. When taken by mouth or by shot, however, corticosteroids should be reserved for more serious cases of nasal allergy with sinus blockage where the acute swelling is beyond the control of topical steroid nasal sprays, antihistamines, and decongestants, or where a more rapid reversal of swelling is needed. When given by mouth in either liquid or pill form, corticosteroids should be taken for as short a period as possible, usually for no longer than 7 to 10 days for an acute problem, and usually with a graduated reduction of dosage to allow the body to recover its own productivity of hydrocortisone. Where prolonged treatment by pill is indicated, you can sometimes follow with low dosages on alternate days, a regimen that has often proven successful and presumably with less suppression of normal adrenal cortical function. If you use a steroid nasal spray in conjunction with the pill or shot form, even when receiving an alternate-day dosage, the added absorption of the nasal spray through the respiratory membranes as well as through the GI tract could increase the total body dosage, sometimes with harmful effects.

The various steroid nasal sprays should be used only as recommended. You should use them selectively in the presence of a bacterial infection and then usually in conjunction with an appropriate antibiotic. Although there are interesting arguments to the contrary, I believe they should generally be avoided with most viral respiratory infections. To control seasonal allergy, you should, whenever possible, start taking them 7 to 10 days in advance, since they sometimes require 3 or 4 days to start working and often up to 2 weeks to produce their maximum effect. It should again be pointed out that excessive or prolonged use of a corticosteroid, even as a nasal spray, can cause a reduction of normal steroid secretion by the body. Moreover, the spray medication as well as its aerosol gas propellant, when included, could both be irritating to nasal membranes, causing mild headache, sore throat, and more nasal swelling with more sinus blockage, and could therefore be counterproductive. In some people, a spray may also cause nasal membrane ulceration with bleeding. Hand-pumping propulsion is frequently provided with steroid nasal sprays to eliminate any nasal membrane irritation by a gas propellant. No nasal sprays of any kind should be used in the treatment of rhinitis or sinusitis if they cause any sustained irritation, bleeding, burning, or additional swelling of the nose or throat.

CROMOLYN Cromolyn, a nonsteroidal nasal spray that inhibits the release of histamine from mast cells in an allergic reaction, is also effective in controlling or preventing allergic rhinitis, which in turn may benefit a superimposed sinusitis. When possible, you should start using Cromolyn several weeks ahead of time for an anticipated extended allergy problem, and you may also require additional help from a decongestant spray or tablet and possibly an antihistamine while getting started. Since Cromolyn has an excellent safety record with very few side effects and doesn't seem to react with other drugs, it is now available over the counter. It has been used successfully for truly allergic rhinitis during pregnancy but only with a doctor's permission. It may occasionally cause sneezing and sometimes excessive nasal irritation and may have to be discontinued. Cromolyn is used by people who have sinusitis for prophylactic and definitive treatment of allergic rhinitis, but it will not reduce nasal or sinus membrane swelling once it develops and unlike steroidal sprays does not appear effective in cooling down nonallergic hyperreactive airways. Because of Cromolyn's slow reaction time, it is usually not recommended for on-the-spot treatment of an acute allergic rhinitis problem, and unlike steroid nasal sprays, it will not diminish nasal polyp formation.

OTHER CAUTIONS AND CONSIDERATIONS When corticosteroids are used in any form, you should be on the alert for evidence of a superimposed fungal infection involving not only the nose, throat, and lungs but any of the body's mucous membranes, nails, or skin. If you have a history of tuberculosis, diabetes, or herpes of the eye, you have to be extremely careful about using the corticosteroids in any form. If you are pregnant or a nursing mother, you should use them only with your OB doctor's permission. Prolonged intake of corticosteroids by mouth in children has been shown to delay growth but apparently only temporarily and while they are taking them. However, children should catch up and resume their normal growth once the steroids are discontinued. They should be used carefully in children under age 12 and are not usually recommended in children under age 6 without a doctor's permission. Again, in some cases of marked nasal swelling, the additional use of a decongestant spray may be necessary during the first 2 or 3 days of steroid spray usage to quickly reduce nasal swelling, open up the nasal passages, and provide more nasal membrane exposure for the steroid spray.

PAIN MEDICATIONS

For sinus pain, acetaminophen or Tylenol, aspirin, and the other nonsteroidal anti-inflammatory drugs (NSAIDs) are all effective. Aspirin as well as any of the NSAID group may sometimes cause GI irritation, ulceration, and bleeding as well as a flare-up of esophagitis. So far we don't know for certain about the NSAIDs, but aspirin should definitely be avoided by young people with chicken pox, viral respiratory infections, and fever because of the danger of developing Reye's syndrome, a very serious, sometimes fatal illness affecting the liver and brain. Here acetaminophen for pain would definitely be the wiser choice. Fortunately, with the many warnings accompanying aspirin medications, Reye's syndrome has become a rare disease. Aspirin and the NSAIDs should never be used if you are suspected of being aspirin sensitive or aspirin intolerant, since taking them could aggravate a rhinosinusitis, encourage nasal polyp formation, and precipitate an asthmatic attack.

Acetaminophen in normal dosage is not generally considered harmful if you have a healthy liver and healthy kidneys unless you consume a significant daily amount of alcohol as well. In such instances, there have been a few cases of liver failure, and a caution to this effect is included with the medication. Fasting or intensive dieting may be a predisposing factor to liver damage in heavy drinkers who may be taking acetaminophen for even a rather short period. There has also been some suggestion that even lower dosages of acetaminophen over many years may possibly increase the risk of kidney failure. The NSAIDs have also been suspected in a few instances of having caused kidney damage, even in relatively low doses, but so far this hasn't been true of aspirin. However, a lifetime dose of 5,000 or more NSAIDs tablets is thought by some doctors to increase the odds of kidney failure.

These are all good medications for sinus pain and headache, but you should not take them in excess or for a very long time without a doctor's approval. Moreover, people with liver disease or significant daily

alcohol intake should exercise care, especially in taking acetaminophen.

CONTROLLING ALLERGENS

If you have allergic rhinitis, are prone to sinus infections, and can
anticipate being exposed to a known allergen such as weeds, grass
pollen, or mold, and especially when you plan to clean the attic, rake
or blow leaves, clean the gutters, sweep the basement, or cut the grass,
by taking a fast-acting non-sedating antihistamine an hour or so ahead
of time and wearing a good dust mask, you might lessen your sinus
problems considerably. Keeping your lawn cut short and cutting it frequently before the grass has a chance to bloom should also help to
reduce the amount of grass pollen in the air. You could still get it from
your neighbor's yard, however, or from up the block if the wind is
blowing in the right direction, but at least you will be getting a lot less
exposure with your own mowing. Taking one of the earlier sedating
antihistamines before driving a lawnmower or cleaning gutters could
of course be dangerous. Even if you are a nonallergic sinus-prone person, you should still wear an effective mask under these circumstances,
since heavy concentrations of almost any dust can irritate your nose
and sinus drainage openings. Desensitization therapy may sometimes
be necessary in some of the more severe cases of allergic rhinitis with
sinusitis, particularly where avoidance and conservative measures fail.

Even if you have no allergies but are sinus prone, sometimes avoiding milk products including cream, curds, whey, casein, caseinate, lactose, lactalbumin, yogurt, butter, and cheese can make a difference in
your sinus problems, even when a true allergy to milk or milk products doesn't exist. You may have noticed very thickened mucous secretions in your nose or chest 30 to 40 minutes after ingesting any of these
milk products, and this could be enough to aggravate an already existing sinus or lung problem.

Once you succeed in identifying your allergies and realize what
works best in treating them, preventative therapy administered well
ahead of exposure will often minimize nasal swelling and sinus blockage with very rewarding results. Antihistamines can be very effective
and very useful in minimizing allergic flare-ups, but to be really effective, they must provide continuous coverage throughout the duration
of the exposure and for a short while afterward. Moreover, antihistamines cannot reduce swelling once it occurs. The 4- to 6-hour sedating antihistamines may be taken every 4 to 6 hours during the day

provided they are well tolerated, but a longer-acting 8- to 12-hour antihistamine would be preferable at bedtime to provide coverage throughout the night, unless of course you plan to get up in the middle of the night at a certain time to take another pill. For this reason, it is always very important to know not only the dosage but how long a medication is effective.

The gradual reduction in the cost of the long-acting non-sedating antihistamines, as well as the marketing of a reduced-dosage pill and liquid for allergic children, has been most helpful in suppressing their allergies, in occasionally improving their dispositions, and in avoiding drowsiness at school or at play. Not only will skating or riding a bike be safer for children now, but the mucociliary cleansing of their nose, sinuses, and lungs should function better with the new generation of non-sedating and less-drying antihistamines.

MEDICAL TREATMENT
DECONGESTANTS
An episode of acute sinusitis that develops in normally healthy sinuses is usually brought on by some form of insult to the nose or upper respiratory tract causing the membranous linings of the nose to swell and block the sinus drainage openings. This is more often the result of a viral infection such as a cold or flu but may also occur from an inhaled allergen as in hay fever or allergic rhinitis, or from breathing a nonallergenic but otherwise very irritating substance in a gaseous, liquid, or powdery form. If it is the result of a viral infection, the treatment would consist of trying to keep your nose open and the sinuses draining well by taking a decongestant pill such as pseudoephedrine hydrochloride (Sudafed), preferably using the 12-hour dosage so that it will last through the night when the nose and sinuses are inclined to swell the most, or by using a nonirritating decongestant nasal spray, but usually for no longer than 3 to 5 days. The latter might also be recommended if the nasal swelling is very marked or very slow in responding to the decongestant pill, and in some instances both may be useful. The oral decongestant does have the advantage of reducing the membranous swelling within the sinus cavities themselves, which the nasal spray cannot do. They may also reduce swelling in some areas of the nose that may be unreachable by a spray.

If you cannot take oral decongestants at night because they keep you awake, or for certain medical reasons such as prostate enlargement or hypertension, a decongestant spray would usually be the wiser choice. However, you should remember that if rebound swelling of the nose does occur within an hour or two after you use a nasal decongestant spray, you should stop using the spray. This is called the rebound phenomenon, and it occurs in a significant number of people who use a decongestant nasal spray, especially when it is used too often or for too long a period. The longer-acting decongestant nasal sprays in particular may occasionally cause too much nasal irritation and even nasal bleeding and may have to be discontinued should this occur.

If you have an elevated blood pressure, thyroid disease, diabetes, epilepsy, or certain heart conditions where the use of a decongestant stimulant such as pseudoephedrine by mouth might be considered unwise, you may sometimes try a mild decongestant nasal spray for a very short period in the half-strength pediatric dosage, even then using it sparingly. Before doing so, however, check with your general medical doctor. The same advice would apply if you suffer from nasal and sinus congestion during pregnancy, and here too you should consult your OB doctor before you take any medication. People taking certain antidepressant drugs, or medications for certain emotional conditions or for Parkinson's disease, or those prone to urinary obstruction from prostate enlargement may have to avoid oral decongestants altogether.

GUAIFENESIN

Guaifenesin, a so-called mucus thinner or liquefier that apparently acts as an expectorant by reducing the stickiness of mucus, thus making it flow more freely and usually making a cough more productive, is frequently recommended for respiratory infections with or without sinusitis. It is also found in dozens of over-the-counter cough, cold, flu, and sinus preparations. It may benefit certain bronchial or lung problems, but whether it will help you with sinusitis is still unproven. The mucous secretions within the sinuses, however, are well protected from the drying effects of the nasal airstream and should flow freely provided the cilia sweeping action is adequate, body hydration is good, and the sinus drainage openings are not obstructed, none of which taking this particular medication is likely to improve. Guaifenesin may, however, be useful for sinusitis infections in some AIDS patients, whose sinonasal drainage may sometimes become very sticky.

ANTIHISTAMINES

Antihistamines, which are also found in many over-the-counter cold and sinus remedies, are generally of no help and not indicated in the treatment of sinusitis unless there is a significant allergic component, and then they should be taken for only a relatively short period. This is particularly true for the conventional sedating kind. In fact, if you are a nonallergic individual who has sinusitis and you take one of the sedating antihistamines even for a relatively short period, it will usually cause some thickening of mucous secretions within your nose and sinuses, resulting in a reduced mucous flow and a less effective sinonasal cleansing action, often prolonging a sinus infection. However, it does appear that the newer non-sedating antihistamines may not alter mucous secretions significantly and might therefore be taken for very extended periods without harm if you are allergic and have sinusitis, but it may take a while to fully determine this.

For some people with sinusitis, especially those with a superimposed allergic problem where it is obvious that the allergic rhinitis is enhancing the sinus blockage, using a steroid nasal spray may be especially worthwhile and may even make it possible to discontinue an antihistamine sooner. Even people with long-standing nonallergic rhinitis may find a steroid spray effective, since it may help to tone down and soothe a very reactive inflammatory response on the part of their nasal membranes to some chronic irritant, often referred to as hyperreactivity. If there is an obvious infectious component, however, you should also be covered with an antibiotic, since corticosteroids, even when applied locally, may tend to inhibit your body's normal defense against infection.

In many cases of acute sinusitis associated with a viral respiratory infection such as a cold or flu and involving mostly healthy sinuses, taking over-the-counter oral or nasal decongestants, exercising good judgment, using a steam vaporizer or a saline nasal spray to keep the membranes moist (especially in cold weather), drinking adequate fluids other than alcohol for the same reason, sleeping slightly elevated, getting adequate rest, and avoiding stress or unnecessary exposure to irritating inhalants, to drafts, and to the elements may result in a normal recovery within 7 to 10 days. This will usually happen without the use of antibiotics, which are not effective against cold or flu viruses anyhow, even though the nasal discharge will usually turn very cloudy by the third or fourth day of the cold due mostly to a superimposed bacterial infection. Fortunately, the normally healthy nose and sinuses have an inherent ability to recover rather quickly from a viral infection, to replace any damaged or destroyed ciliated hair cells, and to begin sweeping themselves clean again in very short order, even in the presence of very large amounts of infected sinonasal discharge, provided they are not completely obstructed and provided their drainage is not too thickened or dried out from low humidity, body dehydration, alcohol intake, fluid pills, or other mucus-drying medications. Replacement of damaged ciliated cells usually occurs within 48 to 72 hours provided their basement membrane cells remain intact and are not damaged by the virus.

ANTIBIOTICS

If you have normally healthy sinuses and should develop an acute bacterial sinusitis, usually in association with a viral respiratory infection, and have tried decongestants but show no improvement within 7 to 10 days, or if any complications should develop such as an ear infection, intensified headache, cheek pain with upper tooth discomfort, a sinus air-fluid level on X ray, a significant fever, or lung infection, then an appropriate antibiotic will usually be necessary. A significantly elevated temperature with cough and chest discomfort may also indicate the need for a chest examination and possibly a chest X ray to rule out an associated pneumonia. The duration of antibiotic treatment for a sinusitis flare-up will depend on how long the sinus infection has been present, the strength and resistance of the infecting organism, the effectiveness of the antibiotic, whether the infection is complicated by allergic rhinitis, AIDS, cystic fibrosis, cleft palate, pregnancy, and so on, the degree and duration of the nasal and sinus swelling as well as how quickly it subsides, how much sinus blockage from old scarring exists, how long antibiotics have been required in the past, and of course whether there are any complications.

Any discussion as to the various kinds of bacteria involved in a sinus infection and especially the different antibiotics considered to be effective against them will have to be limited, since this may change from time to time. Any antibiotics recommended now may turn out to be useless or possibly even harmful at some point after this writing. For the present, however, the antibiotics most commonly used for sinus infections belong to the penicillin, macrolide, cephalosporin, and sulfa groups, and their newer and less bacteria-resistant forms are often preferred in troublesome cases. The proper selection of an appropriate antibiotic by your doctor will usually depend on what antibiotic allergies or sensitivities you have, whether there could be serious side effects, how long you will have to take it, the overall cost, and many times on what success your doctor may have had with a particular antibiotic in the treatment of similar infections in the past. He or she will try to choose one that will not only eradicate the infection but also be safely tolerated for a very extended period should that prove necessary. The doctor's decision in this regard may also be influenced by any culture and antibiotic sensitivity studies available and by the prevalence of certain bacteria in your community or workplace, as well as their antibiotic resistance levels. At the same time, your doctor will take into consideration your own general health as well as your body's usual response to infections in the past, which may be very poor for a diabetic, an immunosuppressed patient, or someone with a chronic debilitating disease. Sometimes the convenience of administration and your daily schedule have to be considered as well.

The most commonly encountered bacteria in acute and early subacute sinusitis at the time of this writing are the *Streptococcus pneumoniae,* the *Hemophilus influenzae,* and the *M. catarrhalis,* all of which seem to have a preference for viral-damaged sinonasal membranes, whereas chronic sinus disease may often attract several of a half a dozen or more respiratory bacterial pathogens including anaerobic bacteria as well as *Staph. aureus, Pseudomonas, Klebsiella, Chlamydia,* and *E. Coli,* some of which may occasionally be found in acute sinusitis as well. Also, the organisms previously mentioned as commonly found in acute sinusitis are sometimes found in chronic disease, and this seems to be especially true for children. A continuously blocked sinus whose lining membrane may absorb the oxygen from any air trapped within its cavity can therefore provide an ideal environment for anaerobic bacteria, which grow and multiply only in the absence of oxygen. At the same time, the production of nitric oxide by the sinus membranes may also inhibit the growth of most bacteria. However, when anaerobic organisms are present, they may require a different and sometimes more expensive antibiotic, which may have to be given intravenously in serious cases.

Large doses of an antibiotic by pill or intravenously, unless the sinus infection is very complicated, are not usually as important as prolonged adequate dosage, and stopping too soon can result in a much more obstinate infection. Moreover, you may be able to tolerate the lesser dosage for a longer period with less GI upset. A few people will even show a lessening of any GI symptoms while still taking the antibiotic, but if you continue taking the antibiotic on that basis, your GI problems could become very much worse, so it is not always a good idea. Some people who experience antibiotic-initiated diarrhea may become seriously ill from intestinal wall invasion by a rather dangerous bacterium called *Clostridium difficile,* resulting in intestinal bleeding with bloody diarrhea and often requiring hospitalization with very vigorous treatment. This has occurred with nearly all types of antibiotics and can range from mild to life-threatening in severity. Stool cultures may be necessary to confirm the presence of this type of colon infection, often referred to as pseudomembranous colitis, which sometimes may not show up for a month or more after stopping the antibiotic.

If you can avoid a GI upset, a more complete absorption of your medications will occur, since inflamed gastrointestinal membranes can't absorb medications as well. If a lesser but adequate dose continues to irritate your GI tract, then it may be necessary to change to another less irritating antibiotic after 2 or 3 days of abstinence to give your GI tract a chance to recover, or it may be necessary for your doctor to prescribe an antibiotic intramuscularly or intravenously if the oral medication is not tolerated at all. However, even this route of administration will sometimes produce GI symptoms, including diarrhea, but at least by the intravenous or intramuscular routes, you do have the assurance that you are absorbing all of the medication.

For acute bacterial sinus infections, if an antibiotic is necessary, your doctor will generally prescribe it for 10 to 14 days, and often twice as long or longer for recurrent acute flare-ups of chronic sinusitis. For sinusitis that develops after flying or deep-sea diving with a head cold or flu, you should receive antibiotics for two or three times as long a period as you would normally. Such cases associated with pressure changes seem to develop a very deep-seated infection and will nearly always require prolonged antibiotic treatment for a cure, especially to prevent a recurrence of the same infection several weeks later. Ear infections associated with flying or diving, which may also represent a deep-seated and very stubborn drainage problem, should be treated in a similar fashion.

In most instances of sinus or ear infections in children, antibiotics should be prescribed for even longer periods because of the tendency for children's nasal, eustachian tube, and sinus membranes to swell excessively and because of their naturally smaller drainage passages. Subacute sinus infections that may have been going on for 4 to 6 weeks or more may require at least 3 or 4 weeks of antibiotic therapy and many times longer, since it is often very difficult to tell just how long the sinus infection may have been present, and this is especially true in a child. Those infected for 2 or 3 months may require several months of antibiotic therapy, and those with chronic disease may often require an antibiotic for an even longer period, many times with prolonged antibiotic treatment for each subsequent sinus flare-up as well. In some cases, changing to a different antibiotic during a long course of treatment on the possibility that the dominant bacteria may have developed some resistance is often worthwhile, especially if there have been interruptions in treatment. Sometimes a culture and antibiotic sensitivity studies may help in determining this. Skipping or crowding of doses may encourage the growth of resistant organisms as well. If a child is on an every 6 or 8 hour antibiotic dosage and because of much-needed sleep has to go for 10 or 12 hours at night on a single bedtime dose, it may be necessary to increase the bedtime dosage if the child shouldn't be awakened. Consulting your physician or pharmacist may be helpful in such cases.

Bacterial resistance to an antibiotic may develop for a number of reasons, but when you are treating sinusitis, resistance probably more often results from stopping the antibiotic before the sinus infection has completely cleared. This may occur from self-treatment with too few antibiotic pills left over from a spouse's infection or from pills you have deliberately saved by stopping them too early during a previous infection, or if you decided on your own that your sinuses were better, and therefore did not refill the prescription, although previously instructed to do so by your physician. Bacterial resistance may also result from taking an inadequate dose, from taking an adequate dose irregularly, or from having to stop antibiotics too soon because of a reaction. It may likewise occur from taking antibiotics for strictly viral infections, for which antibiotics are of no use, or from using them prophylactically in too small a dose over a prolonged period to prevent infections. It may even occur in a few individuals by transference of an antibiotic-resistant organism from someone else with a sinus or respiratory infection.

Although 7 days of an effective antibiotic may be sufficient for many soft-tissue infections elsewhere in the body, it is usually inadequate for most sinus or ear infections. With both of these infections there is nearly always a drainage problem requiring a reduction in swelling with reestablishment of drainage and a nearly complete expulsion of the infected discharge from their respective cavities before the antibiotic can be stopped. The longer this obstructive swelling has been present, the longer it will usually take to disappear. The ethmoids, which are the most commonly infected sinuses, are said to have a somewhat reduced blood supply, which could also cause an even slower resolution in their membrane swelling. As previously mentioned, children will often take longer for their sinus infections to clear up, not only because of their smaller sinus drainage openings and smaller nasal passages, but especially because of a greater tendency for their sinonasal membranes to swell and to remain swollen.

When you are on prolonged antibiotic therapy, taking a multivitamin is a good idea, since antibiotics, by killing off some of the susceptible normal bacteria in the intestines, may disrupt some of your vitamin synthesis. Eating yogurt several times a day may help with this problem unless you are taking a medication incompatible with milk products. If so, it is usually stated on the prescription bottle, many times along with a warning to avoid excessive exposure to sunlight or ultraviolet light, since they may cause severe sunburn if you are taking certain antibiotics. It is always very important to read all the labels on a prescription bottle.

The intestinal tract normally contains millions of mostly harmless bacteria—as well as more than 500 different types. Many of them may serve as barriers to invasion of the body by harmful bacteria and also aid in breaking down and absorbing complex carbohydrates from fruits, whole grains, and vegetables, as well as playing a role in the synthesis of vitamins. These bacteria also aid in the digestion and absorption of the mucous secretions from your sinuses, nose, and lungs, which you are normally swallowing constantly in the amount of 2 pints or more a day, and which you can't afford to lose. An encouraging note is that this intestinal bacterial flora, which is obviously important to your body but is sometimes depleted by taking antibiotics, will usually recover and resume its normal function once the antibiotics are no longer interfering. Some normal intestinal bacteria may even take on some antibiotic resistance of their own over a period of time. However, bacteria in general do breed out their generations very rapidly, and many may in time also breed out their resistance to certain antibiotics. Unfortunately, this is not something we can count on for the immediate infection, although it may help with some others later on.

If you must be on very prolonged antibiotic therapy, periodic blood studies may be indicated for any evidence of bone marrow suppression such as sometimes noted by a drop in the hemoglobin or especially in the white or red blood cell counts, or by a reduction in the blood-clotting platelets, and sometimes for signs of diminished liver or kidney function. Some special antibiotics may also affect your hearing or balance centers. If evidence of such suppression or malfunction is noted, the antibiotic therapy will have to be changed or sometimes discontinued altogether.

When treating a very prolonged sinus infection, it is often wise to keep up the antibiotic for a week or 10 days after the discharge no longer appears cloudy, since hidden infected discharge may still be trapped within a sinus cavity, poised to reinfect the sinus as soon as you discontinue the antibiotic. Should the sinus infection show up again several weeks later, you and sometimes your physician may assume it is a new episode of sinusitis, when most of the time it is simply a resurgence of the same infection. Each time there is a resurgence, you should be given 10 days to 2 weeks of either the same antibiotic that was successful before, especially if it is the only one you tolerate, or a different antibiotic, which may also be necessary to combat any newly created antibiotic-resistant bacteria. Sometimes recurrences of the same infection can be more difficult to treat, since the residual swelling has then been present for a much longer period, will have become more indurated, and will therefore take longer to subside. Moreover, any surviving bacteria may now represent a much tougher or more resistant strain. In people who have subacute or chronic sinusitis, this regimen may have to be repeated a third or even a fourth time, and in rare instances sometimes more, before you can completely recover from a particular sinus infection.

With sinusitis, it is important to remember that immediately after completing an adequate course of an effective antibiotic, you may be completely symptom free, and at the time, everything may even appear normal to the examining physician. The inflammation and any really impressive swelling in the nose will many times have disappeared, and no cloudy infected discharge may be seen even with the examining endoscope; but your sinuses could still be infected, and cloudy discharge could still be trapped within a sinus cavity. That is why it is more important and usually more revealing for your physician to see you a week to 10 days after the full course of antibiotic treatment, when any lingering infected discharge indicating a persistent infection will usually be more obvious, rather than a day or two after you complete your medication. Even a limited CAT scan taken then may not show if your sinus infection has completely disappeared, since swelling of a sinus lining will often persist for 6 weeks or longer after the infection has departed. Sometimes the persistence of a nasal tone to the voice, especially in a child, may be the only clue that a sinus, especially a maxillary sinus, is still blocked and therefore potentially still infected and might therefore require further antibiotic therapy.

PROLONGED ANTIBIOTIC THERAPY
No doctor, knowing the many pitfalls, ever likes the idea of prescribing antibiotics so frequently and for such long periods as is often necessary to prevent or cure a subacute or chronic sinusitis. The otolaryngologist, however, can sometimes shorten that period and speed up recovery by puncturing and irrigating a sinus cavity filled with pus, by excising an obstructive polyp, or by endoscopically enlarging a chronically blocked sinus drainage opening. However, the sinus specialist also realizes that if efforts to cure the problem surgically or medically are unsuccessful, you could end up taking many times that amount of antibiotics for repeated sinus flare-ups and for any complications thereof during the rest of your life, with many more opportunities to create more antibiotic-resistant organisms. Because subacute and chronic sinus disease can be so totally lacking in outward signs of illness, sinus specialists have always had a very difficult time in justifying their insistence on prolonged antibiotic therapy, not only to the patient and the patient's family but also to a referring doctor. In the meantime, you will often have become so frustrated with lack of progress with medical therapy alone that you might welcome any offer of expediency through surgery.

NASAL SURGERY FOR SINUSITIS
SINUS IRRIGATION (MINOR SURGERY)
A simple, safe, effective, and very commonly performed sinus operation that will usually shorten the course of antibiotic therapy is the puncture and irrigation procedure often performed on a completely blocked sinus cavity partially or completely filled with pus, which is usually reported on X ray or CAT scan as an air-fluid level. With the patient under local anesthesia, the surgeon, using an irrigation needle, or trocar, will enter the nose, penetrate the very thin bony sinonasal wall, and gently flush out the sinus, along with its infecting contents, using a sterile normal salt solution. The entire procedure takes only a

few minutes and may occasionally have to be repeated in a few days, particularly if the natural drainage opening of the sinus is markedly swollen or badly scarred. Although this minor surgical procedure is sometimes necessary for people who have acute sinusitis but otherwise fairly healthy sinuses, it may be required periodically if you have chronic sinusitis and especially for the sinusitis patient with AIDS or fungal sinus disease. Performing this rather minor operative procedure promptly can be effective in relieving sinus pain or headache as well as in curing the sinus infection. Failing to do it when indicated could result in a more prolonged sinus infection with more pain, more antibiotic therapy, more loss of time from work or school, and more permanent damage to the sinus lining as well as to its drainage opening from more scarring. In a few rare instances of total sinus blockage, a rupture of the sinus wall has resulted from pressure buildup within the sinus cavity. The extra drainage openings into the nose found in the medial walls of some maxillary sinuses would be considered a very minor example of such a rupture but would be of very little significance compared to a devastating rupture of infected sinus contents into the brain or an orbit.

This sinus irrigating procedure has also been used diagnostically to obtain cultures, especially from the maxillary sinuses, and also to see if there is some retention of infected discharge in an inadequately draining sinus cavity that may not be obvious with a sinus X ray or a CAT scan. It is also useful for flushing fungal matter out of a sinus cavity as well as for postoperative irrigation of a maxillary sinus to remove blood clots and other debris. Suctioning infected discharge from the nose or sinus opening can sometimes be beneficial, but it is not a substitute for puncture and irrigation of an infected and totally obstructed sinus cavity.

Irrigation of a maxillary or sphenoid sinus through their natural openings is sometimes performed but in some instances could traumatize the opening to cause more scarring with more obstruction. With regard to the maxillary opening, the surgeon could also be probing one of the most sensitive areas of the nose. Completely avoiding the natural opening is more important when it comes to the frontal sinuses, especially in the 20 to 40 percent of the population who have elongated and sometimes tortuous frontal sinus ducts. They, like the very long eustachian tubes leading to the ears, should never be probed, stretched or dilated, since doing so will nearly always result in more scarring with more narrowing and more blockage. Most young sinus doctors are repeatedly cautioned by their professors very early in their training to respect the virginity of the frontal sinus duct, and this would apply to the eustachian tubes as well.

A rather similar puncture-and-irrigation procedure is sometimes carried out on the other two larger sinuses, namely, the frontal and sphenoid, for similar reasons. Their respective locations in the forehead and the back of the nose, however, make the procedures a little more difficult. With regard to the frontal sinus, in order to drill through its thicker bony wall, a surgeon will usually make a skin incision through the eyebrow, although some may prefer to go through the thinner bone in the roof of the orbit just beneath the brow. This procedure can be done under local anesthesia but can sometimes be uncomfortable, so a general anesthetic may be preferred. Here a short drainage tube is usually inserted into the frontal sinus cavity for subsequent daily saline irrigations. Once the irrigating solution flows freely into the nose, the tube is removed, and the skin opening will close very quickly. The puncture-and-irrigation procedure for treating sinus infections has been around for a very long time and has much the same general effect as surgically draining an abscess or pocket of pus elsewhere in the body as far as expeditiously eradicating a localized, sealed-off area of infection.

OTHER OPERATIONS

There are also a number of surgical procedures on the nasal passages, some very simple and some more complex. The surgeon may carry out some individually to see how much improvement is noted, while others may be combined with more definitive sinus surgery. Straightening your nasal septum or removing a septal spur can correct a misdirected nasal airstream that may be contaminating or drying out a sinus or eustachian tube opening. Surgical removal of a benign growth, cyst, or polyps from your nose may also improve nasal airflow as well as sinonasal drainage and prevent pooling or stasis of mucus with its enhancement of bacterial growth. Surgically trimming an enlarged or misshapen turbinate or shrinking it with cryosurgery can also improve sinonasal blockage and nasal airflow. Correcting a nasal valvular or nostril deformity (often as part of a septal procedure), trimming away excessive erectile tissue in the front of the nose, or removing excessive scar tissue or adhesions may also improve nasal function as well as airway resistance, which in the long run may also benefit the sinuses.

The use of an external nasal dilator device for better breathing may benefit certain individuals, particularly during sleep or when performing slight to moderate exercise, by improving airflow through the nasal area. However, any intense exercise will nearly always require constant mouth breathing for adequate oxygen intake, and there is no evidence so far that the use of such a device will in anyway benefit a sinus problem. With most surgical procedures on the nose, it is very important that the surgeon resist the temptation for too much enlargement of the breathing passages, as this can lead to excessive drying out of nasal membranes as well as to bleeding, scab formation, stagnation of mucus, infection, more sinus blockage, and more sinusitis. On the other hand, an overzealous effort on the part of the surgeon to obtain a near-perfect cosmetic improvement of a nose or a nasal tip can sometimes result in too much restriction of a nasal airway and subsequently lead to more obstructive problems with more sinus problems.

DENTAL TREATMENT FOR SINUSITIS

In a few cases of chronic or recurrent maxillary sinusitis, dental surgery to remove an infected upper tooth or an embedded infected tooth root left behind in an extraction and sometimes acting as a foreign body may be necessary to eliminate the sinusitis completely. The penetration of dental filling material beneath the membrane of a maxillary sinus in performing a root canal on an upper tooth can sometimes lead to a chronic sinusitis problem. Dental cysts arising from an upper tooth may also invade a maxillary sinus and obstruct its mucous flow, thereby causing a persistent sinusitis and requiring surgical removal of the cyst along with the responsible tooth.

Whenever a maxillary sinus infection refuses to clear up after more than adequate treatment, or if it should keep recurring, and especially if there is a sensitive upper tooth just beneath it, or even one that has had a root canal, a crown, or a bridge indicating a previous extraction, the physician must view this area with suspicion and as a possible cause of the persistent maxillary sinus problem. Dental X rays and a dental consultation will often be necessary, and a very suspicious tooth or retained root may have to be removed before the sinus infection will clear up completely.

EXTERNAL SINUS SURGERY

If a chronically diseased frontal sinus can't be adequately and permanently drained through the nose and its function restored, or if there is an associated bone infection or a chronically infected frontal ethmoid sinus adjoining the frontal sinus that likewise can't be reached through the nose, or if there is a benign growth or large mucocele in a frontal sinus that can't be removed or drained through a nasal procedure, then the frontal sinus may have to be opened up externally through a brow or scalp incision. Then, depending on what is found, the lining membrane may have to be removed and the cavity obliterated with a fat graft or sometimes with a synthetic material so that it may no longer exist as a sinus cavity or harbor disease.

SINUS SURGERY FOR CHILDREN

Surgery on children's sinuses is something the endoscopic sinus surgeon would like to avoid, but unfortunately this is not always possible. A child may sometimes need nasal polyps excised for better drainage, a maxillary sinus punctured and irrigated, occasionally a drainage orifice enlarged, a window made, a growth or cyst removed, an obstructive malformation of a nasal passage corrected, or a large, chronically infected adenoid mass excised. As to whether more extensive endoscopic sinus surgery (ESS), often so successful in older adolescents and adults, will be consistently feasible on a child's still-developing sinonasal structures, we have yet to learn. So far we don't really know the full effects of operative intervention and postoperative scarring on nose and sinus development in the very young patient. Some studies suggest that the effects on facial growth and development may be greater with sinus surgery performed before age 9, and the more extensive the sinus surgery, the greater the effect. Endoscopic sinus operations carried out on young pigs have supported these findings. Working with such comparatively small structures as a young child's nose and sinuses, in such a confining area, somewhat devoid of good surgical landmarks and so close to certain vital structures, requires exceptional expertise gathered from long hours of study, training, and experience. Also, having to put a child to sleep for the very necessary postoperative treatments following endoscopic sinus surgery can complicate the picture immensely.

SURGICAL AIDS

The role of surgery in the treatment of sinusitis has become more important in recent years with the introduction of very delicate and more efficient operative instruments, better magnification, and more effective fiber-optic lighting, making it possible for the endoscopic sinus surgeon to work in a very narrow area with greater skill and far greater safety. More recent innovations have also made it possible to see and work around corners should it become necessary. Operating room TV monitors providing computer-guided displays for three-dimensional spatial orientation of operative instruments within a nose or sinus cavity coordinated with a preoperative CAT scan and live endoscopic vision make it possible for the sinus surgeon to know within a 2-millimeter range exactly where the tips of those operative instruments are and where the dangers lie. These technologies also make it possible for the experienced endoscopic surgical instructor to closely monitor nearly every operative move of a still-learning resident. Fairly simple periodic checks during surgery may still be necessary to correct any drift in the 3-D coordinates due to headset movement or displacement. The use of fixed anatomical reference points with the introduction of continuous computerized three-dimensional guidance monitoring of the operative dissection itself may not be that far away.

The availability of preoperative CAT scans, MRI, bone scans, and 3-D imaging have also greatly improved the sinus surgeon's ability to identify the full extent of the sinus disease and the proximity of any rather vital structures such as the optic nerves, internal carotid arteries, orbits, and brain as well as the presence of any anatomical anomalies that might complicate the procedure.

FUNCTIONAL ENDOSCOPIC SINUS SURGERY (FESS)

The endoscopic sinus surgeon has two main goals. The first is to preserve as much of the potentially healthy sinus lining as possible so that once the infection, swelling, and blockage have cleared, it may effectively proceed with sweeping the sinus cavity clean again. Even rather severely diseased sinuses can often be restored to this functional state if not too badly scarred.

The second goal is to restore adequate sinonasal drainage and sinonasal air exchange for any chronically obstructed sinus cavities either by enlarging their natural drainage openings or, where indicated, by completely removing a portion of a sinus wall, keeping in mind that the cilia sweep and mucous flow along its remaining walls will continue in the general direction of the natural sinus opening.

Meeting both of these goals will provide the very best chance of surgically eradicating a chronic sinus infection as well as restoring sinus function, and the operative technique employed is therefore called functional endoscopic sinus surgery, or FESS, now often referred to by its shortened form, endoscopic sinus surgery, or ESS.

To accomplish this, the endoscopic sinus surgeon must have an intricate knowledge of sinus anatomy, have carefully reviewed the preoperative CAT scan to determine the extent of the sinus disease as well as to identify any unusual structural abnormalities that might jeopardize the operative procedure and harm the patient. The sinus surgeon must also be able to control bleeding for good operative visibility as well as for identifying surgical landmarks. Even so, the very complex anatomy of the ethmoid sinuses and the almost complete lack of uniformity in their development make orientation within these structures, particularly with regard to surgical boundaries and their relationship to vital structures, one of the most difficult problems the endoscopic sinus surgeon has to face. He or she must know precisely where the tips of those dissecting instruments are located at all times, use good surgical judgment, and know when to quit.

In both adults and children, since the maxillary and ethmoid sinuses are far more often involved with chronic disease than the frontals or sphenoids, most endoscopic sinus surgery has to do with them. This is especially true of the more vulnerable anterior ethmoidal group, since their drainage openings are the smallest and therefore more easily obstructed, their blood supply is generally considered to be the poorest, and there are also usually more of them. Since each one has its own drainage opening, the odds for one of them becoming obstructed and infected and then infecting others are far greater.

Since the drainage openings of the anterior ethmoids and maxillary sinuses are situated so close together in what is known as the ostiomeatal complex, or anterior OMC, a persistent infection of one may very easily involve the other. Consequently most endoscopic sinus surgery performed for chronic sinusitis will involve both and will usually entail exploring the ostiomeatal complex, enlarging the natural drainage opening of the maxillary sinus, and opening up the anterior ethmoids, also for better drainage. In some instances, the dissection may have to be carried toward the back of the nose and superiorly to include posterior ethmoids and posterior OMC, but a preoperative CAT scan will often indicate the need for this. It is in the back of the posterior ethmoids that the endoscopic sinus surgeon would more likely encounter the optic nerve to the eye, since it has been found exposed there and possibly vulnerable in 6 percent of the Caucasian population. Just as the frontal sinus may have to be approached through the anterior ethmoids, the sphenoid sinus may sometimes be entered through the posterior ethmoids, the latter occasionally bringing the endoscopic sinus surgeon into close contact with another very vital structure, namely, an exposed internal carotid artery to the brain. The bone overlying this internal carotid artery, as well as that covering the optic nerve, may be very thin or even absent in about one-fourth of the population.

When surgically exploring these various sinus cavities, unless their membranous linings are so badly diseased and scarred that they can't recover their normal function, the surgeon should leave them mostly intact. This is where sound surgical judgment as to what to take and what to leave plays such an important role. From experience with earlier and more radical sinus surgery, we have learned that whenever we completely removed a partially damaged sinus lining, it would often be replaced by a more extensively scarred membrane with less cilia and fewer mucus-secreting glands, usually resulting in a greater loss of function. Also requiring good surgical judgment would be the decision to continue or to stop the procedure in the face of excessive bleeding, poor visibility, an unsure surgeon, a drug reaction or anesthesia problem, an uncooperative patient, a disturbing vital sign, or an orbital or central nervous system intrusion. Areas of missing bone between a sinus cavity and the orbit, the optic nerve, the internal carotid artery, or the brain, or an infected sinus cavity impinging on any of these structures, could complicate the operative procedure very significantly and in some instances even endanger the patient's vision or life. However, these anatomical abnormalities, one or more of which may be found in more than 50 percent of people with chronic sinusitis as opposed to about 10 percent of the general population, can often be demonstrated on preoperative CAT scans, thus avoiding a surprise encounter in most instances and again emphasizing the importance of close cooperation between the endoscopic sinus surgeon and the radiologist. Operating on someone with distorted or missing landmarks due to previous sinus surgery, especially when performed by a different surgeon, could also lessen the chances of success with a second or third operation. Here the use of the computer-assisted three-dimensional guidance system for endoscopic sinus surgery could prove very helpful.

SURGICAL DISCIPLINES

To eradicate a chronic sinus infection, reestablish good sinonasal function, and avoid complications, there are certain basic disciplines that the endoscopic sinus surgeon usually follows:

1. Obtain and thoroughly review the CAT scan before surgery.

2. Provide adequate anesthesia, reduce swelling, and control bleeding.

3. Look for surgical landmarks and avoid vital structures, as well as certain important nerves and vessels. Know where you are at all times, and above all know when to stop.

4. Limit the sinus surgery to the extent of the chronic disease whenever possible.

5. Establish adequate drainage and adequate sinonasal air exchange for all chronically obstructed sinus cavities.

6. Avoid injury to normal nasal or sinus membranes, which could result in excessive scarring or adhesions.

7. Be especially careful not to elevate, strip, or remove the membranous walls of the maxillary sinuses.

8. Avoid removing any healthy or potentially healthy membrane from any sinus walls except when necessary to establish good drainage or excise a growth.

9. Remove as little of the turbinates as possible and avoid traumatizing them unnecessarily.

10. Avoid too much enlargement of a nasal passage, which can cause drying, crusting, and bleeding.

11. Avoid creating too small or too narrow a nasal passage when cosmetically reducing the size of a nose, and maintain adequate support for the nasal bridge.

12. Refrain from enlarging any sinus drainage openings that don't need enlarging.

13. When possible, avoid creating a second permanent opening into a maxillary sinus, since it can cause recirculation of mucus within the sinus cavity, resulting in stagnation of mucous flow with more infection.

14. Avoid leaving behind exposed cartilage or any large areas of exposed bone as well as any sharp bony projections or bony fragments. The latter may act as a foreign body, and bony projections will cause granulation tissue formation as well as delayed healing.

15. Avoid unnecessary injury to the olfactory area containing the end organs of smell and to the lacrimal duct that transports tears from the eyes to the nose.

16. Look out for signs of a breakthrough into the orbits such as eye changes or the presence of orbital fat as well as for any evidence of an intrusion into the central nervous system resulting in a cerebrospinal fluid leak. Recognize and treat all such complications early.

17. Try to avoid postoperative nasal and sinus packing, but when required for bleeding control or structural support, pack as loosely as possible and remove as early as practical.

18. Provide frequent and continuous postoperative care until healing is complete, all sinus infection has cleared, and function is restored.

When possible, endoscopic sinus surgery is performed under local anesthesia and with adequate sedation. Children should be done under general anesthesia and will usually require more general anesthesia for postoperative care. Topical decongestants and injectable vasoconstrictors before and during surgery are used to control bleeding and shrink membranes, thereby providing better visibility for the surgeon. The patient's eyes are usually kept uncovered during the surgery so that the operator or anesthesiologist may observe them for any subtle pupil, eye, or lid changes suggestive of orbital intrusion or orbital hemorrhage. Postoperative nasal packing is avoided whenever possible, but when necessary, it is usually applied fairly loosely, since too tight a packing may also cause excessive pressure on an exposed orbit or eye. A protective gelatinous film has been used postoperatively to prevent adhesions from forming between the turbinates and the lateral nasal wall, but some feel it may cause more granulation tissue with more delay in healing and more scarring. However, there is a strong suggestion that some tissue-compatible silicone stents may work better. Granulation tissue, also known as proud flesh, has a granular-appearing surface and usually forms in open infected wounds during the process of healing. Adhesions result when opposing tissues are bound together by scar tissue. Children seem to heal faster following endoscopic sinus surgery, but they also seem to have more granulation tissue and a higher incidence of adhesions, especially children under age 7.

Carefully regulated postoperative visits following endoscopic sinus surgery are necessary and almost as important as the surgery itself. You will usually have to see your doctor frequently at regular intervals beginning only a few days after surgery, and you will usually require repeated nasal and sinus suctioning, and sometimes nasal irrigations, division of adhesions, and regular forceps cleaning of the operative field under local anesthesia. This includes forceps removal of granulation tissue, especially from sinus drainage openings, along with bloody scabs, clots, mucous crusts, bone fragments, and bony spicules. In a child, this usually has to be done under general anesthesia.

Repeated endoscopic exams may be necessary to determine the progress healing and the persistence of any infected sinus discharge as well as any complications such as a clear cerebrospinal fluid leak. The latter seems to occur more often following ethmoid surgery on the right side, and when a leak is present, you will usually become aware of a very thin clear drainage from a nostril or down the throat. Antibiotics are usually prescribed until healing is complete and no evidence of an infected cloudy discharge is noted. Steroid nasal sprays may be necessary to control any allergic rhinitis and to calm a reactive nasal airway. A CAT scan may be necessary if you fail to get well or stay well, remembering, of course, that postoperative swelling in the operated area as well as in any nearby normally healthy sinus cavities may persist as long as 6 weeks or more after healing and any associated infection has cleared. Your own healing powers, tendency for scar formation, resistance to infection, and the lack of postoperative complications may all play an important role in the results.

Unfortunately, a second or third endoscopic sinus operation may sometimes be necessary and may at times be even more extensive than the first. Besides the continued presence of disturbing sinusitis symptoms, the most important findings suggesting the need for further sinus surgery are the persistence of an infected discharge on endoscopic exam in spite of prolonged antibiotic therapy as well as the progression of the sinus disease on follow-up CAT scans. With each course of antibiotic therapy or with each surgical procedure, the chronic sinusitis patient usually has high hopes of finally obtaining a complete cure and may eventually become very discouraged or depressed if it doesn't happen.

Surgical failures seem to be mainly due to inadequate, incomplete, or interrupted surgery, excessive bleeding, excessive scarring, inadequately treated postoperative infection, unsuccessful surprise encounters with anatomical abnormalities during surgery, previous sinus surgery, the absence of (or failure to identify) surgical landmarks, delayed recognition and therefore delayed treatment of any complications, and sometimes even inadequate follow-up care.

People who have active nasal allergy, asthma, immunodeficiency diseases, bilateral nasal polyps, or mucociliary problems such as cystic fibrosis or Kartagener's syndrome seem to have the highest percentage of failures. Those with multiple bilateral nasal polyps may enjoy a marked improvement in sinusitis symptoms initially, but some may have a recurrence of their nasal polyps along with their sinus symptoms.

Even so, some endoscopic sinus surgeons have reported very low failure rates of 10 percent or less and with at least a 50 percent improvement in sinus symptoms nearly 18 months or more after surgery in almost 90 percent of their cases. Especially encouraging have been reports of close to 50 percent of the latter being essentially symptom free. However, people who have undergone previous surgical procedures on their sinuses may end up with less improvement in their symptoms, especially with regard to headaches, which in some instances may be related to the effects of additional surgical scarring around nerve endings.

Although the results in most instances of endoscopic sinus surgery have been impressive, the overzealous surgical pursuit of extensive chronic disease, especially by an inexperienced endoscopic sinus surgeon, can result in serious complications, particularly with regard to a patient's vision or central nervous system. At the same time, an incomplete excision of permanently diseased tissue, failure to restore adequate drainage, or having to limit or abort a sinus operation only partially completed could result in even poorer sinus function.

In spite of more extensive training of endoscopic sinus surgeons, the number of major complications from endoscopic sinus surgery is increasing, but so is the number of endoscopic sinus surgeries being performed and the number of surgeons being trained to do them.

We must remember, however, that sinusitis, whether acute, subacute, or chronic, is still primarily a medical disease, and that surgery should be reserved for those cases where more than adequate medical treatment has failed or where it may be an adjunct to medical treatment by establishing better sinus drainage, and of course for those cases where there is suspicion of malignancy, or where some acute or complicated sinus problem may require rapid surgical intervention.

CONCLUSION

In the overall treatment of sinus disease, you should now realize that preventative care is of major importance, and that by working together with your physician as a team, it may be possible for you to learn what precipitates your sinus attacks, what makes them worse, how best to treat them, and most importantly how to prevent them. If you also have allergic rhinitis, you should find out what causes it, and if you can't avoid it, you should minimize the symptoms with early and appropriate treatment. You should also make an earnest effort to reduce your exposure to viral respiratory infections when possible through good hygiene and good judgment, to stay completely away from primary and secondary tobacco smoke, and to monitor your own living and working conditions and to maintain them in a healthy state.

You should avoid excessive stress and exhaustion and unnecessary exposure to dampness, air pollution, and cold, all of which could make you worse. You should seek early medical attention for stubborn respiratory infections or sinus flare-ups long before they have a chance to become chronic. Finally, you should make every effort to take your full course of sinus medications as prescribed, provided that they are well tolerated. It should be emphasized once again that when taking an antibiotic for a sinus infection, whether it be acute, subacute, or chronic, you should continue it until well after your cloudy sinus discharge has cleared and until the inflammatory swelling blocking your sinus drainage openings or interfering with their mucociliary flow has subsided sufficiently to restore adequate sinus drainage, an adequate sinonasal air exchange, and an adequate sinonasal cleansing action.

It is also important for you to realize that in spite of frequent and prolonged medical treatments, and even with extensive and repeated endoscopic sinus surgeries, a complete cure of your sinus problem may not always be possible and that you may continue to require periodic medical care.

CHAPTER TEN

What Are Antihistamines?
How Do They Affect Your Sinuses, and How Useful Are Over-the-Counter Cold, Flu, and Sinus Medications?

ANTIHISTAMINES

Antihistamines, which have been around for more than half a century, are chemical compounds used to counteract histamine, a powerful substance normally released in small amounts mostly by mast cells within the body and in accelerated amounts often as a result of tissue injury or an allergic reaction. (A detailed discussion of histamine and the histamine reaction is provided at the end of this chapter.)

Since their discovery, antihistamines have had a tremendous effect on the practice of medicine as well as on the pharmaceutical world in general. They have been used not only in the treatment of all kinds of allergic problems but also in the care of numerous medical conditions often considered unrelated to allergy, such as nausea and vomiting, seasickness, vertigo, gastrointestinal inflammation, bleeding from the GI tract, gastric and duodenal ulcers, esophagitis or heartburn, persistent cough, chronic itching, diminished appetite, insomnia, alcohol withdrawal symptoms or DTs, emotional problems, some types of vascular headaches, as an adjunct to anesthesia, and also to stabilize certain brain pathways to lessen some of the symptoms of Parkinsonism. Paradoxically, some antihistamines may even cause a tremor or gait problems suggestive of Parkinsonism, especially with excessive dosage and especially in the elderly. Antihistamines have always been very unpredictable and may cause the opposite reaction in different individuals, such as drowsiness in some but nervousness or insomnia in others, dizziness in some but as a cure for dizziness in others, tremors in some but as a tremor relief for others, and even asthmalike bronchial spasm in a few with occasional relief of bronchial spasm in others. Some children taking the earlier sedating antihistamines for allergic rhinitis may exhibit agitation, irritability, and even temper tantrums, which could present behavior problems at home and at school. Some children may become argumentative and antagonistic even after a single dose. If your child experiences these symptoms, taking one of the non-sedating antihistamines should solve the problem. At the same time, it might even improve school productivity for your child if he or she is suffering from the distracting symptoms of allergic rhinitis or from a classroom drowsiness problem due to a sedating antihistamine.

If the results from taking one of the sedating antihistamines should prove unsatisfactory, either from the standpoint of no improvement in symptoms or because of some untoward reaction such as drowsiness, changing to an entirely different antihistamine can often make a difference. Many times it becomes a question of trial and error to find the right antihistamine for the right person, as well as for the right medical condition. Sometimes you may find after a week or two of taking a sedating antihistamine that the drowsiness problem may be considerably reduced, but unfortunately that may be true for the drug's effectiveness as well.

BENADRYL

Two of the earliest antihistamines that many may remember were Benadryl and Pyribenzamine (PBZ). They are still around and are still used, although the newer longer-acting non-sedating ones are becoming more popular but may require a prescription and are also more expensive. Benadryl, or diphenhydramine (DPH), has many other useful properties that have made it popular in the past as a cough suppressant, a treatment for itching, or urticaria, and as a substitute for strong sleeping pills. This latter use has occasionally been worthwhile for people trying to break the sleeping-pill habit, since Benadryl is not considered habit-forming, but may cause very significant drowsiness in some. Benadryl is also the main ingredient of Sominex and Nytol, two well-known over-the-counter sleeping preparations. Another unique property of Benadryl is that when given intravenously, it has been found to block the brain pathways that are responsible for the very frightening symptom of lockjaw, or trismus, sometimes seen in people taking compazine, a nausea-relieving medication.

COLD, FLU, AND SINUS MEDICATIONS

Today there are several hundred over-the-counter (OTC) cold, flu, and sinus preparations, including a large number recommended for nasal congestion, runny nose, allergies, rhinitis, cough, nasal swelling, chest congestion, and itching. Many of these preparations contain one of the early-generation antihistamines. Diphenhydramine, or Benadryl, is usually one of these, and another early one frequently found in these OTC preparations is chlorpheniramine, which you might remember as Teldrin or Chlortrimeton. These two early-generation antihistamines or their derivatives now make up more than 70 percent of the antihistamine components of the over-the-counter flu and cold preparations.

Although each over-the-counter cold, cough, and flu preparation is presented to the public by a multitude of different brand names, most of them are basically made up of varying combinations of the same five or six generic drugs. You should therefore read the labels, and especially the active ingredients, since you may very well find out you are paying nearly twice as much for the same product. Besides containing one of the early-generation antihistamines, these OTC flu, cold, and cough preparations often include a decongestant such as pseudoephedrine (Sudafed) or phenylephrine, along with a cough suppressant such as dextromethorphan, and a pain reliever such as acetaminophen or more recently one of the NSAIDs such as ibuprofen. Occasionally an expectorant, or so-called mucus liquefier, known as guaifenesin will be included in place of an antihistamine, especially if the preparation is recommended for sinusitis or bronchitis, since the sedating antihistamines especially, because of their mucus-drying effects, are not usually recommended for nonallergic sinusitis or bronchitis and certainly not if they are to be taken for an extended period. Also, their tendency to suppress a cough is not considered beneficial for bronchitis or chronic lung disease, especially if you have a cough productive of a cloudy infected discharge that should be coughed up.

PSEUDOEPHEDRINE

Pseudoephedrine, or Sudafed, has also been around for a long time and is still highly effective as an oral decongestant for colds and sinusitis. It is also very often encountered as a single medication. Unfortunately, many of the kitchen laboratories used for manufacturing illegal drugs have discovered how to make methamphetamine, a powerful stimulant also known as crank, ice, or speed, from pseudoephedrine, and this practice has already required curbing of bulk sales, since it takes a thousand tablets to make an ounce of "meth." Although pseudoephedrine has been banned by the Olympics, it is hoped that over-the-counter sales will continue, since it is extremely effective in treating sinusitis and in diminishing the sinus problems that usually follow colds or flu. People suffering from colds, flu, or sinusitis are also more inclined to take a medication if it is sold over the counter than if they have to see a doctor for a prescription.

Both of the decongestants, pseudoephedrine and phenylephrine, have their drawbacks of sometimes producing a fast heartbeat, nervousness, inability to sleep, and a slightly elevated blood pressure. Unfortunately, in some hypertensive individuals, even a slight increase in blood pressure can lead to serious problems. Decongestants should also be avoided by individuals taking certain antidepressant drugs and by those with Parkinsonism, as well as those with certain thyroid diseases, or diabetes, some types of heart disease, seizure problems, as well as those with an already elevated blood pressure. Decongestants may occasionally cause difficulty urinating, especially in men with enlargement of the prostate gland. This urinary complication usually results from muscular constriction at the bladder's neck, but it is also this same undesirable effect that makes decongestants sometimes very useful in controlling urinary incontinence or lack of bladder control, not only in humans but also in some house pets.

If you are unable to take an oral decongestant, for nasal or sinus congestion, a decongestant nasal spray is usually very effective, but it should not be used excessively or for more than 3 to 5 days at a time. If there is a pediatric strength available, adults may find it just as helpful, potentially less irritating, and probably less inclined to cause rebound swelling in the nose. The oral decongestants, of course, work systemically and therefore have the advantage of reducing swelling within the sinus cavities, which a nasal spray usually cannot do. Unfortunately, decongestants by spray or pill will not relieve the sneezing, itching, or excessive watery nasal discharge of allergic rhinitis, and it may take an antihistamine spray or pill to accomplish this. It is important to realize that antihistamines don't cure allergies, but with regular usage, most people who suffer from allergic rhinitis will experience at least a 50 percent reduction in allergic symptoms, and some may be completely relieved. Since antihistamines do not reduce nasal swelling or sinus congestion, the additional use of a decongestant pill or spray may be necessary. It is mainly for this reason that decongestants, either by liquid or pill, are often found in combination with antihistamines in over-the-counter preparations.

Another advantage for combining the two is that decongestants are stimulants and will often counteract the sedating effect of some of the older first-generation antihistamines. This combination may be a little safer during the day if you are driving or if you are performing a hazardous job and require an antihistamine because of an allergy problem, provided of course that the stimulant and the sedative effects are of the same duration. This sedative-stimulant combination is also good if you want a good night's sleep and still need a decongestant to breathe freely or to keep your sinuses open and draining well.

Some pharmaceutical companies now promote daytime and nighttime cold and flu preparations, each containing a decongestant, but with the nighttime dose also containing a sedating antihistamine to counteract the stimulating and insomnia-causing effects of the decongestant. Decongestants are especially important during the night with colds, flu, or sinusitis, and this combination can be helpful if you are unable to tolerate a decongestant alone. However, some people will tolerate a decongestant alone at night and still sleep comfortably, so it is often worth a try, since most physicians agree that using only one medication is nearly always better than taking several medications to accomplish the same thing, especially when the continued use of a sedating antihistamine may prolong a sinus infection. A few individuals, especially children, may become drowsy when taking a normally stimulating decongestant at night and sleep well, however.

GUAIFENESIN

Guaifenesin, a mucus liquefier and expectorant used in more than a hundred different OTC flu, cough, and cold preparations, as well as for sinusitis patients with coughs, has so far revealed no serious side effects, and the chances for toxicity are very low. It is said to increase mucous output as well as mucous flow, usually resulting in a thinner mucus, more easily moved by the cilia sweep in the respiratory tract, and also more easily coughed up. So far there is no evidence that guaifenesin inhibits cilia activity, but also no proof that it can benefit sinusitis either. Although no serious reactions, complications, or drug interactions from taking guaifenesin have been noted so far, it should be pointed out that it was 15 years or more before doctors began to realize that prolonged use of antihistamines could make some sinusitis patients worse, and that was after using them rather extensively and sometimes for a very long period. As to the effectiveness of guaifenesin in people with sinusitis and bronchitis, only time will tell.

ACETAMINOPHEN

Acetaminophen, the active pain reliever in Tylenol, Anacin 3, Excedrin, Sominex 2, and Contac Flu and Cold preparations, as well as in some of the other over-the-counter cold and sinus medications, is not generally considered harmful or toxic in normal dosage if you have a healthy liver and healthy kidneys. There has been some speculation, however, that normal and even lower daily dosages of acetaminophen, when taken over many years, may possibly increase the risk of kidney failure. This is sometimes difficult to prove, however, especially in the elderly, because of the many other medications consumed by the older generation that might also prove toxic to their livers or kidneys over a very extended period. A study at Johns Hopkins and the University of Geneva did, however, strongly suggest that taking more than one acetaminophen pill a day for a lifetime accumulation of more than 1,000 pills could double the odds of a person developing kidney failure. This doesn't necessarily mean that taking only one pill a day over a very long period is entirely safe, since it would depend on the age and size of the individual as well as the size of the dose, whether it is the extra-strength kind, and whether there is any existing kidney or liver damage. It has also been estimated that acetaminophen may be responsible for at least 5,000 cases of kidney failure in the United States each year. This is not too surprising, since it is apparently a metabolite of phenacetin, which was the middle component of the famous APC capsule used widely as a pain and headache medication for many years until it was finally taken off of the market because of being toxic to the kidneys.

There have also been instances of liver failure in people taking high but still normal daily doses of acetaminophen for relatively short periods but who also admitted to a significant daily alcohol intake, and a warning to this effect now accompanies the medication. Since acetaminophen is included in so many over-the-counter preparations, and since it may be found singularly in almost everyone's medicine cabinet, if you have a bad episode of flu, cold, or sinusitis with significant pain, you could inadvertently take it both ways and thereby take too much. Also, when administering liquid medications, a parent may sometimes exceed the dosage recommendations for a very small child by using a tableware teaspoon because it is often larger than a measuring spoon or the spoon sometimes included with the medication. Infant Tylenol is provided in a concentrated liquid form that is three and a half times stronger than Children's Tylenol, and you should therefore carefully measure each dose to avoid possible liver damage. Two or three times the normal dose over a period of time could even destroy a child's liver.

Overdosage of acetaminophen or Tylenol may produce early symptoms of nausea, vomiting, profuse sweating, and extreme tiredness, but laboratory evidence of liver toxicity may not show up for two or three days. This fact could prove very unfortunate for those who would prefer to wait for the lab report on the status of the liver before beginning specific medical treatment for an overdose.

Children's livers may sometimes survive an overdose of acetaminophen with less permanent damage than adults. As to whether such damage will predispose them to future liver deficiency, possibly from further insult by alcohol or other liver toxic drugs, only time will tell.

With the tremendous increase in over-the-counter medications, with medicine cabinets becoming overloaded with out-of-date prescription drugs, and with patients seeing different doctors or trying different pharmacies, hopefully to save money, we all have to become more concerned about the potential toxicity of excessive dosage, incomplete records, out-of-date drugs, drug interactions, and long-term dosing. Although no accurate accounting can be given as to the overall damaging effects to the general population from the use of over-the-counter medications, it is thought to be rather extensive, since even drugs ordered by prescription for older people are considered to be responsible for at least 25 percent of hospital admissions. The computer has been a great help with this problem, but it would also be a very good thing for the head of the household to keep an up-to-date memo book on the medication history of each family member listing the medication, the date, for what it was prescribed, for how long, and then list any problems that may have occurred while taking it. Doing this could very possibly save a life.

Even with the aforementioned potentially serious side effects from acetaminophen, especially when taken in excess or with alcohol, or even by people who have existing liver or kidney damage, it would still appear to be one of the most popular pain relievers for head and face discomfort associated with sinusitis. According to Johnson and Johnson, acetaminophen is used for various reasons by more than 55 million Americans each year.

ASPIRIN

Aspirin, another very effective painkiller and fever reducer, has its drawbacks, too, with its tendency to produce severe gastric irritation and ulceration, GI bleeding, and aggravation of an esophagitis, as well as to cause problems for some asthmatics and for sinusitis patients with aspirin intolerance. Aspirin should also be avoided in children and teenagers who develop respiratory infections with fevers or rashes, such as noted with flu and chicken pox, because of the possibility of their developing Reye's syndrome. It is primarily for this reason that aspirin is usually omitted in the over-the-counter cold and flu preparations for children.

NONSTEROIDAL ANTI-INFLAMMATORY DRUGS (NSAIDs)

Even the newer aspirin-like drugs called NSAIDs and derived mostly from ibuprofen, flurbiprofen, indomethacin, piroxicam, oxaprozin, naproxen, and ketoprofen and more commonly known as Advil, Motrin, Daypro, Ansaid, Nuprin, Indocin, Feldene, Naprosyn, and Orudis, to name just a few, and all very similar to aspirin in their action, are not without their own hazards. Their abbreviated name, NSAID, stands for nonsteroidal anti-inflammatory drug, and they are used to treat a multiplicity of inflammatory conditions usually associated with pain, swelling, and fevers. Some are sold in OTC combinations with other medications for relief of colds, flu, and sinus symptoms. So far there has been no evidence that the NSAIDs, like aspirin, might predispose a child or adolescent to Reye's syndrome, even though it may still be too soon to tell. Reye's syndrome was first described in 1963 by Dr. R. D. K. Reye, an Australian pathologist. At that time, more than a third of the children who came down with the disease died. Three years later, the connection between aspirin and certain acute viral illnesses such as chicken pox and flu in causing Reye's syndrome was realized. Since then, an intensive public education program has reduced the incidence of the disease by more than 90 percent.

NSAIDs also have the same aspirin-like tendencies to cause GI ulceration and bleeding or a flare-up of esophagitis and heartburn even in normal dosage. Like aspirin, they should be avoided for 10 days to 2 weeks before surgery, since they can cause bleeding, and the same advice would apply to anyone taking blood-thinning or anticlotting medications. Bleeding from taking anticoagulants can usually be controlled by blood testing and regulating the anticoagulant dosage, but this may be more difficult if aspirin, NSAIDs, or even Tylenol is being taken as well. Also like aspirin, NSAIDs are generally not recommended for asthmatics, nor should they be given during the last 3 or 4 months of pregnancy. During early pregnancy, they should only be given on your doctor's advice. Nursing mothers should also avoid them. When NSAIDs are combined with alcohol intake, the tendency for GI bleeding and ulceration is accentuated. Insulin-dependent diabetics, when taking any of the NSAIDs, including aspirin, over a prolonged period, may sometimes require an adjustment in their insulin dosage. Kidney damage can occur with overdosage of NSAIDs, and a few people may have experienced kidney damage even with relatively low dosages, but again possibly influenced by other factors. A lifetime dose of more than 5,000 tablets is said to increase the odds of kidney failure to some degree, and of course taking these preparations with existing kidney damage could make total kidney failure all the more likely. Prescribing them for people who have congestive heart failure could also increase the chances of kidney failure.

So far, none of this has been found true for aspirin. NSAIDs may sometimes reduce the effectiveness of antihypertensive medications resulting in an elevated blood pressure, but again this has not been found true of aspirin. It should also be mentioned that one of the NSAIDs may give a positive drug screening test for Valium, so if you are undergoing such a test for an athletic event or applying for a job, you should report this even if you have taken only one pill within 3 or 4 days of testing, since it could prove embarrassing and may even damage your chances for employment. More recently, some people have noted skin rashes on exposure to sunlight while taking NSAIDs, but these rashes usually involve only the exposed areas, and discontinuing the medication usually corrects the problem.

Acetaminophen or Tylenol might offer another possible advantage over the NSAIDs for people with sinusitis, especially since it is not an anti-inflammatory medication. Inflammation is a complex effort by the body to control infection, and we don't really know if suppressing it with an anti-inflammatory drug could also depress the body's natural immune response or even inhibit the healing process. NSAIDs and aspirin, by reducing pain and especially inflammation, may block the formation of prostaglandins, a naturally occurring body chemical that plays a significant role in the body's response to infection. Histamine, on the other hand, is considered in its normal role to be a stimulator of prostaglandins, and this might be another reason to avoid antihistamines in sinus infectious when unrelated to significant allergy. Still another factor that might be considered in treating sinusitis with NSAIDs is that they may also inhibit the release of lysozyme or muramidase, an enzyme found in mucous secretions and considered to be destructive to the walls of certain bacteria.

Since NSAIDs, like aspirin, can be very irritating to the stomach as well as to the esophagus, it is extremely important when taking any of these pills to thoroughly wash them down the esophagus and into the stomach with a half or preferably a full glass of water. If allowed to dissolve in the esophagus, they can cause severe irritation resulting in esophagitis or heartburn, and even ulceration. You should be especially careful to swallow these pills completely when taking them at bedtime or during the night, and that advice applies to other pills as well. Saliva secretions are reduced during sleep and even more so in people age 65 and older. This plus the loss of muscle tone in the walls of the esophagus usually starting in the sixties will further diminish the effectiveness of the swallow reflex. During sleep, you also lose the gravitational effect on swallowing because of the lying down position; but more importantly, in deep sleep, you may lose a lot of the stimulus for further swallowing during the night, and a pill may therefore remain in the esophagus, to very slowly dissolve and to inflame the esophageal wall.

You should also remind yourself that aspirin is acetylsalicylic acid and that the esophagus doesn't tolerate acids well. Drinking sufficient water and thereby diluting the concentration of a medication will reduce its irritation of both the esophagus and the stomach lining. In addition, you should remember that anyone who says he or she is allergic to aspirin or has aspirin intolerance, and who then takes one of the NSAIDs preparations, could likewise develop a severe reaction. An impressive number of asthmatics are very hypersensitive to aspirin as well as to the NSAIDs, and many of them also have rhinosinusitis with nasal polyps. This combination of aspirin intolerance, asthma, and nasal polyps is often referred to as the aspirin triad, or Samter's syndrome, but very often the polyps may take a while to show up. Since polyps usually obstruct sinus drainage even when very small, however, sinusitis nearly always accompanies them. Anaphylactic shock, sometimes with fatal consequences, may occasionally occur as a result of taking aspirin or NSAIDs.

DEXTROMETHORPHAN

The fourth common ingredient frequently included in over-the-counter cold and flu medications, many times in combination with an antihistamine, is the cough suppressant dextromethorphan. This ingredient has the ability to raise the cough threshold in the brain and is about equal in effectiveness to another frequently prescribed cough suppressant, codeine, or its synthetic derivative hydrocodone, both of which are addictive, prone to cause abdominal cramps as well as constipation, and not recommended for asthmatics. Even though dextromethorphan is a synthetic morphine derivative, it is considered to have no depressant effect on the brain and no addiction liability. Occasionally, it may cause some release of H_1 histamine, which could present a problem, especially in children prone to allergic asthma or allergies in general.

Dextromethorphan has not been found to suppress cilia sweeping activity in the sinuses or respiratory tract, a problem frequently encountered with chronic tobacco smokers and cocaine snorters. People taking certain antidepressants called MAO inhibitors should avoid over-the-counter flu, cold, and cough preparations containing dextromethorphan, as well as those containing decongestants and antihistamines, since the combination may intensify and prolong the mucus-drying effects and add to central nervous system depression. Apparently as a result of a FDA ruling, dextromethorphan has now replaced Benadryl as a cough suppressant in most over-the-counter preparations for colds and flu.

OTHER CONSIDERATIONS WHEN TAKING ANTIHISTAMINES

LABELING

Now that physicians and most pharmaceutical companies have become aware that antihistamines are generally not helpful in treating nonallergic sinusitis and that the sedating kind in particular, if continued for more than a few days, may even tend to make sinus infections worse due to their drying effects on mucous secretions, most drug manufacturers have become more particular about the wording in their advertising and labeling. When an antihistamine is included in a preparation for upper respiratory tract infections, the label will more often use such general expressions as "relieving colds clear down to your sinuses," or "for the treatment of colds and allergies in association with sinusitis." This avoids saying that the antihistamine is effective for the treatment of sinusitis, which is certainly a step forward, since only a few years ago, drug companies—as well as some physicians—were frequently recommending antihistamines even for rather long periods for sinus infections and even when unrelated to any allergy problems.

DROWSINESS

Since most of the early-generation antihistamines have for most people the very unpleasant side effect of producing drowsiness and even causing some people to fall asleep, they have to be taken with considerable caution in any combination with alcohol or other sedating medications, especially if you drive automobiles, trucks, buses, trains, motorcycles, snowmobiles, golf carts, boats, land-moving and farm equipment; or if you pilot planes, sky jump, ski, use saws or drills, climb ladders, and work on buildings or bridges. Even children who bicycle, water ski, or roller blade should use antihistamines cautiously, especially when jet ski boating, where a slow reaction time might also endanger others. We truly have no way of knowing just how many accidents, falls, hip fractures, and other injuries or deaths can be attributed to the use of antihistamines, since many preparations containing them are now sold mostly over the counter in drugstores and can be purchased in convenience stores, gas stops, and food markets. With on-the-job accidents, it would be unlikely for the victim even to think of or blame antihistamines unless questioned specifically, thus making it even more difficult to determine how often they are at fault.

So far I have yet to hear anyone blame them for causing an automobile, boat, or plane accident, and yet it has been estimated that sleepy or drowsy automobile drivers may cause as many accidents as drunken drivers. In many states, it is against the law to drive under the influence of any drug or medication that impairs driving performance, and this may be one reason antihistamines are not blamed by defendants in court cases. Some accident investigators feel that 1 out of every 20 drivers in the United States has caused an accident by nodding off at the wheel, and that in some heavy-traffic areas more than one-third of all the fatal accidents may be attributed to not just lousy but drowsy drivers. The National Transportation Safety Board (NTSB) has estimated that driver fatigue may be a factor in 30 to 40 percent of all heavy truck accidents.

Complaints by people who have taken antihistamines and general observations of their muscular coordination and mental activity have suggested that a somewhat sluggish hangover effect the next day may occur in some individuals after ingesting one of the shorter-acting sedating antihistamines or a cold preparation containing them, even though their true effectiveness is generally considered to last only 4 to 6 hours. This seems to be even more likely with the elderly as well as in some individuals known to have low thyroid function. It should be emphasized that if you drive or engage in any other potentially hazardous activity while taking the conventional supposedly short-lasting sedating antihistamines alone or in combination with other medications, and even if you are not obviously drowsy (like some heavy drinkers who may not be obviously drunk), you may still have some impairment of coordination and mental alertness 12 to 24 hours after taking the last dose. Hopefully, computer-based skill testing will eventually be available and required of commercial drivers, perhaps at truck weighing stations. Such tests could even be made available as coin-operated machines for the concerned everyday automobile driver who after testing may decide that it is safer to pull over or to let someone else drive. Stricter adherence to the federal regulation limiting commercial drivers to 10 consecutive hours behind the wheel at a time should also be enforced, especially since the effects of sleep deprivation can be cumulative. We might consider the example set by the United Kingdom, where a driver who falls asleep and causes a fatal accident could be charged with vehicular homicide.

Since a significant number of people who take over-the-counter first-generation sedating antihistamines may show performance deficits, and because this may be further enhanced by the use of alcohol, tranquilizers, or addictive drugs, the resulting combined effects on that individual and even on anyone nearby could be extremely hazardous. A driver on the highway who is hopped up on drugs and also taking an antihistamine compound for a cold or flu becomes even more deadly, and the same might be said of some jet ski boat operators as well. If you are involved in a potentially hazardous job or sport, and if you study, lecture, operate, or do anything requiring very alert brain function or dexterity, and you must take antihistamines, you would be wise to take the newer non-sedating kinds, which are reputed not to cross the blood-brain barrier, and therefore very rarely produce any impressive drowsiness. However, when you take any antihistamine, whether it be sedating or non-sedating, you should never exceed the recommended dosage or take doses too close together.

OVERDOSAGE

Unfortunately, overdosage of all medications occurs all too frequently, especially with the over-the-counter preparations. With them, people are inclined to think that since the medication doesn't require a prescription, it must be rather harmless. Most people abhor reading the detailed instructions on the labels, especially in such fine print, and may therefore take medications too often or in combination with other incompatible medications. Finally, as with all medications, prescriptions or otherwise, some people feel that if a teaspoon or a tablet will help, two will help twice as much. With both the sedating and the non-sedating antihistamines, this kind of thinking could get you into serious trouble.

Overdosage may easily occur and without warning if you are already taking a prescription antihistamine on a fairly continuous basis for chronic rash, chronic itching, persistent hives, or hay fever and then you develop a flu, head cold, or cough requiring an over-the-counter preparation containing another antihistamine. One must be reminded that many antihistamines have a very strong sedative potential including those sold over the counter, and that a significant overdose could prove fatal. The short-acting ones in particular are absorbed rapidly into the body system, and therefore inducing vomiting or pumping the stomach for an overdose must be done quickly to be effective. Keeping a bottle of syrup of ipecac in the medicine cabinet to induce immediate vomiting as well as some activated charcoal in liquid suspension to absorb any excess medication in the GI tract could be lifesaving, but directions as to their use and contraindications must be followed closely. Here a quick call to an emergency room or a poison control center could be very helpful.

OTHER SIDE EFFECTS

Conventional antihistamines are usually recommended with caution in people who have an enlargement of the prostate, since these medications may also increase obstructive urinary problems, although decongestants seem to be greater offenders in this respect. Conventional antihistamines should not be used by people with a certain type of glaucoma or in conjunction with certain antidepressant medications. When taken with any skin photosensitizing medications such as certain antibiotics, antihistamines may occasionally intensify the symptoms of a bad sunburn. Their extensive prolonged use may also inhibit saliva flow, which may sometimes encourage gum and dental problems as well as fungal infections of the mouth or even salivary gland infections in the elderly. In elderly people, antihistamines are especially inclined to cause a drop in blood pressure, incoordination, blurred vision, dizziness, and drowsiness. These symptoms may of course become accentuated markedly if the older person is at the same time taking alcohol, narcotics, tranquilizers, or sleeping pills. Such combinations may cause injuries, accidents, or falls and may be responsible for some of the hip fractures occurring rather frequently in older people, especially when they get up at night. Substituting the newer non-sedating antihistamines for the older conventional type, particularly for the elderly, would seem worthwhile in most cases provided they are not taking a conflicting cardiac or fungal medication. Some older people, especially when taking the conventional sedating antihistamines, may become slightly delirious, falsely suggesting early senility or even Alzheimer's, and temporary personality changes even after one dose are not uncommon.

CHILDREN AND ANTIHISTAMINES

In infants and small children, although very rarely, the older conventional antihistamines may produce hallucinations, convulsions, and even death. For this reason, and also because it is difficult to regulate their safe dosage accurately in a child or to know exactly how the child's system will respond, antihistamines are infrequently recommended in children under age 12, and practically never in those under age 2, without professional consultation and very careful follow-up. For similar reasons, they should be avoided during pregnancy and by nursing mothers. Children ages 6 to 12, if required to take an antihistamine, should have the dosage regulated according to their size and tolerance, preferably on a physician's advice. Generally speaking, with regard to most medications, children from ages 6 to 12 are usually given half the adult dose with exceptions for certain medications and also for very small 6 year olds or for very large 11 and 12 year olds.

NON-SEDATING ANTIHISTAMINES

If the more recent non-sedating longer-acting antihistamines should continue to show very minimal drying effects on mucous secretions, then their prolonged usage for sinusitis or bronchitis patients with allergic problems could prove very worthwhile. They can also be very effective in relieving persistent sneezing, tearing, sniffling, and sometimes a runny nose, as well as ocular, nasal, and palatal itching, but not in reducing nasal or sinus swelling or congestion. As far as the lower respiratory tract is concerned, antihistamines can suppress allergic reactions, occasionally act as a bronchial dilator, and possibly afford some protection against exercise asthma, but they would not be expected to diminish bronchial hyperreactivity unless there is an allergic component. However, even then, their usage is not entirely without its complications, especially if the recommended dosage is exceeded or if there is impaired liver or kidney function. Serious consequences, including cardiac fatalities, have been reported when some of the long-acting non-sedating antihistamines were combined with certain heart medicines, antifungal drugs, or specific antibiotics, particularly those belonging to the macrolide group such as erythromycin and biaxin. However, antihistamines' once or twice a day dosage does allow for a more convenient and more closely regulated regimen with less chance of gaps or overlaps, provided that you take them on an empty stomach and at the same time each day, but never with grapefruit juice, since it can cause increased blood levels not only for certain antihistamines but in other medications as well. The non-sedating claims for some antihistamines are not totally accurate, since in rare instances they may cause some drowsiness. Although they work fairly rapidly, one reportedly as quickly as in 20 to 30 minutes, and others in 1 to 3 hours, they need not at this time replace the earlier, less expensive sedating antihistamines in many instances unless one of the aforementioned incompatibilities exists or unless, of course, there is a significant drowsiness problem with the conventional type. The effectiveness of the newer non-sedating antihistamines is about the same as some of the earlier conventional ones as far as reducing the symptoms of allergic rhinitis.

THE HISTAMINE REACTION

Histamine is a powerful substance normally released in small amounts mostly by mast cells within the body and in larger amounts often as a result of tissue injury or an allergic reaction. Once released, histamine may bind with certain receiving sites in the body known as H_1 and H_2 histamine receptors, which may in turn cause a body response specific for that particular receptor. An antihistamine does not prevent the release of histamine within the body but rather serves as an H_1 histamine receiving site antagonist, since it competes with histamine for these specific binding sites. Normal binding and stimulation of receptor sites by histamine is helpful and necessary for various body functions, but an excessive histamine release with overstimulation of receptors can produce unpleasant as well as unhealthy body changes. Such is the case with the excessive membrane swelling in the nose and sinuses, which may be initiated by an allergic reaction with histamine release that can lead to sinus blockage followed by infection. Histamine, as the good guy, is a vigorous stimulator of stomach acid, a producer of body mucus, a constrictor of bronchial wall muscles, a factor in intestinal, gallbladder, and uterine contractions, an enhancer of pancreatic and salivary secretions, a promoter of tissue swelling and healing, a partner in nerve transmissions within the brain, an accelerator of heart rhythm, a factor in cellular growth, as well as a dilator of small arteries and capillaries, and is therefore capable of affecting in some way every organ in the body.

Excessive histamine release and binding with H_1 receptors to initiate an allergic response, if unopposed by an antihistamine, or certain other medications such as epinephrine or one of the corticosteroids, can produce certain very unpleasant allergic manifestations such as hives with itching of the skin, headache, rashes, nasal congestion and sinus blockage, lung congestion, shortness of breath, itching of the nose, throat, palate, and ears, sneezing, red and watery eyes, swollen lips, face, and eyelids, swollen tongue and larynx, obstructive breathing, hoarseness, excess mucous secretions, runny nose, and asthmatic bronchial spasm with wheezing. This swelling of the lips, face, eyes, tongue, and larynx, often noted in serious allergic reactions, is called angioedema. It represents a noninflammatory localized buildup and retention of tissue fluid beneath the surface, whereas hives are an even more localized small rounded swelling on the surface, and both may occur together in an allergic reaction. Histamine may also bind with H_2 receptors in the gastrointestinal tract, and excessive amounts may cause abdominal cramps, vomiting, and diarrhea. Severe allergic reactions with excessive histamine release can lead to a fall in blood pressure, swelling of the brain, hallucinations, disorientation, respiratory failure, cardiac arrhythmias, circulatory collapse, shock, and cardiac arrest. Some individuals experiencing a severe reaction may even describe an overwhelming feeling of impending doom. This arrangement obviously gives the body its own built-in means for self-destruction.

You have most likely either known or heard of someone who died or nearly died from a bee sting, from a shot of penicillin, from an injection of a dye for an X-ray study, from taking a pill, from diving into ice-cold water, or from eating something to which the person may have suspected he or she may be allergic, such as seafood or even a small piece of nut that the server didn't realize was in the salad. Unfortunately, some commercial salad dressings may have invisible nut particles or compressed nut oils, and a busy server may not have had time to read the label. If the misinformed diner doesn't die instantly from cardiac arrest, then his or her face may suddenly become flushed, followed quickly by generalized body itching and hives. The lips, face, and eyelids may swell, and the nose may become congested. He or she may also notice swelling of the tongue and larynx with progressive hoarseness, difficulty breathing, and wheezing from bronchial constriction.

Under such circumstances, the sudden onset of hoarseness or wheezing would usually be considered a major warning sign of a possible airway collapse. Nausea, vomiting, and abdominal cramps may develop as well. The blood pressure may drop precipitously, and the heart may race to pump more blood to an oxygen-starved brain. A fairly intense headache may accompany this, but it, like most of the other symptoms, may be completely overshadowed by the breathing problems. The individual may begin to feel faint and have to sit down or lie down to keep from passing out.

ANAPHYLAXIS

The result may be a very sudden life-threatening and very frightening series of occurrences caused by a massive histamine release and called anaphylaxis, or in its most severe form, anaphylactic shock. The name is derived from two Greek words meaning "away from protection" and denotes an unprotected hypersensitivity reaction within the body. A more graphic description would be a veritable star wars brought on by an allergic reaction of considerable magnitude with a systemwide histamine release from mast cells and basophils, and with showering of very potent histamine particles everywhere. The H_1 and H_2 histamine receptors may be overwhelmed, and their target sites, especially in the crucial cardiopulmonary systems, may be markedly activated. The shock organs and systems more commonly involved in anaphylaxis or anaphylactic shock are those that are the richest in mast cells, the major producers of histamine. Basophils, which are members of the circulating white blood cell family, also secrete histamine. They are not attached to tissues like the mast cells but travel throughout the body in the circulating blood and are more often involved in the delayed part of an allergic reaction.

Anaphylaxis or anaphylactic shock may also occur unrelated to a typical allergen-antibody reaction and not always as a response to histamine release. Drugs derived from opium such as morphine, codeine, and heroin may bypass the allergen-antibody stimulus and act directly on mast cells or basophils to release massive doses of histamine. Aspirin and the other NSAIDs including ibuprofen, indomethacin, and naproxen may take a different route with other mediators than histamine but are capable of the same end result. The shower of histamine particles provoked by diving into cold water, called cold allergy by some but often classified under the physical allergies, can also cause anaphylactic shock with fatal results.

In such instances, the patient should be rushed to a hospital emergency room, where a potentially lifesaving shot of epinephrine (adrenaline) will probably be administered. In the worst-case scenario, the doctor will perform a tracheotomy or insert an airway intubation tube. The latter may sometimes be difficult to accomplish if the larynx is markedly swollen. Obviously, you should never attempt a tracheotomy at home except under the very gravest of circumstances. A penknife thyrotomy, or stab incision, made in the palpable indentation just beneath the skin in the midline of the neck and a finger's breadth below the Adam's apple may be more successful but still should be done only as a last resort.

If the anaphylactic reaction is extreme, then histamine-blocking medications sometimes including both H_1 and H_2 histamine antagonists will very likely be given intravenously in the emergency room following the epinephrine shot, since the H_1 and H_2 receptor antagonists cannot cover for each other and both may be involved with anaphylaxis. Intravenous Benadryl and intravenous Tagament or Zantac are now considered very good choices, which may come as a surprise, since the antihistamine Benadryl has been around for more than half a century. Intravenous or intramuscular cortisone preparations, which may take 3 or 4 hours to become completely effective, are helpful in prolonged or delayed reactions but will not act fast enough in an emergency situation, especially when you may have only 10 to 30 minutes and sometimes much less. Antihistamine or cortisone preparations by mouth are likewise far too slow in treating or preventing pending anaphylaxis, and to delay going to the emergency room in order to see if they work could be a very grave mistake. However, taking them in adequate dosage after the ER visit might prevent or modify a delayed reaction, which usually occurs within 4 to 6 hours and can also be quite serious.

If the patient survives this crisis, the important thing then is to accurately identify the cause of the reaction whenever possible so that it doesn't happen again. If it can't be avoided, such as with bee stings, you should make certain that emergency treatment is always available. That means keeping a bee or wasp sting automatic syringe kit containing epinephrine in the car, another in the house, or one on your person if you are inclined to take long walks in the woods or fields during bee season. This shot medication should be kept in a closed kit or in the dark, since epinephrine deteriorates much faster on prolonged exposure to light. You should always avoid walking in the grass barefoot if you are allergic to bee stings. Wearing shorts, bright-flowered clothes, or a sweet-smelling scent that might be alluring to bees is also unwise. If the ER is a long distance away, the use of a tourniquet above the sting may temporarily reduce venom absorption into the circulating blood, but the tourniquet would have to be released momentarily and periodically. It is never a substitute for early or immediate treatment, however. Desensitization shots are worth considering if you are highly sensitized to the protein in bee venom.

Even some of the drops used in the treatment of glaucoma can, in rare instances, precipitate an attack of anaphylaxis, and this possibility should be considered if no other obvious cause is found. A slow pulse will nearly always rule out anaphylaxis or anaphylactic shock, and in such cases, another diagnosis and another treatment will usually have to be considered. However, this may not be true in someone wearing a fixed-rate pacemaker.

Most of the cases of anaphylaxis or anaphylactic shock can be traced to some medication the patient received or to a food he or she ingested, and many of the victims are atopic, which means they have a genetically related family history of allergies. The NSAIDs and certain shellfish seem to be the most common drug and food instigators of anaphylaxis. Wearing a medic alert bracelet identifying the problem will make the diagnosis much easier and can be lifesaving, especially if there is a syringe of epinephrine such as EpiPen or EpiPen Jr. nearby.

The visible skin evidence of histamine activity is in plain view much of the time. You can see it in hives and red rashes brought on by drugs, foods, chemical contacts, infections, insect bites, injuries, sunburn, mental and physical factors, stings, inhalants, or just plain scratching;

as well as its assertiveness in the initial redness of scars, in the disfigurements of keloids, and even in the fascinating designs of dermatography, or skin writing.

These are just some of the symptoms and signs that may result from the release of histamine, mainly by the mast cells that are located throughout the body, and especially in the connective tissues that bind together the supporting framework for most of our body structures.

CHAPTER ELEVEN

When Do You Operate for Sinusitis?

WHEN TO OPERATE is sometimes a difficult decision even for the sinus surgeon, and needless to say, it will likely pose a dilemma for you, since you must give your permission, many times after hearing a somewhat confusing explanation of the surgery in medical terms as well as a long list of things that could go wrong. This is what is called "informed consent." This chapter presents a comprehensive list of conditions that usually indicate a need for nasal or sinus surgery, followed by a discussion of the many factors both you and your doctor will need to consider in making this important decision. Later in the chapter, I have provided a brief description of some of today's surgical methods and approaches, as well as a section on possible complications that might occur from surgery.

INDICATORS FOR SURGERY

Nasal or sinus surgery, and sometimes both, would be generally indicated in most of the following instances:

1. Where there is a subacute or chronic sinus infection that exhibits persistent or repeated obstruction to sinus drainage and to sinonasal air exchange and that fails to respond to prolonged medical therapy, namely, extended courses of more than one antibiotic, environmental controls, and allergy treatment when indicated.

2. Where a sinus is completely obstructed; contains entrapped pus as noted on X ray, usually with an air-fluid level; is causing considerable

discomfort; and refuses to drain on its own and obviously needs to be drained. More definitive surgery on the nose or sinus might be recommended following such an episode, and very definitely after a second occurrence involving the same sinus.

3. Where there is a single polyp, multiple polyps, or an enlarged misshapen turbinate that obstructs sinonasal drainage or air exchange and that will not clear up with medical treatment.

4. Where there is a mucocele, benign tumor, or drainage-obstructing cyst, since most of them will usually continue to enlarge, not only causing further sinus obstruction but also possibly destroying surrounding bone and impinging on certain vital structures such as the orbit, optic nerve, certain vascular structures, and the brain. Visual loss from optic nerve compression by an expanding mucocele should be surgically relieved within 24 hours for best results.

5. Whenever there is the possibility of a malignancy in the nose or sinuses or even a mass that might become malignant.

6. In most instances of repeated acute sinus flare-ups requiring extended antibiotic treatment each time and occurring more than three or four times a year, especially in an adult and not just with viral respiratory infections and not just as a recurrence of the same sinus infection that may have been inadequately treated.

7. When a sinus infection involves the bony sinus walls as in osteomyelitis or has extended beyond their bony confines to involve certain vital structures such as the orbits or the brain.

8. Where a persistent sinus infection might be causing recurrent infectious flare-ups in distant organs or body structures including heart valves, the urinary tract, the prostate, and so forth and does not clear up completely with medical treatment.

9. Where a sinus infection is contributing to an asthmatic condition or an infection in the lower respiratory tract or lungs and either or both fail to clear up and remain clear with medical treatment, often indicating that better sinus drainage is needed.

10. Where there is a very serious or life-threatening disease such as meningitis, septicemia, brain abscess, orbital abscess, orbital cellulitis, or cavernous sinus thrombosis suspected of arising from a sinus infection or sinus fracture.

11. Where there is a fistula or persistent opening from the mouth into a maxillary sinus, usually the result of an upper tooth extraction, permitting food or liquids to continuously contaminate and infect the sinus.

12. Where there is intractable sinus disease, especially in an immuno-suppressed individual who may be compromised by an opportunistic disease such as a fungal sinusitis and who therefore needs better sinus aeration and drainage.

13. Where there is a badly displaced sinus fracture needing realignment, or where retained bone fragments from the fracture might act as a foreign body within the sinus and need to be removed.

14. When there is any other retained foreign material in a sinus cavity such as a bullet, shrapnel, shot, tooth or tooth root, dental filling, fungus ball, broken scissors points, knife tips, glass, rocks, and wood splinters (all of which I have at one time been called on to remove).

15. Where there is a dental cyst invading a maxillary sinus and has to be removed along with its tooth of origin.

16. And, finally, where there is a nasal airway deformity or obstruction that might be contributing to a persistent sinus or lung problem, sleep apnea, snoring, insomnia, headaches, improper airway function, chronic hoarseness, or eustachian tube blockage with diminished hearing or a loss of sense of smell and taste.

FACTORS TO CONSIDER

In most cases of sinus infection, unless it is an emergency or semi-emergency situation, surgery should be postponed until you have tried conservative treatment with antibiotics, decongestants, and sometimes various allergy treatments and have corrected any living or working conditions that might be causing or aggravating your sinus problem. Making such an important decision may also include several return visits to your physician's office, since after seeing you a second or third time and observing your response to various medications, the sinus surgeon will often come up with a different idea as to the major source of the problem, which sinus or group of sinuses is primarily responsible, and, if surgery is still indicated, what kind would be more beneficial. A CAT scan and sometimes an MRI may be very helpful in deciding what should be done. Sometimes surgically improving the drainage and air exchange for one sinus or group of sinuses may, with the help of antibiotics, permanently relieve an infection in other nearby sinuses, especially in those that occupy the same side of the nose and have adjoining drainage openings, thus avoiding what at first seemed to require surgical correction of both sets of sinuses. Whenever possible, surgery on the sinuses should be kept to the very minimum necessary to restore function and achieve a cure. This is even truer in a child, whose sinonasal structures are still very small; doctors cannot totally predict what effect surgery or postoperative scarring will have on the development of these structures, as well as their ability to handle infection later on. Of course, at times, functional endoscopic sinus surgery (FESS) will still be necessary in a child when environmental controls, allergy evaluation, and prolonged medical treatments fail.

If a child has a persistent sinusitis somewhat resistant to treatment, and especially if it keeps recurring after extensive and more than adequate medical treatment, and if there are no contributing sinonasal blockage problems such as polyps, nasal structural abnormalities, a foreign body in the nose, or allergic rhinitis, your doctor should investigate the possibility of chronically infected adenoids serving as a source of infection to the back of the nose and subsequently to the sinuses. Chronically diseased adenoids can harbor infection indefinitely, and although sinusitis is seldom cited as an indication for an adenoidectomy, in some cases, their removal can make a significant difference in the health of a child's upper respiratory tract as well as the sinuses. The sometimes overlooked triad of chronic sinusitis, chronically infected adenoids, and recurrent ear problems in the child, often influencing each other, is important to keep in mind and will usually require treatment of all three.

Although the sinus surgeon may speak in strong terms of doing only as much surgery as necessary to restore sinus function, even with extensive surgery, it may not always be possible for him or her to eradicate all of the disease; and the extent of the scarring following sinus surgery can be very unpredictable, sometimes itself being responsible for limited surgical success and for the persistence of a sinus problem. In some instances, the best approach for minimizing the extent of the sinus surgery as well as the amount of postoperative scarring is to do it in a steplike fashion by surgically correcting some of the more obvious minor problems first. Frequently, something relatively simple such as puncturing and thoroughly irrigating a maxillary sinus, enlarging a sinus drainage opening, or removing a small obstructive polyps, along with prolonged antibiotic therapy or allergy treatments when indicated, may be all that is necessary in the way of surgery.

If your sinus problems are primarily on only one side and you have an obstructive nasal deformity on that side, correcting a bad septal deviation, reducing the size of an enlarged or deformed turbinate, trimming away excessive erectile tissue in the front of the nose, correcting a collapsed nasal valve, or excising scar tissue or nasal adhesions can be done without directly invading the sinus structures themselves and could make a difference. In other words, the surgeon might decide to correct some of these contributing factors and withhold any significant surgery on the sinuses until he or she can evaluate the results of the lesser surgery. A CAT scan before surgery, followed by another limited one after you have been thoroughly treated and allowing at least 6 weeks for sinus membrane swelling to subside, will help the surgeon to identify a persistent sinus problem and to evaluate the success of the surgery.

Deviations of the nasal septum are commonly found in almost two-thirds of older adolescents and adults, but only a very small percentage of deviated septums may cause significant nasal or sinus problems or need surgical correction. The nasal septum is a vertical, thin-walled partition about an eighth of an inch thick, composed mainly of cartilage in front with bone behind, enclosed in a tough fibrous envelope and dividing the nose into two separate nasal passages. Septal deviations are found more frequently in males than in females, probably due to their suspected injury origin. Except for a slight invagination of nostril skin in front and a strip of membrane along the top of the septum on each side containing some of the organs of smell, the nasal septum is mostly covered by a ciliated mucus-secreting membrane like the rest of the nose and the sinuses. It is sometimes thickened to twice its normal size, occasionally S-shaped, but more often curved to one side. Instead of a smooth curve, the septum can have sharp angulations, projections, and spurs, often due to old injuries. Although rotation of the head in the birth canal has been blamed by some, the two most likely reasons for a septal deviation appear to be injury and growth, with abnormal growth following a nasal injury in childhood being the most likely cause. Even though an early injury might stimulate the septum to grow abnormally, it rarely causes any obvious problems until after puberty. Since the nasal septum doesn't usually reach full growth until age 16 in girls and 17 in boys, it is usually not operated on before then, since the trauma of surgery could interfere with normal bone and cartilage development. However—as nearly always in medicine—there are exceptions to the rule.

The various reasons for surgical correction of a deviated nasal septum, other than to lessen sinus problems, are to improve nasal breathing, to restore upper-airway function, to improve sleep apnea, to relieve headaches due to septal pressure, to correct the flow of a misdirected nasal airstream along with its many irritating pollutants, to improve your sense of smell, sometimes to protect a eustachian tube opening from a deflected airstream, and occasionally to provide a better functioning total airway if you have chronic lung problems. A septal operation may also be performed as part of a nasal or sinus operation to provide more working room and better visibility for the surgeon, especially in excising tumors of the nose, sinuses, and pituitary gland. Septal operations are also frequently included with cosmetic surgery on the nose to facilitate realignment of nasal structures.

If a maxillary sinus has a recurrent or persistent infection that fails to respond to treatment, a simple enlargement of the natural drainage opening by endoscopic sinus surgery for better aeration of the sinus as well as for better drainage can often make a big difference in clearing up a persistent infection and preventing future flare-ups. This surgical procedure has mostly replaced the long-used window operation, which was very useful in improving the sinonasal air exchange for a maxillary sinus but was not so effective in restoring functional drainage, since any cilia sweep along the sinus walls would still continue in the direction of the natural sinus opening. In superimposed fungal infections of a maxillary sinus, where good air exchange and repeated irrigations are so very important, a window procedure, in addition to enlarging an obstructed natural drainage opening, can sometimes prove very helpful.

The procedure may also be worthwhile for removing sinus packing after the reduction and fixation of a maxillary sinus fracture or as a safety valve after closing a fistula or opening into the maxillary sinus from the mouth. An additional window that remains open, however, may sometimes create a recirculation of mucous flow between the two openings, causing stagnation of mucus within the sinus cavity and the persistence of a sinus infection. This problem can usually be very easily corrected by combining the two adjacent maxillary sinus windows into one. Too large a window, however, may sometimes impair arterial circulation within the maxillary sinus and even damage the tear duct on that side. In very stubborn cases of maxillary sinusitis, a dental consultation and dental X rays may be worthwhile in revealing a chronically infected upper tooth or an embedded, broken-off upper tooth root from a previous extraction or injury, either of which may be acting as a source of infection to the maxillary sinus and may therefore require dental surgery to permanently cure the sinusitis. Upper teeth that have previously undergone root canal surgery for infection, and that lie directly below an infected maxillary sinus that has failed to clear up with more than adequate treatment, should be investigated as a possible source of continuous infection to that sinus. If found guilty, the tooth may have to be extracted in addition to any proposed sinus surgery in order to permanently clear up the maxillary sinusitis.

If these rather simple procedures plus fairly intense and prolonged medical treatment are unsuccessful, then the more complicated surgery involving the sinuses themselves may be warranted. In some instances, however, the more extensive and complicated sinus surgery may have to be carried out initially, especially for extensive chronic disease as well as in individuals with associated bone infection, tumors, or other complications. Even for these people, getting the sinus infection under control, correcting any environmental factors, and suppressing any nasal allergy before surgery are all very important.

Certain sinus infectious problems may occur as more of an emergency, and surgical delay could be costly, although a doctor will consider each case individually and on its own merit. A case of meningitis or brain abscess thought to be arising from a sinus infection or from a fracture of a sinus wall may require, in addition to intensive medical therapy, early surgical drainage of the sinus and usually more definitive sinus surgery later to avoid a recurrence of the problem. A similar surgical emergency could arise where a sinus infection has invaded the orbit or eye and might permanently damage vision. A fracture of a sinus wall with a large blood clot filling the sinus cavity, especially in the case of the frontal sinuses, might in rare instances require surgical drainage, especially if it becomes infected and is incapable of draining itself. Also following a maxillary or frontal sinus fracture, the bony walls may have to be realigned, and any loose bone fragments may have to be removed lest they act as a foreign body and cause a persistent infection. A fracture through the back, or posterior, wall of a frontal sinus can lead to intracranial infections such as meningitis and brain abscesses or even a mucocele many years later if surgery to correct the problem is disregarded. A fracture through a frontal sinus drainage duct may permanently seal off that sinus cavity and require surgery for an alternate drainage opening into the nose.

Occasionally a frontal ethmoid sinus arising from the anterior ethmoid group may develop within the uppermost regions of the nose, sometimes within the partition between the two frontal sinuses, or along the inner orbital rim, just above the eye; and either through growth enlargement or by becoming infected, it may interfere with the drainage of the frontal sinus duct, causing a persistent frontal sinusitis. Most of the time, these misplaced and diseased frontal ethmoid sinuses can be surgically uncovered or drained through the nose and the drainage of the frontal sinus itself likewise restored. In some cases, however, the infected frontal ethmoid sinus may extend too far forward or outward over the roof of the orbit to be reached through the nose and may have to be approached externally through the brow. Fortunately, a CAT scan can usually identify this problem for the surgeon ahead of time.

Sinus air-fluid levels, where pus and air are trapped in a completely blocked sinus cavity producing the characteristic air-over-fluid appearance on X ray, often require early surgical drainage to minimize scarring, especially to a sinus drainage opening, and thereby reduce the chances of future sinus trouble. Again, however, the decision to do this, and how soon, would have to be considered on an individual-case basis. One episode of acute frontal sinusitis with an air-fluid level on X ray is usually sufficient reason to surgically correct any nasal problem that might be contributing to the frontal sinus blockage such as a significantly deviated nasal septum, an enlarged or malformed middle turbinate, or an obstructive polyp. In such cases, attention should also be directed to correcting any ethmoid or maxillary sinus problems on the same side as the diseased frontal sinus, since all three drain into the middle meatus in very close proximity to each other and an infection of one may cause infection, swelling, and blockage of the other. Following an attack of frontal sinusitis, especially when there has been complete sinus blockage with an air-fluid level shown on X ray, if nothing is done to correct the problem more permanently, then this rather serious frontal sinus infection will very likely recur, and it may do so in some instances even after any contributing factors in the nose or nearby sinuses have been corrected.

If you have valvular heart disease or a history of bacterial endocarditis and an infected discharge is trapped within a blocked sinus cavity, early surgical drainage or needle irrigation of the cavity accompanied by intensive antibiotic therapy would be important, since bacteria may sometimes enter the bloodstream from an obstructed infected sinus and subsequently infect an already damaged heart valve. Suction or aspiration of infected discharge from a nose, which some patients seem to interpret as draining the sinuses, is rarely a substitute for surgical drainage or needle puncture and irrigation of an obstructed sinus cavity containing pus.

When a solid mass other than a polyp is found in a sinus on X ray and confirmed on a CAT scan, even if it is not yet causing obstruction to drainage, bleeding, persistent infection, or bone destruction, surgical investigation should be very strongly considered early, since the mass could be a malignant tumor. A history of recurrent bloody discharge from that side of the nose would make such a procedure even more urgent, and any sign of adjacent bone erosion on CAT scan would make it mandatory. If on further studies the mass is determined to be a polyp or cyst and is asymptomatic, in many cases, the initial examination can be followed with another X ray in a few months to see if it is enlarging. If it is found to be enlarging with the prospect of blocking sinus drainage or is producing symptoms, then it should be surgically removed. Some polyps, especially in a maxillary sinus, may occasionally cease to enlarge and remain entirely asymptomatic. Cysts, especially those noted in a maxillary sinus, may also stop growing altogether and remain asymptomatic, and a few of them may spontaneously rupture and disappear, though you should never depend on that.

When a cyst is noted to be arising from the floor of a maxillary sinus just over the root of an upper tooth, especially if the cyst appears on CAT scan to be fairly thick-walled, a dental consultation and dental X rays may be necessary to determine if the cyst is of dental origin, arising from the base of an upper tooth, and breaking through into the sinus. In such cases, the sinus will have to be opened up, the cyst removed, and the responsible upper tooth extracted at the same time. If only the dental cyst is removed and the tooth is left in, then the cyst will nearly always recur, and so will the sinusitis. At the same time, an enlargement of the natural opening to the maxillary sinus or at least a window procedure may be necessary for better drainage and aeration, especially during the healing period.

Cysts or polyps developing in a frontal sinus may have to be removed early, especially if they are located near the sinus drainage duct to the nose, since here, even when very small, they may cause marked obstruction to the mucous flow as well as to sinus air exchange with the nose. A benign bony growth, called an osteoma, may occasionally develop, especially in a frontal sinus, and if the growth obstructs drainage, it will likewise have to be removed. Mucoceles, which are usually fairly thick-walled cysts arising from mucous membrane-lined cavities such as a sinus, can sometimes be very difficult to deal with. They are more commonly found in the anterior ethmoid and frontal sinuses. They frequently continue to enlarge and erode surrounding bone and can invade the brain or orbit and cause double vision and sinus obstruction. They will either have to be excised or opened up and incorporated in the drainage flow of the adjoining sinus or sinuses. If nothing is done, due to their obstructive and destructive nature, mucoceles will gradually become more symptomatic, possibly permanently damaging vision and nearly always causing a persistent or chronic sinusitis. They should be treated early and whenever possible before there is significant damage to surrounding structures and before irreversible chronic sinus infection develops.

FUNCTIONAL ENDOSCOPIC SINUS SURGERY (FESS)

In recent years, endoscopic sinus surgery (ESS) using improved magnification through very small telescopes, brighter lighting, and delicate specialized instruments, has in experienced hands been very successful in removing diseased sinus tissue, improving drainage, and restoring adequate sinus function. This is especially true if you have subacute or chronically diseased sinuses, and provided you also have a good immune response, healthy mucous secretions, and adequate cilia motility. The so-called functional endoscopic sinus surgery (FESS) has provided an important addition to the successful treatment of sinus disease. The more recent introduction of three-dimensional image guidance tracking systems allowing the endoscopic sinus surgeon constantly to visualize on a screen the boundaries of the surgical field as well as the nearly exact location of the operative instruments has also made endoscopic sinus surgery easier, faster, more effective, and much safer. In most cases, by using such techniques, the surgeon may reach all four groups of sinuses on each side of the nose by operating through the nose, open up their cavities, remove diseased tissue, and in most instances restore adequate drainage. Occasionally, to correct the problem completely, it may be necessary, particularly with regard to the frontal sinuses and a few far distant ethmoid sinuses behind, above, or below the eye, for the surgeon to also enter through the brow or sometimes externally beside the nose. An external approach to the maxillary sinus from under the upper lip may some-times be required as part of a combined procedure through the nose, especially when there is extensive maxillary sinus disease or a need to remove a tumor, infected bone, a mucocele, a dental cyst, a foreign body, or bone fragments; or to reduce a fracture, tie off an artery in back of the sinus cavity for excessive nasal bleeding, and sometimes just for a better telescopic visualization of the entire sinus.

The external brow approach to the frontal sinus may still be neces-sary at times for emergency drainage of a totally obstructed and infected sinus cavity. It may also be required if there is evidence of a large polyp, cyst, bony growth, or tumor within the sinus cavity that can't be removed through the nose, or if there is an unreachable infected frontal ethmoid sinus cavity above the eye, or if there is a sinus fracture with depressed or retained bone fragments requiring treat-ment. Bilateral brow incisions or a forehead incision within the hair-line may occasionally be required to completely obliterate one or both frontal sinuses because of chronic bone infection known as osteomyelitis, as well as for the excision of certain tumors, or because of repeated failure to otherwise restore frontal sinus drainage through the nose. If the bone is not infected, then fat grafts or implants may be immediately used to obliterate a frontal sinus cavity and still retain the bony contour of the brow. If the bone is diseased, it will have to be excised, and corrective cosmetic surgery may have to be postponed until the surgeon can be certain that all infection has cleared and the surrounding bone is healthy. For some of the more distantly located and diseased ethmoid sinuses behind the eye, which may not be totally accessible through the nose, occasionally opening up the more proxi-mal ethmoid sinuses through the nose may afford adequate drainage for the more distant ones and hopefully effect a cure. However, the procedure could in some instances invite mucocele formation later.

In performing endoscopic sinus surgery, the surgeon often works in a very confined area, particularly so in a child, sometimes with visi-bility partially obscured by membrane swelling or excessive bleeding, and often in very close proximity to some rather vital structures such as the eye, the optic nerve, the pituitary gland, the anterior and poste-rior ethmoidal branches of the ophthalmic artery, the internal carotid artery to the brain, and sometimes even the brain itself. Therefore great care and a very conservative approach is necessary to avoid a cerebrospinal fluid leak into the nose, meningitis, brain damage or abscess formation, pituitary injury, uncontrollable bleeding (especially behind the eye), or permanent damage to the optic nerve, eye muscles, and vision. This is especially true because these very important or rather vital structures are not always situated in their predicted locations with regard to the sinus cavities and may sometimes be separated from a sinus cavity not by bone as the surgeon would expect but sometimes only by a very thin layer of soft tissue. Because of this, it is of the utmost importance that the surgeon obtain a CAT scan, and in some instances an MRI, before significant sinus surgery. Such complications, although fairly rare with endoscopic sinus surgery, still have to be considered by you and your doctor in deciding when to operate, how far to go into these somewhat dangerous areas, and whether the anticipated but sometimes uncertain results will justify the risks. Fortunately, the great majority of people who have sinusitis, and even a large number of those who have chronic disease, may not require surgery to get well and stay well.

COMPLICATIONS FROM NASAL OR SINUS SURGERY

The complications you might expect from sinus surgery are mostly minor, but a few can be serious, debilitating, and even fatal. Of course, any surgical complications mentioned here are in addition to those that could result from a local or general anesthetic, from any transfusion or drug reactions, or from body system failure such as a heart attack, renal shutdown, respiratory failure, and shock, or from hyperthermia, a life-threatening elevation in body temperature experienced by 1 in 20,000 patients undergoing a general anesthesia.

SWELLING AND INFECTION

The most common early complications of sinus surgery are infection, bleeding, and swelling. Swelling of surgically traumatized tissues is always expected to some degree, but here it can sometimes be excessive and externally involve the face, lips, cheek, nose, and orbital tissues. More often, however, it is internal, involving the nasal passages, turbinates, sinus membranes, and their surrounding tissues.

The presence of some infection in the operative field following sinus surgery is also to be expected, since many people undergoing surgery already have a chronic infection and the raw areas created by the surgery are completely exposed to all kinds of bacteria, including those normally present within the nose or inhaled with almost every breath. Any packing or stents temporarily used for support or to prevent adhesions or to control bleeding will act as foreign bodies and encourage more infection. Antibiotics are often prescribed postoperatively to control infection during the healing period and to prevent localized infection from spreading to the orbits, cavernous venous sinuses, and the central nervous system and brain, which fortunately is a rare occurrence.

BLEEDING

Bleeding from the operative field is usually minimal but can be excessive and on rare occasions may even require blood transfusions as well as arterial ligation. It is usually fairly easily controlled by packing. The most common of the potentially serious complications you might encounter is bleeding into the orbit. This is even more serious when it occurs behind the eye. It may result from injury to the anterior or posterior ethmoid arteries or from inadvertently breaking through the thin bony plate separating the orbit from the sinuses. As previously mentioned, this bony plate may be partially missing, and this increases the chances of an orbital intrusion. If it should happen, there is usually urgent need for early recognition and treatment to avoid permanent loss of vision. The surgeon will carefully observe your eyes during surgery, especially for any signs of bleeding beneath the orbital skin, since this may be the first clue.

SEPTAL ABSCESS AND HEMATOMA

A few postoperative patients may develop black eyes from minimal extravasation of blood under the skin similar to a bruise, and a rare case may experience bubbles of air also beneath the orbital skin, known as subcutaneous emphysema, which is usually absorbed rather quickly. Persistent pain, headache, or sometimes an area of localized numbness may develop in your forehead or cheek following sinus surgery but are usually temporary. In rare instances after nasal septal surgery, you may develop an abscess within the nasal septum or a large hematoma or blood clot next to nasal cartilage or around a cartilaginous implant, sometimes resulting in deformity or melting of the cartilage. When a clot begins to dissolve, its contents or breakdown products can be very irritating to cartilage and therefore may have to be evacuated before damage can occur. Bone grafts, as well as cartilaginous implants in the nose or sinuses, are likewise very vulnerable to infection, which could jeopardize their survival.

SEPTAL PERFORATIONS

On rare occasions following septal surgery, a perforation or hole in a nasal septum may occur especially if there is a superimposed infection.

Small holes in the back part of the septum usually present no problem, although a few may cause a whistling noise with deep breathing. However, those in the front of the septum, especially if they are large, may cause problems with crusting, scabbing, bleeding, occasionally a nasal breathing problem, and sometimes an odor. A chronic rhinitis may occur as a result and could initiate a sinusitis. Large perforations in the front of the septum may also weaken support to the front of the nose and sometimes cause a flattening known as a saddle nose. Many years ago, instead of straightening a septal deviation, the custom was to remove it entirely, which usually created serious problems with nasal support. Nevertheless, this was a step up from the practices of the ancient Egyptians, who would amputate the entire nose, including the septum, of anyone found guilty of adultery.

Septal perforations may also result from other types of trauma including nasal fractures, infection around rings placed in the nose, finger trauma, too vigorous insertions of a nasal spray nozzle, as well as from stabbings and bullet wounds. Other causes of nasal septal perforations not resulting from trauma include tuberculosis, syphilis, malignancies, septal abscesses, as well as breathing mercury fulminate, arsenic, or chromate fumes and caustic chemical dusts or vapors; the use of caustic solutions by boxers, wrestlers, and other athletes to stop nosebleeds; sniffing crack or cocaine, and the frequent use of any very strong irritant in the nose.

Surgery to close septal perforations, if they are small, may meet with considerable success, but rarely for the larger ones, where surgical removal of any irregular margins or exposed cartilage around the perforation may provide some relief from scab formation, bleeding, and rhinitis.

Occasionally, following nasal or sinus surgery, there may be blockage of one of the tear ducts to the nose with tears running down your cheek, but most of the time this is temporary and sometimes even the result of a very tight nasal packing used to control bleeding. Occasionally, a reverse flow of blood up a tear duct from the nose to an eye from a tightly packed nose may also occur, but this should disappear with loosening or removal of the packing.

LOSS OF SENSE OF SMELL

With nasal and sinus surgery, some people may also lose their sense of smell and consequently their sense of taste temporarily, and a few may even lose it permanently from extensive nasal or sinus surgery. Of course, nasal and sinus surgery may also improve a sense of smell and therefore the sense of taste as well. Many times people over age 60 may already have a significantly reduced sense of smell.

CEREBROSPINAL FLUID LEAK

A few people may experience a leakage of clear cerebrospinal fluid from the intracranial cavity or brain into the nose or down the throat following nasal or sinus surgery. This seems to be more common now than in the past, probably because sinus surgery is more frequently performed today and generally more extensive with the use of more delicate instruments, magnification, and better lighting. It is nearly always a correctable problem, however, and sometimes may correct itself. In very rare instances, even a spontaneous cerebrospinal fluid leak into the nose, totally unrelated to surgery or injury, may occur. You should be suspicious of this complication if there is a fairly constant drip of clear fluid, especially from one nostril on tilting the head forward.

MENINGITIS AND BRAIN ABSCESS

Meningitis and brain abscess are very rare complications of nose and sinus surgery but can occur.

DOUBLE VISION AND BLINDNESS

Double vision, which is usually temporary and more often noted immediately following surgery, may occasionally occur if the orbit is inadvertently entered, particularly during ethmoid surgery. Even permanent loss of vision in one or both eyes has occurred in extremely rare instances following sinus surgery. When it does occur, it is usually following sphenoid or posterior ethmoid surgery with resulting damage to the optic nerve, since both of these sinus structures may lie next to, and in some cases may even surround, the optic nerve, sometimes with only soft tissue between them and the nerve. In very rare instances, damage to the internal carotid artery supplying the eye and brain could also result from surgery in this area, since here the bony covering of this artery as well as the optic nerve may be very thin or absent in about one-fourth of the population. Here also the presence and surgical removal of a fairly large posterior ethmoid sinus called the Onodi cell may sometimes damage the optic nerve, whereas a preoperative CAT scan identifying this anatomical varient might avoid this.

SCARRING AND ADHESIONS

Excessive postoperative scarring or adhesions, usually a later complication of sinus surgery, may rekindle a sinus problem and even seal off a sinus cavity, causing a mucocele or cyst to show up years later.

CRUSTING AND SCABBING

Too much dryness in the nose, with postoperative crusting, scabbing, and sometimes bleeding, may occasionally occur from excessive enlargement of a nasal passage by removing or trimming too much of a turbinate. Too little nasal breathing space may occasionally result from too vigorous an effort to make a nose smaller or narrower cosmetically, sometimes resulting in a collapse of the nasal valve as well.

TOXIC SHOCK SYNDROME

Toxic shock syndrome (TSS), also a rare complication, may develop within 24 to 48 hours of a nasal or sinus operation. TSS may occur in both adults and children and usually causes a high fever, a sunburn-like rash, and a significant drop in blood pressure, often to the point of shock. There can be multiorgan failure often accompanied by vomiting and diarrhea. Toxins released by certain staphylococcal bacteria within the nose or sinuses, or sometimes by strep bacteria, and taken up by the circulating blood are generally held responsible. In addition to the presence of these organisms, other contributing factors to TSS are the foreign-body reaction to nasal or sinus packing, the blockage of sinonasal mucous flow by swelling as well as packing, inflammation with increased blood flow to the area, and finally increased bacterial toxin absorption from a snugly packed cavity. Similar episodes of toxic shock syndrome have occurred from the use of tampons during menstruation and for many of the same reasons.

When TSS does occur, you should immediately be hospitalized if not already so and given emergency treatment for shock. If there is a bleeding problem, your doctor will remove or loosen any nasal packing. The nose and sinuses should be suctioned or irrigated if practical. Blood and nasal or sinus cultures should be obtained, and you will be started on appropriate intravenous antibiotics. Once the fall in blood pressure has been corrected, the possibility of further bleeding from the operative site has to be anticipated, especially if the nasal packing has been loosened or removed. Since so many patients are now being discharged on the same day, or within 24 hours, of nasal and sinus surgery, TSS is mentioned here so that you may quickly recognize the symptoms at home as well as the very serious need for immediate emergency care.

PART THREE

Possible Contributing Factors

CHAPTER TWELVE

Commonly Encountered Allergens That Could Affect Your Nose and Sinuses

THE COMBINATION OF allergy and sinusitis can be very distressing to you and sometimes discouraging to the doctor responsible for keeping your sinuses healthy. Even people who have perfectly healthy sinuses but develop an uncontrollable sensitivity to a specific allergen, especially when it is one they can't avoid, may in time join the ranks of chronic sinus sufferers. In such instances, the allergy will keep the nasal membranes swollen and the sinus drainage openings obstructed. The sinuses then become infected because they can no longer drain adequately or properly flush themselves out. Taking an antibiotic and decongestant may render the sinuses temporarily free of infection, but as soon as these medications are discontinued, the cloudy infected discharge and unpleasant symptoms may begin all over again unless the sinonasal swelling and its obstruction to drainage can be more permanently relieved by successfully treating the allergy as well.

This is when you and your doctor should put your heads together to come up with the best means of avoidance or preventative care and the best possible combination of drugs or desensitization shots, better known as immunotherapy, to maintain a healthy nose and healthy, freely draining sinuses. To accomplish this, you must become very much aware of your surroundings, both at home and at work. You must be tuned in as to what makes you feel better and what makes your nose and sinuses worse; whether you feel worse because of the pollen, dust, or mold in the air; or from being around the office secretary who wears the strong perfume, the carpooler with the aftershave or deodorant, the food and drink consumed in the restaurant the night before, the cat or dog who sleeps on the bed, the trip to the barn and horseback ride over the weekend, the bug repellent sprayed on the ankles and probably inhaled just before playing golf, or possibly from the scented hairspray or shampoo used by a spouse each morning.

You will also have to pay close attention to the foods you eat, especially milk and milk products, soy, wheat, eggs, fish, mollusks, crustaceans, some fruits, various nuts (especially peanuts), as well as what happens when you eat them. Remember that added spices, stabilizers, emulsifiers, thickeners, natural flavorings, and preservatives can also be a factor in some suspected food allergies and may tend to confuse the picture as to the exact cause of the allergic reaction. Food cross-contamination by salad bar utensils, ice cream scoops, deep fryers, blenders, and meat slicers, which are often used for slicing cheese, may also provide misinformation. Someone who thinks he or she is allergic to wheat flour might really be allergic to the mealworms in flour or even to the dust mites that sometimes frequent the flour bag as well. Even more confusing, an allergic reaction to a specific food may produce different reactions in different areas of the body in different individuals.

Elimination diets, in which certain suspected foods are removed and then reintroduced into your diet, one at a time, to see if they will cause symptoms, may require careful scrutiny on your part. Challenge testing with food extracts in capsule form administered under the supervision of a physician will help to confirm your findings. You must truly become a Sherlock Holmes and report every observation to your physician, who unfortunately can't follow you around taking notes like a Dr. Watson.

The physician must then put all these findings together and, with the aid of lab studies, blood testing for IgE antibodies, skin tests, nasal smears for eosinophil cell counts, a thorough physical examination, and sometimes a consultation with a sinus specialist or allergist, try to identify the guilty instigators and decide what can be done about your allergies now and what can be done to control them in the future. To help your doctor accomplish these goals and to restore your nose and sinuses to their original healthy state, it is important for you to have some basic knowledge of allergy, especially how it can affect the nose and sinuses.

WHAT ALLERGIES ARE

Allergy is a genetically induced or otherwise acquired sensitivity on the part of our bodies to something in our immediate environment, whether it is breathed in, eaten, or physically contacted. Allergy represents an exaggerated reaction, often called a hypersensitivity reaction, on the part of your immune system to an offending substance designated as an allergen, which means "allergy-producing." Any subsequent contact with this same protein substance or a very similar one can result in a myriad of allergic symptoms ranging from itchy skin rashes and hives to sneezing, runny nose, itchy palate, nasal and sinus congestion, red itchy watery eyes, blocked eustachian tubes, swollen face, eyes, and lips, upset stomach, cramps, and diarrhea, wheezing, swollen tongue, hoarseness, lower airway obstruction, shock, and even death.

With the first exposure to a potential allergen, no such symptoms should occur, but after a few days to a few weeks, the body and its immune system may have become sensitized, usually resulting in a significant allergic reaction of some kind on the very next contact. In a few instances where residual allergens from that first contact may have been left behind within the body, such as can occur with a shot of long-acting penicillin, an allergic response may then develop as soon as the several days to several weeks needed by the body to produce enough sensitizing antibodies to that initial contact have passed. In such instances, a person will not require a second exposure but only a prolonged first exposure to develop an allergic reaction.

During the sensitizing period, antibodies are formed for a particular allergen because our immune systems are programmed to react in this way to foreign proteins entering our bodies, especially invading bacteria or viruses. Many times our immune systems can't distinguish them from noninfectious foreign proteins such as those found in pollen, in the saliva, excreta, and body parts of dust mites and cockroaches, in molds, in bee venom, in certain complex chemical compounds, and in animal danders. The latter represent tiny flakes of the animal's skin resembling dandruff, often coated with skin oil or sebum, as well as with saliva, urine, and fungi, the latter often considered a favorite meal of dust mites.

These antibodies, created by your immune system on exposure to a potential allergen, belong to a type called immunoglobulin E, or IgE, which can be specifically identified and measured from a blood sample and are also the basis of the so-called RAST blood test for antibodies to specific allergens. B cell lymphocytes, which are white blood cells derived from bone, with the aid of cytokines, a kind of body hormone, are mainly credited with the production of these IgE antibodies after having been warned of the foreign protein invaders by another group of white blood cells, the very alert and well-known helper T cells, which also belong to the lymphocyte family and, as the prefix T would indicate, are derived from the thymus gland in the upper chest.

Because of the role they play in our cell-mediated immunity, these particular T cells are often referred to as the Paul Reveres of the immune response. If the invader happens to be a virus, these helper T cells will alert the killer T cells, who will then proceed to seek out the viral-infected body cells and to puncture their membranes, thereby disrupting the viral takeover, but unfortunately at the same time sacrificing the body cell. That is why the helper T cell, as the body's lookout scout and whistle-blower, is considered to be a number one enemy of the AIDS virus and is the cell deliberately tracked down and destroyed by it.

With the allergic process, these IgE antibodies generated by B cells attach themselves to mast cells and to circulating white blood cells known as basophils. Mast cells are found throughout the body, but especially in the tissue linings of the airway, stomach, and skin, those areas where the main signs and symptoms of an allergic reaction are so frequently observed. With any subsequent exposure of the unsuspecting victim to the same allergen or sometimes to a very similar one, this body-invading protein will bind to these IgE antibodies attached to mast cells and basophils to cause the release of certain chemical mediating substances.

Prominently included among them is a very potent mediator called histamine. This newly released histamine is picked up by specific receiving sites called H_1 histamine receptors on target cells located in various parts of the body, which in turn initiate the various responses we identify as an allergic reaction. Histamine is normally released in regulated minimal amounts to perform specific stimulatory tasks within the body and is therefore responsible for numerous necessary bodily functions, including many of those within our enormously complex immune systems. One of histamine's many important functions is to cause dilatation or expansion of small arteries as in inflammation, which if unregulated and excessive may cause excessive swelling, rashes, inflamed and swollen membranes, oversecretion of tears, red eyes, an overproduction of mucus in the nose, sinuses, bronchi, and lungs, as well as itching and hives.

Hives, or urticaria, are small fairly circumscribed slightly raised white to pinkish skin eruptions sometimes called wheals or welts that itch profusely. Although they are usually initiated by an allergic systemic reaction, they are mainly the result of localized histamine release from mast cells within the skin. They may develop as a result of a sensitivity response to inhalants, food allergens, insect stings, drugs, chemicals, cosmetics, bacterial, viral, or fungal infections, serum sickness, and psychic disorders, as well to certain physical stimuli such as heat, cold, trauma, exercise, sweating, skin pressure, friction, vibrations, water contact, breathing certain odors, and exposure to sunlight. Recent studies have indicated that chronic hives may develop from an allergic sensitivity to your own tissues, known as an autoimmune response.

Histamine release also plays a role in the contraction of smooth muscle in the walls of the bronchial tubes, which, if excessive, can result in asthmatic-like wheezing. These sometimes rather unpleasant histamine-induced reactions within or on the surface of the body should make us more aware of some of the benefits fairly often derived from taking an antihistamine to counteract them.

No one knows for certain why some people react to a foreign substance in such a hypersensitive manner and others don't; nor do we really know why an individual can be exposed to a foreign substance on an almost daily basis for years and then suddenly become sensitized to it. The best thinking for the present is that allergies are mostly genetically induced. We do know that at least 17 to 20 percent of the U.S. population has some form of nasal allergy; and well over 50 percent of those have a positive family history of allergies, suggesting a rather widespread inherited predisposition for allergy, called atopy, and this seems to be increasing among the general population. If one parent has a positive history of allergies, then an offspring has at least a 25 percent chance of developing allergies and better than a 50 percent chance if both parents have it. It is thought that at least 10 genes may be related to this inherited tendency, and several of them have already been identified. The body's development of an allergy may in some cases follow an intense or prolonged exposure to a potential allergen, a protracted illness, hormonal changes, and some types of stress and may occasionally result from certain emotional factors. It is also suspected that frequent exposure to potential allergens or possibly to respiratory viruses in very early life, especially in infancy, may be significant factors in a person's developing allergic rhinitis or asthma at a later date.

THE ALLERGIC REACTION

When an allergic reaction occurs from exposure to one of the many different possible allergens in your environment, even though it may appear to be seasonal, it could still be difficult for you and your doctor to decide if your allergy is due to grass pollen, tree pollen, dust, molds, or certain flowers, or even which grass or tree, or whether several may be responsible, since all may be stirred up by the wind or air currents, with many of them floating in the air at about the same time. Flower and shrub pollens, however, are generally larger and heavier and seldom cause trouble, since they fall to the ground rather quickly. They therefore depend more on the bees, birds, butterflies, and other insects, rather than the wind, to do their pollinating. By the same token, what was once called rose fever is now mostly attributed to windblown grass pollen collecting on the roses, since uncontaminated greenhouse roses have generally failed to produce allergic symptoms.

The allergic reaction you experience, however, could be due to none of these but to something entirely different in your household or working environment, or even to something you ate. For this reason, you will often end up having skin or lab testing for allergies, and sometimes both. Skin testing by pricking or by needle injection often reveals other allergies of which you may be totally unaware and with which you may recall no problems in the past. Thus the careful measurement of the extent of the reaction to skin testing with each allergen is important in determining the degree of sensitivity, and this may be measured further by systematically reducing the strength of the testing solutions. Fortunately, children under age six seldom show significant pollen sensitivities, but they may sometimes be very responsive to perennial allergens such as animal danders, cockroaches, and dust mites, which, like sinusitis, may sometimes cause a nighttime cough. It has also been estimated that 75 to 85 percent of children with bronchial asthma in early childhood are allergic to dust mites even though their asthma may originally have been triggered by a viral respiratory infection. For children living in the inner city, this figure may be just as high or even higher for cockroach allergen and the development of asthma.

Once you become sensitized to a particular allergen in the air, reactions to any subsequent contact can be almost immediate, usually within the first 20 to 30 minutes following exposure, with sneezing, itching of the nose and eyes, and a clear watery nasal discharge. This is often followed by a delayed reaction, usually developing within the next 4 to 6 hours and frequently manifested by inflammatory swelling of nasal membranes. If the early reaction is very minimal and goes unrecognized, it could make it even more difficult to identify the allergen or exposure responsible for the delayed reaction.

Allergic reactions may vary not only from person to person but also with the different kinds of allergen exposure as well as its route of entry into the body. One person may react with hives or swelling of the lips, tongue, larynx, eyes, and face from something he or she has eaten, whereas someone else who had eaten the same food may respond with an allergic rhinitis or an asthmatic attack. Cross-sensitivity reactions may sometimes occur in the same individual for pollen of different origins as well as for different foods. A person allergic to ragweed pollen might also experience an allergic reaction to melons, and one allergic to birch tree pollen could have an allergic reaction to apples, although he or she might still tolerate cooked apples. Unfortunately, the latter is not necessarily true for eggs, nuts, fish, shellfish, and crustaceans, whose protein allergens seem to be mostly heat stable. A cross-sensitivity may develop in some individuals between ragweed and dahlias, daisies, or chrysanthemums, as well as between latex rubber and chestnuts, bananas, kiwis, or avocados.

A few unlucky individuals, especially if they are atopic and therefore have a predisposition for allergies, might develop multiple sensitivities, which might include various foods and pollens as well as dust mites, cockroaches, molds, and animal danders. Not infrequently, one child from an allergic family may show up with asthma, whereas a brother or sister may develop allergic rhinitis. Fortunately, most allergic individuals—and even those with a genetic predisposition—seem to keep their really troublesome allergies down to a few. One still has to wonder about a common denominator in some food and inhalant allergies, since most inhaled allergens are caught in the mucous flow from the nose and lungs and subsequently swallowed, thus ending up in the same digestive tract as the food allergens.

FOOD ALLERGIES
Some people who have food allergies may gradually become turned off on food and no longer enjoy eating, especially if they are allergic to such common foods or food ingredients as eggs, milk, wheat, seafood, nuts, and soy. Milk products, eggs, and soy may be particu-

larly insidious as hidden ingredients in many foods, and severe allergic reactions may occur from ingesting even very small amounts of them. Food-allergic individuals never know when other foods may have to join their forbidden lists, and they often find themselves spending more and more time reading contents labels in food markets, which can sometimes be difficult to do without a magnifying glass. Being invited out to dinner can create major problems if you have food allergies and can also prove embarrassing when you have to turn down a special dessert or even the main course because of the heavy cream sauce. Although it can be annoying, the time you spend reading food content labels could save someone's life, be it your own or that of a family member or even a guest invited to dinner who may sheepishly ask if there are any nuts in the pie or cookies, not even guessing that there may be a nut oil in the salad dressing.

Further complicating the problem has been the introduction of new genes into certain crops in order to increase their productivity, rate of growth, resistance to disease, and sometimes their nutritional values, and it is important for people with food allergies to realize that this new, often unlisted addition may represent something to which they have a known allergy. This was aptly demonstrated when the Brazil nut gene was introduced into the chromosome pattern of soybeans for greater nutritional value. When this soybean product was consumed later, it caused an allergic reaction in people sensitive to Brazil nuts.

SOY ALLERGY Soy, a product of soybeans, has become a rather common allergen in everyday life, since it is now an ingredient of so many different foods, including all kinds of sauces, milk, baby formulas, baby foods, cereals, margarines, tofus, soups, broths, mayonnaise, ice creams, gums, starches, emulsifiers, stabilizers, salad dressings, processed meats, hot dogs, canned tuna, hamburgers, cooking oils, cakes, cookies, candies, puddings, pastries, and breads. Further problems may be created when some of these ingredients containing soy are added to other foods, where many times the soy content will not even be listed. It is easy to see that for the allergic individual to avoid soy entirely could be exceedingly difficult and might require a rather extensive study of all possible forms and compositions. This again emphasizes the importance of reading content labels, being aware of possible "hidden ingredients," and making certain that manufacturers clearly identify all the ingredients.

SERIOUS OR FATAL REACTIONS Allergic reactions to drug injections can be instantaneous, severe, and even fatal, and yet reactions to ingested drugs, food, and drink can occur almost as quickly or be just as serious, and the same would often apply to inhaled allergens as well. It has been estimated that more children and adolescents die in the United States each year from food allergies than from insect stings. A typical example is the person who knows he or she is allergic to nuts and unknowingly swallows even a very small piece in a salad, cake, or cookie and almost immediately begins to notice swelling of the lips, eyes, and face, followed sometimes by swelling of the throat, tongue, and larynx. Hives with generalized itching and severe bronchial spasm with wheezing may develop as well, sometimes requiring a shot of adrenaline or epinephrine as a lifesaving measure. Similar reactions, including abdominal cramps, airway obstruction, a drop in blood pressure, and shock, may occur with other foods as well, especially seafoods, eggs, and milk products.

Peanuts and peanut butter as well as eggs and milk all have a strong tendency to produce allergic reactions in very young children, especially under age three. Unfortunately, peanut allergy is not as likely to disappear at an early age, as often noted with egg or milk allergy, and may often persist throughout adult life. To further avoid this problem, nursing mothers and perhaps even pregnant women should avoid peanut products, and they should certainly never be given to very young children. Daily or even weekly ingestion of peanut butter in an allergic individual could keep a rhinosinusitis going indefinitely.

PEANUT ALLERGY Peanuts, a common cause of death from anaphylactic shock or allergic airway obstruction, may also cause other serious problems if a young child eats them and subsequently aspirates any part of them into the lungs. There they may block the airway of the trachea or bronchi to cause respiratory distress and asphyxia, and the peanut oil can work its way further down into the lungs to cause pneumonia. These nuts may also tend to crumble when the bronchoscopist tries to remove them, resulting in multiple smaller foreign bodies in the lungs, which may be even more difficult to remove and may cause even more areas of pneumonia or pneumonitis. Some of these patients may go on to develop a very distressing chronic lung infection with destruction of the bronchial wall, known as bronchiectasis. Since peanuts are available in most stores and have become a frequent staple at sporting events as well as on airline flights, they can easily find their way back into the home and into the wrong hands. A wise reminder on the kitchen bulletin board should read: "No Peanuts, Please—Small Children Live Here!" I recall a number of instances in which parents wished they had been so forewarned.

It should be of special interest to those with peanut allergy and rhinosinusitis that the peanut allergen has been demonstrated clinging to the circulating air filters of airplanes. The dry air of the plane also provides for easier penetration of the protective mucous coating of the respiratory tract by the peanut allergen. Once you inhale it, however, just swallowing the peanut allergen caught up in the mucous flow could be just as troublesome to a highly allergic individual as breathing it.

Peanut butter is often used in Oriental cooking, and peanut oil is found in many processed foods as well as in some milk formulas. It may often go unrecognized as a hidden ingredient of many food products. Although properly prepared peanut oil is often considered to be allergy safe, full processing information is not always available.

MILK PRODUCTS Some individuals may show a different kind of sensitivity to milk products, also a very common food allergen to which most of us are exposed almost daily, and which of course would include cheese, ice cream, most sherbets, butter, cream, buttermilk, nonfat milk, whey, and yogurt. Instead of the typical allergic rhinitis response to the milk protein with sneezing, a watery nasal discharge, itching, nasal swelling, and blockage that you might expect, some may notice only an increased flow of a very thick, clear mucus within the nose or throat and sometimes from within the bronchi or lungs, usually developing within 30 to 40 minutes of ingesting a milk product. Since it differs somewhat from the usual IgE-mediated allergen-antibody response with histamine release, this reaction could be due to other mediators or to the production of a different immunoglobulin. For such individuals, it may seem very difficult to blow this thickened mucus out of their noses, as well as to clear it out of their throats or even to cough it up. If it occurs at night, it is usually more obvious when you are lying down.

The problem will often disappear during the night and well before the next morning but may recur following exposure to more dairy products the next day. Although it is not usually considered serious or dangerous, this reaction could aggravate an existing episode of sinusitis or bronchitis. People with chronic sinusitis should note this, and if they do experience an increased accumulation of a rather thick mucus in their nose, sinuses, or chest after consuming milk or milk products, they might consider avoiding all milk products for a while to see if it improves their sinus problems. I can recall a number of sinus patients who volunteered the information that milk products seemed to thicken their nasal and sinus secretions and who subsequently benefited from avoiding milk products. If you think you have a problem with milk, you should carefully read all food labels to avoid ingesting any of the hidden milk products such as curds, artificial butter flavoring, certain margarines containing whey, lactalbumin, lactoglobulin, lactose, lactulose, caramel flavoring, nougat, casein, caseinate, yogurt, and whey. A "D" on a label next to a "K" or "U" in a circle may also indicate the presence of milk protein. Milk products amounting to less than 2 percent of the entire package may sometimes be included under the vague term of natural flavors or flavoring, as well as possibly in some dough conditioners, and could cause a problem for the unsuspecting allergic person. Chocolate, once thought of as a major food allergen, is now considered much less important, and the real problem with it in many instances may be the milk it often contains. Food and medicine dyes or colorings have apparently taken a similar fall from grace but should not be entirely overlooked if you are allergic and have sinus problems.

LATEX ALLERGY

Another increasingly common allergic reaction, and one of special interest to most medical personnel, is an allergic sensitivity to natural latex rubber, as in rubber gloves. Natural latex rubber, sometimes called India rubber or gum elastic, is the milky juice that flows from the rubber tree after the bark is punctured or sliced. Once cured, its flexibility, strength, and elasticity make it a very important ingredient of thousands of manufactured products we encounter in our everyday lives. Some of it is hardened into crinkled sheets called crepe rubber, as used in crepe soles for shoes as well as in rubber tires, where a very hardened resistant nonskid surface is essential. The softer product, liquid latex, is preferred for other materials where stretch and elasticity are important, as in bathing caps, rubber bands, and surgical gloves. It is with this form of latex that most of the recognized allergic reactions occur. It has been estimated that up to 10 percent of health care workers may be allergic to the liquid latex incorporated into rubber gloves and tubing.

Allergic reactions to latex products may occur immediately within minutes, be delayed for several hours, or sometimes may not develop for several days. The much-delayed reaction is usually a skin rash sometimes with blisters and more often resulting from hand, skin, or clothing contact with a chemical ingredient used in processing the rubber. The early reaction is nearly always due to skin or membrane contact with the latex allergen, especially through touching or inhaling the latex protein dust.

Rubber gloves, a frequent instigator, were first introduced to the surgical world at Johns Hopkins in the nineteenth century when Caroline Hampton, an operating room supervisor and later the wife of the renowned surgeon Dr. William Stewart Halsted, developed a skin allergy from bichloride of mercury sterilizing solution seeping through her cotton gloves. Dr. Halsted then asked Mr. Charles Goodyear, a patient of his, as a favor, to make her a pair of fairly thin rubber gloves. They worked for Mrs. Halsted and were then tried by Dr. Halsted himself, at the operating table, with great success. After that, their use in operating rooms soon spread throughout the world.

Today, with such great emphasis on the dangers of contaminated blood, especially from AIDS and hepatitis patients, and with the vast number of medical and nonmedical personnel wearing rubber gloves because of this, we are beginning to see a marked increase in mild to severe allergic reactions to latex rubber. These reactions include rhinitis with nasal congestion, inflammation and swelling, eyelid swelling, asthma-like wheezing, obstructive breathing, hoarseness, swollen larynx, tongue, and lips, hives, skin rashes, low blood pressure, and on some occasions even anaphylactic shock and death. Here again a shot of epinephrine or adrenaline, given immediately, can be lifesaving. Even then, following a usually dramatic improvement in symptoms, you should hasten to a hospital emergency room, since the allergic reaction could return in full strength once the epinephrine wears off, and sometimes even following a second shot. More than 15 deaths have been noted so far from latex allergy, and this can be expected to increase yearly.

Repeated exposure to the latex allergen for someone already sensitive often increases the chances of a severe reaction. Some people who have had to undergo repeated operations may in some instances become allergic to the surgeon's rubber gloves and could subsequently develop serious problems, including multiple abdominal adhesions from an allergic reaction within their abdominal tissues followed by scar formation and even bowel obstruction. During the surgical procedure, the latex-sensitive patient could also develop an unstable blood pressure, cardiac arrhythmias, an asthmatic attack with wheezing and a compromised airway, as well as anaphylactic shock. Some people born with spina bifida are often more inclined to develop latex allergy, and this may be due in part to the multiple surgical procedures they usually require and their repeated exposure to rubber gloves.

Those exposed to latex rubber on an almost daily basis such as health care workers and some lab technicians are generally considered more vulnerable to latex allergy, especially if they have a predisposition for allergies, known as atopy. Perhaps some infants exposed to latex bottle nipples and rubber pacifiers in early life and who may be atopic might conceivably become allergic to latex in later life and might even develop asthma. Now an increasing number of individuals who come in contact with latex products in their daily lives, including rubber balloons, latex condoms, diaphragms, rubber toys, rubber stoppers, some sporting equipment, rubber balls, tires, inner tubes, rubber bands, electrical insulation, bungee cords, rubber catheters, and hoses, may eventually develop mild to severe allergic reactions. Other rubber products that are often overlooked and that could cause a similar problem are diving masks, snorkels, goggles, watch bands, rubber mats, rubber sheets, rubber-soled shoes or shoe covers, hot-water bottles, latex paints, heating pads, light cords, douche and enema tubings, rubber nozzles, water beds, underwear and clothing containing elastics, bra straps, ace bandages, teeth protectors, elastic stockings, pantyhose, blood pressure cuffs, wheelchair tires, tourniquets, jar openers, gaskets, and swim caps.

Allergic reactions to vaginal and rectal exams with latex gloves have also occurred. Rubber-factory workers can develop similar problems through skin contact with the basic latex product or from inhaling or ingesting latex dust. Rubber tire residue on the road, rendered airborne by passing cars or trucks, may blow into a car window or air exchange vent to harm a latex-sensitive person. Since latex tire dust is everywhere, it could also be responsible for some unexplained asthmatic attacks as well as for some year-round cases of allergic rhinitis with sinusitis. Some specialized inks have a latex base that could present a problem for the allergic printer and perhaps even for the reader should it flake off and be inhaled. Some people may react severely from inhaling even very minute amounts of latex dust in a room containing decorating rubber balloons, in a car transporting them, or from just being around a tank or pump inflating them. The simple act of blowing up balloons for a party could provide a heavy dose of latex protein dust, and popping them could produce even more. You should again be reminded that the greater part of any particle matter inhaled is likewise ingested, since it is swept down from the nose or up from the lungs in the mucous flow and subsequently swallowed, making it possible that some of these allergies could be initiated by the digestive system rather than the respiratory tract, where a totally intact mucous blanket might occasionally limit allergen contact with the underlying tissues.

Laboratory studies and skin testings will usually identify the latex allergy, but in someone severely allergic, even skin testing could be very dangerous and should only be done under careful supervision and with great caution. Intradermal testing by needle injection just beneath the skin could cause shock in a latex-sensitive person and probably should be avoided altogether. If you are known to be allergic to chestnuts or to certain fruits such as avocados, bananas, or kiwis, you could be allergic to latex, since there appears to be an occasional cross-sensitivity with them. Some have even found a similar relationship between latex rubber and the four Ps, namely, pineapples, pears, papayas, and passion fruit. In people found to be allergic to latex, avoiding the product is the treatment of choice, with additional standard therapy for any rhinitis, skin rash, asthma, or shock as indicated. These would include topical cortisone preparations and antihistamines for the skin rash; antihistamines, decongestants, and steroid nasal sprays for the rhinitis; and steroid inhalers, bronchodilators, occasionally antihistamines, and sometimes cortisone preparations by mouth or injection for the asthma. If rhinosinusitis should result from prolonged exposure, then antibiotics may be necessary. A fast trip to the emergency room including an epinephrine shot may be required if there is a sudden onset of hoarseness, any signs of lower airway obstruction, or lightheadedness and a fast pulse suggesting impending anaphylactic shock. Although polyurethane condoms may be a little more likely to tear, people allergic to latex should strongly consider using them. Safer and more reliable substitutes will very likely be available in the near future. So far, immunotherapy shots for latex allergy have not been considered safe or practical.

Another source of latex contact, and one of grave concern, is the rubber balloon. Balloons make wonderful decorations and great markers for driveways and are fun for children and adults alike, but they can be fatal to a child. According to an article in the *Journal of the American Medical Association* in December 1995, balloons have been responsible for 131 choking deaths in children over the 20-year period from 1972 to 1992, killing more children than any other toy except for riding toys and bicycles, and representing 29 percent of all choking fatalities in children, other than from food products, as reported to Consumer Safety during that same period. Those figures certainly make the Mylar balloon a far more sensible substitute, and using it may even prevent some children from developing latex sensitivities that might endanger them later in life.

ANIMAL DANDER

Another very common inhalant allergy that frequently produces asthma, hives, or rhinitis, the latter sometimes initiating a flare-up of sinusitis, is allergy to house pet dander. Nearly 5 percent of the general population is allergic to dogs or cats, but this may increase 5- to 6-fold in the atopic or genetically predisposed group. The old idea that shorthaired dogs or cats are better for the allergic patient could provide a false sense of security, since animal dander is not hair but consists of dead skin scales and their skin oils, urine, and saliva contaminants, often clinging to fallen hairs. Having a smaller dog could make a difference in the total dander shed in a 24-hour period, and perhaps some animals do shed fewer skin scales than others, but a lot can accumulate in a house or car over time, sometimes influenced by how frequently the animal is bathed. It may also take a comparatively small amount of dander to initiate an allergic reaction. The idea that the breed of the animal can make a difference is held by some but questioned by others and so far hasn't been proven. The best policy if you are allergic and have sinusitis is still to find another happy home for the pet. If unsuccessful or refused, they should a least be kept out of the bedroom and bathed frequently. It is important to realize that even after a pet is removed from a household, it may take more than just a month or two to eliminate most of the dander allergen from the house or car. The idea that Bashkir horses are nonallergenic is also questionable and so far unproven.

Cats are fast becoming the major contributor to house pet allergies. They have become very popular and usually offer a greater exposure to their dander. Unlike dogs, they are more inclined to sleep in your lap, around your neck, on the squashy pillow or sofa, in the easy chair, in the bedroom, on the bed, and even in the baby's playpen, which a cat can easily climb over or sometimes squeeze through. Cats secrete an allergenic protein called Fel d 1 from the sebaceous glands in their skin, which then coats their fur. Smaller amounts of the protein are also found in their saliva and even in their urine. Saliva deposits from licking their fur and the oily sebum secreted by their skin glands will stick to their hairs and to their skin flakes, thus forming the main components of dander.

Animal dander literally means anything shed by their skin and fur other than hairs but many times along with the hairs. Cat dander is constantly shed and easily distributed throughout the entire house by the animal and scattered by the other occupants when moving about, sweeping, dusting, and vacuuming, as well as by air currents, fans, and ventilating ducts. Dander is very light compared to dust mite or cockroach particle matter, and since dander so readily floats in the air, special high-efficiency particulate air (HEPA) filters are even more effective in collecting it. It is frequently found stuck to the floors and walls of every room in the house as well as in houses and cars that never had cats, a fact that can make dander difficult to avoid, especially since it is so easily transported on shoes and clothing. It also means that your doctor can't always exclude cat allergy as a cause of your allergies just because you don't have cats or if you have no known exposure to cats. Those who are allergic to this protein should likewise find another equally good home for the cat if they want their allergy and sinusitis problems to improve, but unfortunately few will follow this advice.

However, if it is any consolation, cats can be of help if you are allergic to cockroaches, since cats find roaches fun to chase down as well as very tasty. A medication being tested at Johns Hopkins and in Boston offers some hope for a shorter desensitization period for cat allergy over a matter of weeks or months rather than the many months or years often required for conventional shot therapy and possibly with greater safety. If this medication is successful, similar short-term therapies may be used for other troublesome allergens, including the dander of other household pets and farm animals, as well as for allergies to mold, pollen, cockroaches, and dust mites.

DUST MITES

Dust mites, discovered in 1964, have nearly always been with us and can be a major cause of year-round allergic problems. These blind denizens of our carpets, upholstery, mattresses, and bed linens are microscopic creatures having the appearance of some prehistoric beast. They are a kind of flesh eater and live off of bits of dead skin, or dander, shed by our bodies and those of our household pets. When we brush our hair, groom our pets, dry shave our legs, remove our socks or stockings, or even scratch our heads, dust mites have a royal feast. Dust mites find the molds or fungi that like to grow on these flakes of dead skin especially tasty. They can cause nasal allergies and asthmatic attacks when an allergic individual breathes their dried salivary secretions or fecal pellet dusts, both of which may be expelled into the air every time we sweep, vacuum, dust, walk on a rug, or just sit down on a bed, sofa, or easy chair. The almost universal popularity of nailed-down wall-to-wall carpeting, central humidification, and well-insulated, tightly sealed homes have all given a big boost to mites' growth and survival. Like many of us, dust mites love stuffed animals, and they multiply best in a warm and humid environment.

Under such conditions, as many as 150,000 or more of them may live in a single mattress. Three different species of dust mites have been found to exist in temperate climates, and it now appears that one species may even prefer the coziness of our beds to the rugs on the floor. Each mite can pass up to 40 fecal pellets a day, and their multitudes enjoy residence in nearly every home, many buildings, some office waiting rooms, and possibly even in the carpeting and upholstery of some planes, cars, cabin cruisers, buses, and passenger trains, especially if the temperature and humidity are consistently above 70. They are often so completely entrenched in our homes that they probably regard us as their guests.

You can reduce their numbers and limit your exposure to their discharges by enclosing mattresses and pillows in zippered plastic covers; by removing drapes, rugs, and stuffed animals or cleaning them with special solutions; by avoiding porous fabric covers on sofas and chairs; and by washing bed linens, blankets, and coverlets in hot water. Vacuuming instead of sweeping, and using HEPA filters in your vacuum cleaner, may also limit your exposure to their fecal dust, dried saliva, and body parts. You can also reduce their growth and multiplication by keeping your living areas, and especially your bedroom, well ventilated, and room temperatures at 70° F or less and by maintaining the humidity in your home at 60 percent RH or below—but not so low that it dries out sinonasal mucous secretions.

COCKROACHES

Cockroaches can be just as much of a problem for many allergic individuals and especially for those who live in the inner city. Roaches are tropical by nature, and all they want is continuous warmth, food, and a place to hide. Unlike dust mites, who must obtain their water from the air, roaches can usually seek and find water. The protein in their fecal droppings, saliva, and body parts is a common cause of allergic asthma, especially in children, and a significant contributor to year-round allergic rhinitis, often a precursor of sinusitis. It has been estimated that a pair of roaches may be responsible for nearly 100,000 offspring over a 12-month period.

FIBER LAXATIVES AND OTHER POWDERS

Just as some milk-sensitive individuals can react to inadvertently inhaling milk powder, some older individuals, in particular, may experience an allergic or sensitivity reaction with eye itching, sneezing, nasal or chest congestion, and sometimes wheezing from spooning out and inadvertently inhaling the very fine powder of some fiber laxatives that are taken daily for bowel regularity by millions of older people. Most powdery substances are not uniform but consist of both coarse and very fine particle matter and, when disturbed by mixing, stirring, dusting, or spraying, often form a very fine dust cloud that will float in the air and can be inhaled. Although this fine dust cloud is usually invisible to the naked eye, it can often be seen if there is a strong background light.

A very fine cloud formation may also result from the use of powdered cereals, body powders, foot powders, soap powders, various chemical powders, fungicides, pesticides, and even the powdery dust created by sanding, sawing, and drilling. Some of these may be very irritating to your eyes and respiratory membranes, especially in concentrated forms, and others may contain foreign proteins capable of sensitizing an individual and causing an allergic response with any subsequent exposure.

Since you could be sensitive or even allergic to one of the ingredients of Citrucel or to the psyllium seed powder in Metamucil, any part of them left floating in the air after dispensing could cause inflammation of the nose with blockage of the sinus drainage openings. Even if you are not truly allergic to them, they could act as a primary irritant when settling on already inflamed respiratory membranes to cause further irritation, inflammation, and swelling. If you should notice sneezing, eye itching, nasal burning, wheezing, or coughing after measuring or mixing them, you should either hold your breath while mixing and then walk away immediately afterward before drinking the mixture or do it with a room exhaust fan turned on. This could be important to the sinus-prone individual or to the patient with chronic sinusitis or chronic bronchitis, since these fiber laxatives are usually taken every day, and daily irritation of the nose or lower respiratory tract could in some instances cause or aggravate a chronic condition. If such is the case, unless you are truly allergic to one of the ingredients, taking it in a wafer form would avoid any irritating inhalant effects and might be a wiser choice.

PRINTER'S INK

A surprising number of individuals may also be sensitive to airborne print dust released by certain newspapers and magazines and may notice eye irritation with itching and occasionally nasal congestion, sneezing, and sometimes sinus blockage with tightness or sinus pressure in the cheeks during or after thumbing through them. The printer's ink dust may be dislodged and ejected into the air as you turn the pages. It may also cling to your fingers, and rubbing your eyes may cause even more itching. Unfortunately, one of my patients finally had to resort to wearing gloves and a mask to enjoy her morning paper and at the same time keep her rhinosinusitis from flaring up.

Fortunately, many newspapers and magazines now use a more stable ink as well as a better grade of paper, and you may gradually learn to identify the ones that you can tolerate without experiencing sneezing, itching eyes, a stuffy nose, or sinus blockage. You can just imagine a commuter train with everyone reading the morning papers and the potential for ink dust in the air. Hopefully, they are all reading quality papers printed with quality ink. A biodegradable substance known as soy oil made from soybeans is now being substituted for petroleum products in some inks and could help in such cases. However, the presence of various pigments in the inks could be mainly responsible for any truly allergic reactions. For the nonallergic individual, printer's ink dust may act as a primary irritant to respiratory membranes, and inhaling it may aggravate or prolong an already existing cold, flu, sinusitis, or bronchitis.

Short-term flare-ups of allergic rhinitis with nasal and sinus blockage lasting for only a day or two will many times be tolerated by normally healthy sinuses without precipitating an infectious flare-up.

However, prolonged untreated seasonal allergic rhinitis and repeated or persistent episodes of untreated perennial rhinitis both stand a good chance of producing chronic sinus disease. As demonstrated on CAT scans and MRI, some membrane swelling with an excessive accumulation of secretions often does occur within the sinus cavities during an episode of allergic rhinitis; and stagnated secretions trapped by a swollen, blocked drainage opening, whether it be due to allergic swelling or blockage from any other cause, may soon become infected, sometimes even within a matter of hours.

If the sinus blockage is from allergic swelling in the nose, a determined effort should be made to identify the responsible allergen and either remove it, block it with medications, or preferably avoid it altogether. At the same time, your doctor should try to reverse your nasal inflammatory swelling by prescribing steroid sprays and oral or nasal decongestants. Antihistamines and Cromolyn nasal sprays will not reduce nasal or sinus swelling, but both may help in preventing further swelling by blocking or suppressing histamine activity. Antibiotics may of course be necessary if there is any evidence of an associated sinus infection such as a cloudy sinonasal discharge. As with all sinus therapy, the basic goal whenever possible is to restore sinus function by reestablishing a continuously effective sinonasal drainage as well as a constant sinonasal air exchange.

CHAPTER THIRTEEN

Rhinitis and Its Effect on the Sinuses

RHINITIS IS AN inflammatory condition of the nose; "itis" means "inflammation of," and "rhino," of course, refers to the nose. Rhinitis may show up in an allergic person after a second contact with a specific allergen, or it may develop in the nonallergic individual, also with the same nasal symptoms, either from something breathed in, such as an irritating vapor or powder, or from something introduced directly into the nose, such as cocaine or an irritating nasal spray, and sometimes even from something taken internally, such as an aspirin or one of the NSAIDs. The allergic kind, for some, may only occur at certain times of the year when grass, weed, or tree pollen abounds and is known as seasonal allergic rhinitis, hay fever, or pollinosis. Others may experience allergic rhinitis throughout the year, largely due to the allergens found in household dust, including fungi or molds, dog and cat danders, as well as the saliva, excreta, and body parts of dust mites and cockroaches. Some unlucky individuals may have both seasonal and year-round allergic rhinitis, and still others may have a very short-lasting flare-up of allergic rhinitis occurring only a few times a year, or not even that often, usually due to an isolated allergen in some seldom ingested food or in some rarely encountered inhalant in the air. Since both allergic and nonallergic rhinitis may cause nasal membrane inflammation and swelling, often followed by sinus blockage, either or both can therefore have a major impact on the development and persistence of a sinus infection.

ALLERGIC RHINITIS

SEASONAL ALLERGIC RHINITIS

Seasonal allergic rhinitis, commonly referred to as hay fever, is, by conservative estimates, contracted to varying degrees by more than 20 million Americans each year and causes workday losses and schoolday losses also in the millions, either directly or through its complications of sinusitis, bronchitis, and asthma. When you consider this as well as the innumerable doctor visits required and the vast supply of drugs sold to treat it, seasonal allergic rhinitis also becomes a significant factor in our socioeconomic way of life.

NONSEASONAL ALLERGIC RHINITIS

Although we may recognize many of these seasonal hay fever sufferers by their red, itchy, and watery eyes, frequent sneezing, nasal stuffiness, and drippy red noses, the nonseasonal or year-round allergic rhinitis group, which is also very large, is usually less conspicuous but many times just as uncomfortable. Their symptoms are especially disturbing, since their allergens are nearly always close by, and some people may require treatment all year. They can many times remove the offenders from their homes, or at least reduce their numbers, but not from the homes of their friends and neighbors, or even from their workplace. Unlike the seasonal hay fever sufferer, they can't predict when their symptoms will occur, and they can't dismiss them with the first frost. Moreover, they can't retreat indoors to avoid excessive exposure, since that is where most of their allergens are found.

Although their symptoms are usually more intermittent and any eye symptoms often less obvious, many may experience the same nasal stuffiness, itching of the nose, ears, throat, and palate, watery nasal discharge, occasional headache, sleeplessness, sometimes asthmatic wheezing, stuffy ears with diminished hearing, diminished smell and taste, and occasional sneezing. These symptoms are sometimes constant but more often tend to come and go with their periodic exposures to household allergens and their often irregular self-treating with over-the-counter remedies. The hearing difficulties these individuals sometimes experience are usually more common in children, with their small eustachian tubes and their tendency for excessive membrane swelling.

CHILDHOOD ALLERGIC RHINITIS

Allergic rhinitis of childhood, with an estimated incidence of 10 to 20 percent, may also cause chronic mouth breathing, facial maldevelopment, diminished taste and smell, a poor appetite, improper feeding, restless sleeping, nervousness, irritability, decreased pulmonary function, excessive adenoid growth, sometimes delayed speech, and often inattentiveness with temporarily impaired learning. It can also cause fluid formation and infections in the ears of young children as well as infectious processes in their lower respiratory tracts and especially in their sinuses, being rather frequently found in conjunction with chronic sinusitis in children and adults. Children with allergic rhinitis may sometimes develop dark circles under their eyes, often referred to as allergic shiners, and may even exhibit a twitching or rabbitlike motion of the nose attributed to itching. Some may acquire the already mentioned allergic salute, namely, an upward sweeping motion of the palm of the hand in wiping the nose, as well as the resultant identifying skin crease across the lower bridge of the nose.

PSYCHIC EFFECTS

Older allergic rhinitis patients may become increasingly annoyed by their symptoms. They may develop mood and personality changes to include irritability, hostility, depression, and sometimes an inability to concentrate, which in turn can affect their social and family relationships as well as their work or their studies. Prescribing an antihistamine for their allergic rhinitis may relieve some of this, but if it is one of the sedating kind, being drowsy at work or falling asleep in class could also have a significant effect on work performance and schooling. The sedating antihistamines are known to cross the blood-brain barrier and can, in some individuals, cause personality or disposition changes, even in children. The drug manufacturers are now providing us with reasonably safe non-sedating over-the-counter antihistamines for children ages 6 through 12 with allergic rhinitis, and this may go a long way toward solving some of these problems, since the prescription kind is not always available when they need it, especially when traveling away from home.

It is not my intention to leave anyone with the impression that taking a non-sedating antihistamine might enhance a child's performance at school or even elicit higher grades, but it could lessen some of the very distracting symptoms of allergic rhinitis, hopefully improving concentration and attentiveness.

Some people with allergic rhinitis sometimes realize that their symptoms are entirely work related and note distinct improvement on vacations and even at home on weekends, or they may find that they are worse at home or in the car. An awareness of this may be especially helpful to your doctor in tracing the cause of your allergic problems.

NONALLERGIC RHINITIS

Not only may both types of allergic rhinitis play significant roles in sinus disease, but there is another fairly sizable group of patients with nonallergic rhinitis who may be troubled by sinus problems as well. Their nasal irritation, inflammation, swelling, and excessive clear discharge may come from innumerable sources including overuse of nose drops and sprays, from taking aspirin or NSAIDs if they are aspirin intolerant, from inhaling certain irritating powders including cocaine and snuff, as well as from breathing tobacco smoke or other chemical irritants in the air. Breathing these irritating vapors, perfumes, paint fumes, irritating chemicals, and certain kinds of dusts, especially over a prolonged period, may cause a nonallergic rhinitis often followed by a sinusitis and may sometimes even initiate asthmatic attacks. Nonallergic rhinitis could also in rare instances result from the use of eyedrops, especially those containing certain preservatives, which may pass into the nose through the tear ducts to occasionally cause nasal inflammation and sinus blockage. A person therefore doesn't have to be allergic to the volatile oils of a perfume or to the protein in a certain inhalant to develop a rhinitis or sinusitis. Some inhalants are just extremely irritating to nasal membranes and even more so in certain individuals whose membranes tend to overreact.

Sinusitis-prone people should avoid such irritants in all forms whenever possible, however. It is difficult to enter some department stores without being sprayed by a demonstrator's perfume or cologne, or to even approach the candle sales department without being almost overcome by perfume or the burning of incense. Sinusitis-prone individuals should take a deep breath and hold it before being doused or, better still, take a circuitous route around the squirter. Perfumes were originally introduced and found very useful when people couldn't bathe often. Now, not too surprisingly, they have been given a romantic or sensual meaning and are applied to many things other than the skin, including paper tissues of all kinds as well as envelopes, stationery, crayons, handkerchiefs, candles, soaps, lotions, shampoos, and even pamphlets and magazine ads. Some scents are also marketed for pet dogs and cats. Unfortunately, when applied to the helpless pet, a perfume tends to neutralize one of the animal's most acute and cherished senses, namely its sense of smell, which could also block its own enjoyment of food. Worse still, a perfume may cause rhinitis and even sinusitis not only in the pet but in other pets, the owner, and anyone else around them. As mentioned previously, sinusitis in a pet can also be transmitted to the owner or to other members of the household. Those who use perfumes or colognes regularly may also develop the so-called fragrance fatigue as far as their own sense of smell is concerned and therefore tend to use them more and more. Sinusitis-prone individuals should avoid using perfumes and colognes themselves and may even have to avoid other people who do.

Alcohol, as well as certain medications, especially some of those prescribed for hypertension, may cause nasal swelling unrelated to any allergy and may subsequently lead to sinus blockage and possibly infection or at least aggravate an existing sinusitis. Individuals with aspirin sensitivity, also not a true allergy, may develop rhinitis, sinusitis, nasal polyps, and asthma from taking aspirin or one of the other NSAIDs, better known as Motrin, Aleve, Advil, Indocin, Nuprin, Ibuprofen, and others. Reflex swelling of the nose may also occur if you are sensitive to cold or drafts, to bright lights, or to certain strong cooking odors, and prolonged exposure might occasionally result in nasal congestion with sinus blockage. For someone allergic to shellfish, and shrimp in particular, just breathing their steam while cooking them can cause a rhinitis or even a severe allergic reaction sometimes terminating fatally. The same problem might be encountered in poaching fish and steaming clams or oysters for someone highly allergic to them.

Nasal irritation with inflammation and swelling may also occur from prolonged use of oxygen catheters or masks, since heavy concentrations of oxygen can cause a very drying and irritating effect on nasal membranes, as some oxygen-dependent patients soon begin to realize, especially during the dry winter months and sometimes even when oxygen is bubbled through a water container to add moisture. Just directing a stream of air toward a small area of nasal membrane will in a very short period cause inflammation and swelling due mainly to the drying effects, and with an even quicker response if pure oxygen is used. A prolonged exposure may even alter some of the nasal membrane cells themselves resulting in a loss of cilia and cellular changes known as metaplasia. Continuous misdirection or deflection of inhaled air to a particular area of the nose by septal deviations or other nasal anatomical abnormalities may cause similar changes in nasal membranes, and this is even more likely to occur if the air is very dry. Swelling and nasal congestion or rhinitis may also occur from certain hormonal changes as noted in menopause, menstruation, taking oral contraceptives, sometimes from sexual arousal, and especially from being pregnant.

RHINITIS OF PREGNANCY

The rhinitis of pregnancy can be particularly upsetting to a woman who may already be feeling generally uncomfortable and at the same time may present a real challenge to her sinus specialist in trying to keep her free of sinus infection without prescribing anything that might endanger the baby, the normal delivery, or the health of the mother. The rhinitis of pregnancy is a nonallergic phenomenon that sometimes develops during the second or third trimester but may occasionally begin during the first. Either way, it may present another long, drawn-out problem for the expectant mother, with nasal discharge, congestion, and sinus blockage often resulting in a sinus infection that may persist or recur repeatedly until after delivery in spite of vigorous treatment. The nasal swelling and sinus blockage is considered to be mainly due to hormonal changes, particularly with regard to estrogens and progesterone, although it may be greatly enhanced by previous sinus problems resulting in scarring, by nasal airway abnormalities, by fluid retention during pregnancy, by breathing irritating inhalants such as tobacco smoke, and even by some superimposed allergy problem that may sometimes become intensified during pregnancy. Examination of a nasal smear for an eosinophile count is a good noninvasive way of determining if there is a superimposed allergic rhinitis as well. A blood sample for specific IgE antibodies would also be helpful with this diagnosis, but skin testing with needle pricks may not be advisable during pregnancy because of the danger of a generalized allergic reaction.

If you have an accompanying cloudy nasal discharge during pregnancy usually indicating sinusitis, neither you nor your OB doctor should assume that the whole problem will just disappear with delivery, because a sinus infection lasting this long may often become chronic. Even though the sinus infection may tend to recur, taking a safe antibiotic each time it develops will usually prevent chronic scarring of the sinuses and their drainage openings. As always, any medications taken during pregnancy should first have the approval of your obstetrician. The use of a decongestant spray or tablet, especially in half-strength pediatric dosage even for fairly short periods, may provide some relief and sometimes enhance or prolong the effectiveness of the antibiotic therapy by affording better drainage. If you buy the decongestant pills over the counter, you should make certain they are a singular medication and preferably do not also contain an antihistamine or other drugs. The tendency for a pregnant woman with rhinitis to use a decongestant nasal spray too frequently and for too long a period should definitely be discouraged. Substituting a saline nasal spray intermittently may provide additional relief and encouragement.

Although no medication can be declared totally safe for everyone, especially during pregnancy, the decongestant oral medication of pseudoephedrine, especially in half-strength dosage, has generally been considered relatively safe for limited periods during pregnancy provided there are no physical contraindications such as high blood pressure in the expectant mother. However, some of the other decongestants have apparently been associated with increased fetal malformations. Since the nasal steroid sprays often used in the treatment of allergic and nonallergic rhinitis can be partially absorbed into the circulating blood and may cross the placental barrier, taking them during pregnancy should be done with caution, as they might conceivably present a problem for the fetus. If you do use them, you should do so only with the approval of your obstetrician and only if the potential benefits to you outweigh any possible risks to the fetus, which at present are considered to be minimal although still mostly unknown. Cromolyn nasal spray, which is very effective in allergic rhinitis and has an excellent safety record, is now available over the counter, and some have found it useful in a truly allergic rhinitis during pregnancy. A minor drawback is having to use it as often as four to six times a day for best results. Here again, it should be used only with your OB doctor's approval and only if clearly needed. Cromolyn will not shrink swollen nasal membranes, so a decongestant spray or tablet may be needed as well. As previously mentioned, the preferred treatment for any superimposed allergy would still be avoidance of the allergen as well as any primary inhalant irritants such as cigarette and cigar smoke.

The expectant mother may obtain some relief of nasal congestion or at least minimize it by sleeping elevated on a 7-inch foam wedge with a pillow on top of that, but again only with the approval of the OB doctor, since this arrangement might crowd the abdomen, particularly in an obese person. This elevated position of the chest and head would improve the drainage of venous blood from the head, which should reduce nasal or sinus swelling and thereby improve sinus drainage. Elevation of the head alone on two pillows is usually not sufficient and may cause positional neck problems from too much flexion.

The expectant mother with rhinitis should also be aware that if a persistent sinus infection can be avoided and any recurrent sinus flare-ups treated each time they occur, then significant sinus damage can probably be prevented, and her nasal congestion should mostly resolve itself within a week or two following her delivery. Unfortunately, I have examined a number of patients whose sinusitis went untreated during pregnancy and who ended up with chronic sinus disease. Needle puncture with irrigation of an infected maxillary sinus containing pus may sometimes be necessary during pregnancy and often results in dramatic relief of symptoms. However, to avoid radiation exposure, the diagnosis and need for this may have to be determined by the history and clinical findings rather than with the aid of sinus X rays or even a limited CAT scan. Diminished transillumination of the sinus, pain in the cheek or upper teeth on that side, sometimes cheek tenderness, and occasionally a sensation of something moving in the cheek on bending over or walking down steps will often make the diagnosis and indicate the need for surgical drainage. Although sonograms are sometimes used to identify fluid in a sinus cavity, this can be expensive and is often not covered by insurance.

If you have experienced the rhinitis of pregnancy, it doesn't necessarily mean that you will have a similar problem with subsequent pregnancies, but preventing permanent sinus scarring with the first occurrence is your best assurance of fewer sinus problems later.

VASOMOTOR OR NONALLERGIC HYPERREACTIVE RHINITIS

Swelling and blockage of the nose may sometimes result from what some believe to be a type of nerve imbalance, not well understood but commonly known as vasomotor rhinitis, although now it is often referred to as nonallergic hyperreactive rhinitis. It usually produces a clear watery discharge with a partial or complete nasal obstruction that may be chronic or intermittent, involve one or both sides of the nose, and may sometimes alternate from one side to the other. With this condition, the nasal membranes may become inflamed, and although quite unrelated to any allergic stimuli, their early appearance would often suggest an allergic reaction due to histamine release. This condition of so-called vasomotor rhinitis has often been blamed in the past for nasal congestion, swelling, sneezing, and a clear discharge when no other cause could be found.

ATROPHIC RHINITIS

Another poorly understood form of nonallergic rhinitis, less debilitating now thanks to antibiotics, but still causing chronic sinusitis and continuous distress to those so afflicted, is atrophic rhinitis. This condition results from an unexplained degenerative process in the nose with wasting or atrophy of the mucous membranes, mucous glands, and even the bony structures and soft tissues of the turbinates, which many sinus specialists consider to be essential to proper nasal function. With atrophic rhinitis, this shrinkage of the turbinates often creates too large a breathing passage, which may accelerate the drying effect on the nasal membranes, frequently resulting in loss of cilia, crusting, scabbing, a greenish infected discharge, occasional bleeding, and often a foul odor called ozena. Self-irrigations with normal saline solution, saline sprays, and periodic antibiotic therapy will often provide some relief, but cures are rare.

INFECTIOUS RHINITIS

Finally, there is a group of rhinitis sufferers whose irritated, swollen, and inflamed nasal membranes are the result of harboring infectious organisms such as viruses, bacteria, and fungi, and this condition is known as infectious rhinitis. These cases are nearly always associated with sinus infections and may even lead to chronic infection of the lower respiratory tract and lungs as well. It is not uncommon for a chronic infectious process in the upper airway, nose, and sinuses, over a period of time, to involve the lower airway's bronchi and lungs, and vice versa, since bacteria may travel from one end of the respiratory tract to the other on moisture droplets and not usually, as some believe, by swallowing or aspiration of an infected postnasal drip.

FOREIGN BODIES

Rhinitis due to a retained foreign body in the nose should also be mentioned because a delayed diagnosis and removal will nearly always cause a protracted sinus infection. This should always be suspected, especially in a child, when an infected cloudy discharge develops on only one side of the nose and fails to respond completely to treatment. It may also cause a very offensive odor, especially if the foreign body has been present for a while. Some nasal foreign objects that children tend to insert in their nostrils—and which I have had occasion to remove—are peas, buttons, lima beans, pearls, pebbles, plugs of wool, cotton, paper, plastic objects, peanuts, popcorn, beads, dimes, sticks, broom straws, small feathers, pencil erasers, and calcified nasal stones called rhinoliths, which usually develop from calcium and magnesium salt deposits around foreign matter or in chronically infected tissue. I have also found and removed a meconium plug from newborn intestinal discharge, fungus balls, a small branch of a Christmas tree, and on one occasion a bean that had been there so long it had sprouted. A doctor should remove all such objects as soon as possible and carefully search both nasal passages for other hidden secrets. In such instances, usually very prolonged antibiotic therapy for the associated sinusitis is essential, again depending on how long the foreign body and its associated sinus infection have been present.

HAY FEVER OR POLLINOSIS

You can see from this discussion of rhinitis that there are many different kinds with many different initiating causes, and any of them is capable of precipitating or prolonging a flare-up of sinus infection. Certainly seasonal allergic rhinitis, or hay fever, as it is often called, is the most heralded, since it strikes so many people at almost the same time, with such obviously disturbing symptoms usually initiated by the same agent, namely airborne pollen, whose daily presence in our environment is monitored by the press and trumpeted on TV. Pollen is the fertilizing element or male seed of flowering plants, grasses, weeds, and trees. It consists of fine, mostly yellowish grains measuring from 3 to approximately 100 microns in size (a micron being one-millionth of a meter, and the average hair measuring approximately 60 microns in diameter). The airborne type of pollen is mostly 15 to 50 microns in size. It is transported to the stigma, or female sex organ, of another plant by insects, some birds, air currents, and the wind, hopefully to the same species if it is to fertilize successfully. A fine steady rain will beat down or diminish the pollen in the air and also dampen its release from the anther, the pollen-bearing part of a plant's stamen. A hot sun will dry out the anther, allowing the pollen to escape and blow in the wind. Cloudy, humid, and windless days, especially after a steady rain, are usually better for the pollen sufferer, especially for outdoor exercising as far as the pollen count is concerned. Bright sunny breezy mornings in pollen season may be especially troublesome, and like ozone, pollen's pollution of the air we breathe is very much weather related.

When the pollen count is high, allergic individuals, especially those prone to sinusitis, should do their exercising indoors with the windows and doors closed. If you have to be outside, wearing an appropriate mask may be of considerable benefit. Of course, the ozone level should also be taken into consideration when you exercise outdoors, since this irritating pollutant can also cause upper or lower respiratory problems and should be avoided in warm weather and bright sunlight, especially during heavy traffic hours. Most people with chronic lung disease will not be happy exercising out of doors under either of these conditions, especially if the humidity is too high or even too low. If it is too high, it will dilute the available oxygen, and if it is low, it will thicken mucous secretions in the respiratory tract and lungs.

The cause of most seasonal allergic rhinitis is limited primarily to the pollens from numerous trees, grasses, and weeds, since the heavier pollens of flowers and shrubs are rarely windblown far enough or in sufficient quantities to cause a problem and must therefore depend on birds, bees, or other insects for their pollinating. Because there are so many different trees, grasses, and weeds scattered throughout the world, injectable allergen extracts, concentrates, and mixtures of the many different pollens used in immunotherapy for seasonal allergic rhinitis number in the hundreds, and as many or more injectables are manufactured for treatment of nonseasonal allergic rhinitis as well.

Desensitizing shots for allergy, now called immunotherapy, may be recommended when avoidance, environmental controls, antihistamines, corticosteroids, decongestants, and Cromolyn and steroid nasal sprays are unsuccessful. This means starting with a very small dose of an allergen, previously identified by skin tests or blood studies, usually given once or twice a week at first, then gradually increasing the dosage as well as the intervals between shots, finally ending with a regimen of a shot every 3 or 4 weeks, with the idea of gradually making the immune system more accustomed to, or more tolerant of, a particular allergen. In response to these shots, the body's immune system may produce an increase in immunoglobulin G (IgG), a blocking or protecting antibody, with a suppression of the common allergen antibody IgE usually following an initial rise at the beginning of therapy. This regimen seems to be effective in 60 to 75 percent of people with allergies to pollen, mold spores, dust mites, and dog or cat dander. It may take 6 months or sometimes longer before you note significant improvement, and the full treatment may require 3 to 5 years or more. If symptoms should recur after that, further injections for sustained relief may be necessary, usually on a monthly basis for an indefinite period. Whenever possible, shots should be given under medical supervision, since in rare instances life-threatening anaphylactic shock could occur. For this reason, some recommend waiting in the doctor's office for at least a half hour afterward and keeping an epinephrine syringe close by on the way home. Immunotherapy for the allergic individual administered by drops under the tongue or by a nasal spray would certainly be more convenient and much safer, but so far, both appear unreliable, just as immunotherapy shots for food allergies have also been mostly unsuccessful.

The term "hay fever," ascribed to seasonal allergic rhinitis, is probably not the best choice, since many use the term to identify any kind of nasal allergy, and especially since it is rarely the result of exposure to hay, nor does it produce a significant fever unless it is complicated by some kind of infection. There is no doubt that some individuals could be allergic to hay, but that usually results from hay dust in a barn or loft, where mold and fungal spores are very prevalent as well.

"Pollinosis," on the other hand, would seem to describe pollen-induced seasonal allergic rhinitis more accurately. Attacks are mostly initiated by airborne pollen during the pollinating seasons starting with various trees in the spring, grasses and some weeds during late spring and early summer, followed by weed pollens, especially ragweed, in the fall, and usually continuing until the first frost. Goldenrod, which blooms at the same time as ragweed, was once blamed for fall allergies until it was realized that goldenrod's pollen is carried mostly by bees or other insects and not so easily borne on the wind as ragweed pollen. The much-maligned goldenrod, on the other hand, has been used since early times for medicinal purposes as a diuretic, digestive stimulant, and fever reducer, as well as to treat burns, rheumatism, and diarrhea.

Some hay fever sufferers who live in the eastern United States temperate zone find it generally easier to associate the onset of their pollen difficulties with major holidays. Tree pollen allergies start around Easter, grass pollen close to Memorial Day, and ragweed on Labor Day or shortly thereafter. Geographical locations and corresponding growing seasons will naturally affect the time of onset and duration of seasonal allergies as well as the types of pollen you encounter. If you are allergic to certain kinds of pollen, you should always consider this in traveling to other parts of the country or from one country to another.

MOLDS AND FUNGI

Occasionally, airborne fungal or mold spores may confuse the pollen picture, especially if you live near damp river bottoms, lake shores, or coastal areas and are allergic to them. A mold is a filamentous fungus and breathing any of their spores could initiate an attack of allergic rhinitis sometimes followed by sinusitis. Fungus and mold season starts mainly with the rainy spring weather, then continues throughout the entire summer and well into the winter months, often not ending until the first snowfall, and many times starting up again after it melts. Compost piles and garbage dumps also serve as outside mold producers and for that reason should be located downwind and well away from the house. Mold or fungal spores are often found inside the house as well. They grow on houseplants, on their dead leaves, and in their damp soil. They may even grow on the flakes of skin or dandruff that we constantly shed from our bodies and scalps. Dark, damp basements, especially those with exposed concrete walls or floors, are particularly attractive to mold growth, and any stagnant water in sump pumps or humidifiers is equally enticing. Molds may be present on old refrigerated food and even on food in the freezer. Unrefrigerated fruits, potatoes, and vegetables attract molds and fungi, and they love cheeses. They grow very actively in the drainage pans beneath some refrigerators. More than a dozen different fungi or molds, including some that resemble very tiny mushrooms, have been cultured from patients with fungal sinusitis.

Although the mechanism for nasal membrane swelling, inflammation, and watery discharge in certain types of nonallergic rhinitis may not be clearly understood, the whole process of an allergic reaction, even though it may vary greatly in different areas of the body, is very clearly recognized. What isn't so clearly understood is why the very same allergen may cause bronchial spasm or asthma in the lungs of one individual, whereas in another it may cause an allergic rhinitis, or in still another, an intestinal upset or sometimes hives on the skin, and with still others, eye, face, and lip swelling, sometimes with wheezing, or swelling of the tongue and larynx, thus creating the frightening possibility of airway obstruction. A few very unlucky individuals may have all of these symptoms occurring at approximately the same time following exposure to a single allergen, and some may even develop anaphylactic shock. However, the intensity of the allergic reaction may vary significantly among individuals and even from time to time in the same individual, often becoming worse with frequent subsequent exposures and sometimes less intense with a prolonged absence from exposure.

Allergic rhinitis can cause an acute flare-up of sinusitis and, if prolonged and untreated for an entire season, may even transform an acute sinus infection into a subacute or chronic one. Its presence should be suspected in any case of chronic sinusitis or in any acute or subacute case that doesn't respond to treatment, especially in children. It is also important that both you and your physician look for the telltale cloudy discharge usually indicating a superimposed sinus infection and not assume that the symptoms are entirely allergic and will therefore disappear some months later when the allergy goes away. Both should be treated vigorously, since the combination of allergic rhinitis and sinus infection can be stubborn and sometimes very difficult to control. If you have a persistent nasal allergy and infected sinus drainage, you should also be checked periodically for possible nasal or sinus polyp formation, which can further obstruct sinus drainage to cause chronic sinus disease as well as loss of the sense of smell. In a few instances, the excessive accumulation of eosinophilic white blood cells in the mucous secretions of a person with allergic rhinitis may create a slightly cloudy discharge sometimes suggesting a superimposed sinus infection and could occasionally confuse the diagnosis.

EOSINOPHILS

Eosinophils are white blood cells that can be identified under the microscope by a special eosin stain. Although they may travel in the blood, they are far more prevalent in body tissues. They are frequently involved in immune disorders, allergic reactions, drug sensitivities, and some tissue-reactive diseases including psoriasis and cat-scratch disease, as well as Hodgkin's disease, malaria, mononucleosis, fungus diseases, some cancers (especially ovarian), as well as certain leukemias. Eosinophils seem to have their own diurnal rhythm levels with high counts during the night and with lows during the day. They are usually acutely responsive in the delayed phase of allergic rhinitis and asthma, as well as some parasitic diseases or worm infestations, and various drug reactions. They kill bacteria, but apparently not as effectively as some of the other white blood cells. They are thought to excrete a toxin against parasites and may congregate locally in body tissues in response to an allergic reaction, especially in the nose, from which they can be smeared and counted. The presence of an abundance of eosinophils in a nasal smear would strongly suggest a nasal allergy, although occasionally they may be abundantly present in some cases of nonallergic rhinitis and may sometimes be relatively absent in a few people who have allergic rhinitis with chronic sinusitis, especially in a child.

NASAL HYPERREACTIVITY AND REACTIVE LOWER AIRWAY DISEASE

Both allergic and nonallergic rhinitis may occasionally initiate or accompany a state of heightened nonallergic upper airway sensitivity known as hyperreactivity. In this condition, the nasal membranes may continue to react excessively with varying degrees of inflammation, swelling, watery discharge, and sometimes sneezing to often very minimal amounts of an irritating pollutant in the air and sometimes long after their priming effects or that of any allergic stimulus may have passed. Such irritants include cigarette and cigar smoke, smog, acid rain, perfumes or other strong odors, and even some that might be introduced locally such as cocaine, snuff, some eyedrops, and certain nasal sprays. Hyperreactivity could present a continuing problem not only if you have allergic rhinitis, but especially if you have nonallergic rhinitis, since if untreated or if the irritant can't be avoided, it could lead to a chronic progressive nasal inflammation, swelling, and sinus blockage resulting in chronic rhinosinusitis.

On the other hand, reactive lower airway disease, which has long been recognized as a factor in many cases of asthma and in some cases of chronic bronchitis, represents a state of increased responsiveness of the membranous linings and surrounding muscles of the lower air passages, or bronchi, in certain susceptible individuals and usually results in a persistent inflammatory swelling, bronchial spasms, wheezing, and coughing, often with a reduction in rapid airflow from the lungs. Once started, it too may continue to develop from repeated but very minimal exposures to certain airborne respiratory irritants or allergens, and the entire process may often originate from a viral respiratory infection such as a cold or flu, especially from those occurring in early life.

This reactive lower airway condition, as well as upper airway nonallergic hyperreactivity, may occur together in the same person. Very often, either condition may be diagnosed by applying measured doses of histamine or a parasympathetic nerve stimulant called methacholine to the upper or lower airway membranes and recording their response. Such a test might also prove useful in detecting latent asthma or in predicting the future development of clinical asthma in some people who have allergic rhinitis or nonallergic hyperreactive rhinitis, especially since a number of individuals with allergic rhinitis, particularly of the year-round kind, will also develop lower airway reactivity. In such cases, sinusitis can be a contributing factor but is probably more often secondary to the reactive airway disease.

CONTROLLING AND TREATING HYPERREACTIVE RHINITIS

For most people, the best means of reducing nasal hyperreactivity would be to conscientiously avoid irritating pollutants as well as any suspected allergens. Steroid nasal sprays are very effective in controlling the nasal symptoms of allergic rhinitis and may also be helpful in soothing hyperreactive nasal membranes as well as in suppressing early nasal polyp formation.

Cromolyn nasal spray, which is now available over the counter for the treatment of allergic rhinitis, is effective in suppressing histamine activity, and even more so in combination with an oral antihistamine, but neither is effective in controlling reactive airway disease, reducing nasal swelling, or in discouraging nasal polyp formation. To be completely effective in allergic rhinitis, Cromolyn spray should be started well before the allergy begins and then used as often as three to six times a day compared to once or twice a day for steroid nasal sprays. Other corticosteroid medications such as cortisone, prednisone, or prednisolone, by mouth or sometimes initially by shot, may be necessary in stabilizing more severe cases of reactive airway disease, especially when asthma-like wheezing with significant impairment of lower airway function is involved. Antihistamines, including the new non-sedating kinds, are not generally considered effective in blocking the irritant factor in nasal membranes, nor would they be expected to improve nonallergic hyperreactive airways. This also appears to be true for the antihistamine nasal sprays, but they can be useful in blocking histamine activity in the nose of individuals with allergic rhinitis, often with a significant improvement in sneezing, watery eyes, itching, and rhinorrhea and usually with little or no burning sensation. In using this nasal spray, some people have noticed a bitter taste, and a few may experience sleepiness or headache.

Even though the benefits from steroid nasal sprays in allergic rhinitis and nonallergic nasal hyperreactivity are very substantial, they are occasionally outweighed by increased irritation of nasal membranes due to the spray's chemical contents, gas propellant, prolonged use, or sometimes just too frequent usage. A slight nasal burning or stinging sensation, sometimes a nosebleed, and occasionally a headache or sore throat may accompany their use. However, if the burning sensation should persist for very long between treatments and especially if bleeding is noted, it could be a warning of too much nasal membrane irritation and could result in tissue erosion followed in some instances by a nasal septal perforation.

Tilting the spray nozzle slightly away from the midline nasal septum and upward in the general direction of the eye may lessen septal irritation and bleeding as well as the chances of permanent tissue damage. Unfortunately, the area away from the septum and beneath the middle turbinate, where the ethmoids, maxillary, and frontal sinuses drain, known as the ostiomeatal complex (OMC), is generally considered to be the most sensitive part of the nose. Directly exposing the OMC to an irritating spray may cause an increase in nasal discomfort or headache and may in the long run be counterproductive. Using a saline nasal spray before or just after spraying with the steroid spray may lessen irritation or bleeding, but it may also tend to dilute the medication. When using or taking any corticosteroid medications by mouth or by spray, you should follow the directions explicitly to avoid overdosage and bodily harm. You should also remember that it takes several days for a steroid nasal spray to begin to work, and often 10 days to 2 weeks for maximum results. Neither the steroid nasal sprays nor any other allergy treatment or medications, however, should be considered a substitute for maximum efforts to control your exposure to known allergens in your environment.

CHAPTER FOURTEEN

Air Pollution and Sick Building Syndrome

POLLUTION

Pollution of the air you breathe often plays a significant role in sinus disease. It can also shorten your life and diminish your quality of life. This includes outside ground-level air pollution as well as the contaminated air inside your home, in the workplace, at school, on planes or boats, and even in the automobile.

Many times breathing polluted air will not only bring on an acute attack of sinusitis but, if the exposure persists, could even convert an acute or subacute sinusitis to chronic disease. A single short-lasting contact with a very irritating dust or chemical in the air might also prolong an existing sinus infection, especially if you have generally unhealthy sinuses. Even a person with healthy sinuses may soon become a chronic sinus sufferer after moving into a heavily polluted area or selecting a home downwind from a chemical plant, an airport, a large parking area, a main thoroughfare, or a grove of oak trees. Choosing a home with improper ventilation, faulty insulation, a drafty heating and air-conditioning system, or possibly one contaminated by mold in the basement, by allergens left behind by a former occupant's pets, by synthetic residue or dust mites in the carpeting, or by wood or plaster dusts in the ventilating system, may sometimes be all that is necessary to bring on a chronic rhinitis and chronic sinusitis. Because knowledge on this subject can be so critical to your health and happiness if you have an active or even potential case of sinusitis, a closer look at the air we breathe would seem important.

It may come as a surprise that something as common and seemingly benign as the daily use of air fresheners and deodorizers, hair sprays, perfumed soaps, scented tissues, perfumes, skin bracers, aftershaves, body lotions, and scented spray deodorants, or even simply turning the pages of a daily newspaper or cheaply printed magazine and breathing the ink dust ejected into the air, can, in some people, cause chronic irritation of the nose with swelling and sinus blockage followed by infection. I recall a number of instances in which a hair spray, even of the hypoallergenic type, kept a sinusitis or a cough going in spite of intensive therapy until the source of the problem was identified and removed. I also noted that some of these same patients, when brushing the dried spray dust from their hair hours later, would often experience another flare-up of nasal irritation, sneezing, congestion, and cough. In some instances, the hair spray also created a similar problem for the spouse from secondhand exposure to the hair spray in the air as well as to the fallout of dried hair spray on the pillow at night. In most instances, it was eventually possible to find a safe, unscented, and nonirritating spray, mostly through trial and error. Once they found one that was safe to use, however, my patients would often need to keep an extra bottle at the hairdresser's, since forgetting their spray and having to use a substitute could start the whole process over again. In selecting a proper hair spray, it is important to realize that hypoallergenic does not mean nonallergenic or even nonirritating to the respiratory membranes and the sinuses.

If exposure to such irritants should continue on a daily basis for certain hypersensitive individuals, chronic rhinitis, chronic sinus infection, chronic eye irritations, and even chronic lung infection could ensue even when no truly allergic problem exists. In such cases, steroidal nose sprays may help to mask the nasal symptoms, and antibiotics may control the sinus infection for a while, but unless the source of daily irritation is removed, this individual could join the ranks of the chronic sinus sufferer.

Pollution of the environment to a large degree means contamination of the air we breathe by noxious gases, all kinds of volatile substances, various molds and pollens, as well as a variety of particulate matter such as dust, powders, soot, chemicals, smoke, volcanic ash, and desert sands. Other mostly household pollutants would include a great variety of sprays, powders, dusts, volatile oils, scented body lotions, deodorants, soaps, detergents, cleaners, solvents, pesticides, smoke, shampoo, and various perfumes. To observe a subtle household pollutant, all you have to do is to tear a paper towel or a piece of double-layered toilet tissue in front of a lightbulb or an infrared lamp or within a bright ray of sunshine to see the tremendous amount of particle matter ejected into the air. Moreover, if the tissue is of the scented type, breathing those particles on a daily basis could cause a rhinitis in the overly sensitive nose.

OZONE AND SMOG

Outside ground-level pollutants, other than pollen, various aerosols, mold, and fine-particle dusts, including sulfates, that should be of particular concern to those with chronic lung disease or sinusitis are nitrogen oxides, which form ozone. Ozone may irritate respiratory membranes to possibly cause or aggravate an existing rhinitis, sinusitis, or bronchitis, as well as to eventually impair cilia function. Ozone is produced mainly from engine exhausts and industrial emissions, which may sometimes travel for long distances on westerly winds before finally settling out. It is formed when volatile organic compounds, or VOCs, mainly from gasoline fumes, solvents, printer's inks, industrial chemicals, and paints, react with nitrogen oxides emitted by the burning of fossil fuels such as coal and petroleum products and in the presence of hot overhead sun rays. Since cold weather, clouds, and rain tend to reduce ozone, it is generally considered to be a weather-related pollutant of our environment.

It would be very helpful, indeed, if our overabundance of this offensive ground-level ozone could be used to replenish our protective ozone layer far above the Earth, but unfortunately it breaks down before it can ever reach the stratosphere. At ground level, however, by combining with moisture in the air and with other pollutants in the presence of bright sunlight during the warmer months, ozone forms the hazy brownish yellow cloud commonly known as smog we often see over our industrial areas or settling into our valleys. "Smog," as you would expect, is a combination of the words "smoke" and "fog," and it forms when moisture vapor condenses on fine particles of smoke or chemical wastes in the air. Although smog is composed of moisture droplets, various particle pollutants, and other gaseous chemical contaminants beside ozone, its concentration, or density, is more accurately measured by the amount of ozone present and is reported as the ozone index or air quality index. Ozone is used as the standard indicator of air pollution in most industrialized or heavy-traffic areas during the warm season. Until recently, a reading higher than 120 parts per billion or 0.12 parts per million averaged over a 1-hour period was considered unhealthy. However, for people with respiratory or heart problems, it is now realized that an even lower reading can be harmful to their health. With this in mind, the upper limit of the ozone safety level has now been lowered to 0.08 parts per million.

INDOOR AND OUTDOOR POLLUTANTS

All of us are exposed to varying amounts of air pollutants on an almost daily basis, but unless we are truly allergic to them, encounter them in excessive amounts, or are exposed to smaller amounts repeatedly over a very prolonged period, our respiratory tracts, when healthy, can usually tolerate pollutants fairly well. However, the accumulated damaging effects on our respiratory tracts and sinuses from repeated exposures to smaller amounts of certain pollutants may take many years to determine. That is why you should preferably use sprays outside, where they will be diluted by the surrounding air, or, if inside, with some form of exhaust system. When using hair sprays, bathroom sprays, oven sprays, and spray deodorants, you should hold your breath, walk away before taking another breath, and then not return to the area until the spray droplets have been exhausted or have had a chance to settle. If the room does have an exhaust fan, by all means turn it on before spraying. Reliable masks should be worn when sawing, sanding, grass cutting, plant spraying, leaf raking, leaf blowing, cleaning gutters, removing ashes, remodeling old buildings, paint spraying, pitching hay, cleaning attics and basements, and with any kind of heavy dusting in general, remembering of course that a different size dust particle or a different spray may require an entirely different mask or filter. If you have sinusitis, and especially if you have a known allergy to mold, do your leaf raking or leaf blowing while wearing a good mask and try to do it very soon after the leaves fall and before they become damp or moldy.

It is always disturbing to see a professional carpenter sanding plaster, fiberglass, metal, or wood without any kind of dust mask, and especially to see someone spraying fruit trees or a grape arbor with a toxic pesticide and wearing nothing but an ordinary "dog mask."

Even when emptying a shop vac, you should wear a reliable mask or at least hold your breath, and you should always empty the vacuum outside and downwind. If there is no wind, you should walk away quickly while still holding your breath. When removing ashes from the fireplace, you should keep the flue open and a window or door cracked to obtain some updraft, and again you should wear a mask.

FINE-PARTICLE POLLUTANTS

Much of the very fine dust or powdered substances that you are exposed to is easily suspended in air, is mostly invisible except when it collects together to form a cloud, and can very readily irritate your nose and sinuses or find its way deep into your lungs to cause future problems. It is now generally felt that fine particles smaller than 10 microns may penetrate the deep recesses of the lungs, and in many instances, the smaller the particle, the more serious the consequences as far as the lungs are concerned. Most mold spores measure from 3 to 10 microns, whereas the larger pollen particles may vary in size from 10 to 100 microns or more. (By comparison, the average human hair is approximately 60 microns in diameter, and a normal red blood corpuscle will measure 7 microns across; a micron is one-millionth of a meter, or 1/25,000 of an inch). Very fine dust particles may measure 2.5 microns or less, and these should be of the greatest concern to us, since they may be responsible for 50,000 deaths a year in this country. Fortunately, much of the fine-particle pollution as well as the heavier gasses in our atmosphere is prevented from layering or settling out near the ground by the constant swirling of air currents that we call weather, the most formidable force on Earth. It should be emphasized, however, that even larger particles floating in the air, especially those that dissolve in water or mucous secretions, can just as easily irritate the nose and cause sinusitis. The larger particles are also more inclined to filter out in the nose or upper airway, being more easily trapped in the nasal mucous blanket and seldom traveling as far as the lower respiratory tract or lungs.

EFFECT ON THE NOSE AND SINUSES

We normally think of the dust and gaseous pollution we breathe as passing through the nose into the throat and lungs without in any way entering the sinuses tucked away in their very protected locations, and this is generally true. However, the nasal resistance to airflow caused by the narrowed nasal valve area in the front of the nose, the turbulence in the airstream caused by the nasal turbinates, and the pressure differences created within the nose by breathing in and breathing out can not only work a plug of mucus that the cilia have been unable to dislodge through a sinus opening and into the nose but also move fine dust particles or irritating fumes in a to-and-fro fashion near to, or just within, a sinus opening, causing it to become inflamed and swollen. A similar problem may arise when membrane-irritating dust particles, caught in the nasal airstream, are deflected toward a sinus opening by a deviated nasal septum or tend to collect behind a septal spur or a misshapen turbinate, not unlike debris collecting behind a rock or log in a flowing river or stream. Such an accumulation of irritating particle matter, especially when close to a sinus drainage opening, can cause inflammatory swelling with sinus blockage and infection.

A healthy nose and sinuses, on the other hand, will usually tolerate irritating contaminants to a greater degree and in larger concentrations, being less inclined to collect them in their nasal passages and also better able to expel them with the mucous flow. Individuals with healthy sinuses are usually nasal breathers with no impressive nasal airway abnormalities, who also have a smooth and fairly even flow of air through both sides of the nose and without the tendency for any irritating particulate matter or fumes to be misdirected toward a sinus opening. Their sinonasal air exchange, although normally rather limited, would be free and uninterrupted. Their mucus production is usually plentiful, flows freely without damming up, is not dried out by a misguided airsteam, and is therefore usually very effective in preventing membrane penetration by bacterial and viral invaders. They also readily expel all foreign contaminants and infective organisms from their nasal passages, sinuses, and lower respiratory tract into the throat to be swallowed and later disposed of by the stomach acid and enzymes. Finally, a healthy nose and sinuses would not contain an excessive amount of scarring from prolonged sinus infections in the past or from extensive sinonasal surgery or injury. Excessive scar tissue makes it more difficult to control infection, since it can block drainage openings and also impair blood supply. Impaired blood supply to a nose or sinus would then make it more difficult to prevent nasal or sinus membrane swelling, or to diminish it once it occurs.

On the other hand, if you have imperfect upper or lower respiratory tracts and sinuses, or have an allergy or hypersensitivity to a certain contaminant in the air, you can usually expect harmful effects from even relatively small doses of a particular pollutant. Some nonallergic individuals may also find that their respiratory tract membranes, especially those within the nose and bronchi, react to almost any persistent irritant with a somewhat progressive exaggerated inflammatory response usually indicative of a condition known as hyperreactivity and frequently resulting in a persistent rhinitis, sinusitis, or bronchitis.

If the lower respiratory tract and lungs are damaged by prolonged pollution exposure to the point of chronic irritation and infection, then the nose and sinuses will very likely become involved as well, since it would be a fairly uncommon occurrence to have a chronic infection in one end of the respiratory tract without it eventually involving the other. Unfortunately, most of the studies with regard to the effects of pollution on the respiratory tract have to do with the lungs and not with the nose or sinuses, but I would like to emphasize that I have observed numerous cases in which pollution of one kind or another played a major role in the development of an acute or chronic sinusitis.

EFFECT ON THE BODY

A very extensive Public Health study from Harvard carried out in the 1980s and supported by others found that people who live and breathe the air in the United States' more polluted cities have a 15 to 17 percent greater chance of dying prematurely from heart and lung diseases than those who breathe the air in the nation's cleaner cities, possibly shortening many lives by several years or more. These studies are mainly concerned with breathing very fine particulate matter often showing an acid ph and including sulfates especially. They usually measure 2.5 microns or less in diameter, and their very small size makes it possible for them to be breathed into the furthermost regions of our lungs, where there may be no cilia or mucous secretions to sweep them out. It is also felt that 15 years or more exposure to this very fine particulate pollution may produce the more serious results. These findings also take into consideration other mortality risks such as alcohol consumption, smoking, hazardous occupations, race, age, sex, and past medical history, with the risks about equal for men and women. Breathing fine-particle pollution has also been partly blamed for an increase in childhood asthma as well as for an increase in heart and lung problems in the elderly or chronically ill. Even the dangerous and harmful effects of smoking, including emphysema and lung cancer, may be greatly magnified by inhaling fine-particle pollution for many people who live in large industrial cities where sulfates, which make up the largest concentration of fine particles, are mainly to blame. For some years, the Environmental Protection Agency has been regulating the emissions of particle matter 10 microns in diameter or larger. Now, realizing the many dangers of breathing even finer particles, the EPA is beginning to regulate fine particles as small as 2.5 microns, or 1/24 the diameter of the average human hair. Unfortunately, there is no safe level for fine-particle pollution of any size.

Fine particles, like many other pollutants, come from industrial smokestacks, from coal-burning electrical-generating plants, from mining and construction work, from the combustion of gas and oil products, from forest, field, and everglade burning, and even from deserts and volcanoes located throughout the world. Fine particles are often present in higher concentrations in warmer air and about the same time that ground-level ozone readings are elevated, which gives a combined effect to unhealthy respiratory tracts or sinuses. In the cooler months, when smog is mostly absent, this fine-particle pollution may often form a light gray to whitish haze over our industrial cities and dwellings compared to the brownish yellow-tinged cloud of smog usually noted during the warmer weather. Moreover, fine particles may unfortunately enter our homes rather easily along with almost any form of airflow through doorways, flues, cracks, and crannies.

With regard to your nose and sinuses, both fine and coarse particles can be very irritating to the membranes of the upper respiratory tract as well. As already indicated, a lot depends on their concentration, the duration of exposure, the efficiency of the mucous flow, where in the nose they tend to collect, if they contain a chemical substance that is very irritating to nasal membranes, whether they dissolve in water and therefore in mucous secretions, and finally whether you have an actual allergy or unusual sensitivity to any part of the particulate matter.

Open fireplaces and woodstoves have long been important sources of indoor and outdoor pollution, not only for carbon monoxide and nitrogen dioxide, but especially for fine particles. During the winter months, residential wood smoke probably produces as much particle pollution over well-populated areas as coal-burning electric power plants some miles away. Indoor particle pollution from faulty stove or fireplace drafts, back drafts, and the sweeping or removal of ashes may also contribute heavily to the unhealthy state of some household occupants by causing nose, throat, or sinus irritation, and the very fine residue may even remain in some people's lungs for indefinite periods. It has also been noted that children living in homes heated by woodstoves seem to have more upper and lower respiratory infections.

CAR ALLERGENS

Dust, pollen, and very fine particle matter may also be stirred up from the floor mats in cars by blower vents and the shuffling of feet. You should keep car windows closed in pollinating season for the same reason. You may not be allergic to pollen, but you may have given someone a ride who is. If you are inclined to keep a dirty car, you should make a point to vacuum it periodically, and by doing so you may save your family and friends a sinus flare-up. Removing pollen and moldy leaves from the automobile air intake vent at the base of the windshield might also benefit an allergic or sinus-prone passenger. Fortunately, automobile companies are now providing special dust-filtering systems that will trap fine particles as small as 3 microns, or approximately one-twentieth the thickness of a human hair. Unfortunately, very fine dust particles may be many times smaller than 3 microns and therefore able to pass through these filters. However, purchasing one of these air-filtering systems for your car could save you money in doctor bills and medications, especially if you are allergic to molds or pollen.

Most of us like the smell of a new car, but for some, it may represent a source of nasal and sinus irritation hidden in the upholstery, carpeting, plastic trim, plastic ventilating ducts, glues, sealants, and insulations. There are very few areas where we spend so much time that have such a collection of plastics and other synthetics in so small a space. Some of the chemicals used in the formulation and processing of these synthetic materials give off a gaseous residue such as formaldehyde, which can dissolve in water or mucus and cause irritation of the nose, lower respiratory tract, and sinuses in some people, especially if they spend long periods in the car.

FORMALDEHYDE

Formaldehyde fumes can also diminish mucous flow by depressing cilia activity. In such cases, introducing fresh air rather than recirculating the same air may be helpful especially until the new-car odor gradually dissipates. Even so, it may be difficult to separate these from other irritants that filter in from the outside, from the gas tank, and from engine exhausts, including the fumes from fresh paint burning off of a new engine.

A somewhat similar environmental problem occurred in some homes years ago when it was very popular to blow foam insulation into the walls. This insulation contained formaldehyde residue, which would sometimes cause irritation in the nose and sinuses of some of the occupants.

SICK BUILDING SYNDROME

On a very much larger scale, but somewhat along the same lines, is the still poorly understood sick building syndrome (SBS). This syndrome represents a complex range of symptoms experienced by a very significant number of office workers in certain fairly modern buildings with central ventilating systems, including central heating, air-conditioning, and humidification; sealed windows or no windows; some with extensive glass walls, and all usually with an abundance of synthetic building and decorating materials on furniture, floors, walls, and ceilings; and also containing various kinds of insulation, corking, weather stripping, adhesives, paint solvents, glues, and sealants throughout. It should be emphasized that plywood, laminated beams, shelving, some wood sidings, laminated doors, particle board, Formica tops, and even the secondary woods in desks, cabinets, and tables usually contain various types of glues and sealants as well. Many of them may emit solvent vapors, volatile organic compounds (VOCs), and formaldehyde fumes for a very long time after installation.

In sick buildings, the occupants' complaints may include irritation of the eyes, nose, and throat; headaches and stuffiness, dryness of the eyes, nose, and skin; nasal or sinus congestion and occasionally nosebleeds; itching and sometimes a rash; excessive fatigue and lack of concentration; and sometimes hoarseness, coughing, and wheezing. A few may complain of nausea and dizziness, and some may experience extreme tiredness and irritability. Although it has been possible to trace some building health problems to microbial contamination of ventilating systems, including fungal infestation, and even to bacterial involvement of the central air-conditioning system (as in Legionnaire's disease), or in some instances to the accumulation of automobile exhaust fumes from lower-level parking lots, many other buildings have so far avoided an adequate explanation for being "sick." Because these are mostly well-sealed buildings, this syndrome has often been attributed to lack of enough outside fresh air, resulting in a gradual accumulation of unhealthy contaminants within. Unfortunately, efforts to remove or dilute these air contaminants by increasing the fresh air exchange for extended periods have not consistently resulted in relief of symptoms for the sick building occupants.

Formaldehyde, a breakdown residue of many synthetic materials, is a known contaminant of many buildings, and every doctor knows how irritating this substance can be to the eyes, nose, throat, sinuses, and lungs from working with it in the tissue laboratory, where it is used as a specimen preservative. Its accumulation, even in fairly small amounts, along with other airborne respiratory tract irritants, could very well be a significant factor in sick building syndrome. Formaldehyde can also cause diminished cilia movement in the respiratory tract leading to rhinosinusitis and bronchitis.

Other possible contributors to sick buildings sometimes mentioned are improper heating and air-conditioning, inadequate humidification, an accumulation of frequently used electronic equipment, and extensive fluorescent lighting. Some have even considered the possibility that fairly insignificant symptoms, many times ignored, may become magnified by psychological factors to cause a kind of tempered mass hysteria, and this is certainly within the realm of human frailties. Worry or grave concern can also lead to nasal congestion and rhinitis or even accentuate an already existing rhinosinusitis. I had ample opportunity to observe this reaction in association with combat anxiety among our troops during the Korean War.

In the United States, sick building syndrome has been estimated to involve millions of workers in more than a million office buildings, making the syndrome a significant economic problem affecting efficiency, productivity, and absenteeism. Similar complaints have been encountered among office workers in many other industrialized nations throughout the world.

Judging from the number of respiratory tract symptoms experienced by most of the occupants of sick buildings, the offending agent or agents would almost have to be airborne and most likely inhaled into the body. Since inhaled airborne pollutants are usually eventually swallowed with the mucous secretions, they could subsequently produce nausea. Some could also settle out on any exposed skin to cause a rash with itching. However, both of these symptoms could also result from a chronic low-grade toxicity due to body absorption of an inhaled pollutant.

Since people who develop symptoms in a sick building are not limited to a particular floor or to a certain area, you might also assume that the gaseous or fine-particle matter responsible for the sickness, even though it may originate in a certain area such as a basement, shower room, or attic, is distributed throughout the building by means of the ventilating system used for heating, humidification, and air-conditioning. In some instances, it may even originate from within the ventilating system itself, having been inadvertently introduced into it during the building's construction, perhaps from the use of the air-cir-culating system on a very hot or cold day before any filters were installed. However, the very remote possibility that the offending sub-stance in some instances could arise from beneath the building, as finally realized with radon gas, or be admitted into the building through the outside air exchange or even from a central air-condi-tioning and humidification unit located on top of the building, as in the case of Legionnaire's disease, should not be totally ignored.

Nevertheless, it still appears that the more likely cause of most sick buildings, as well as most of the symptoms noted by their occupants, is the accumulation of some form of fine-particle matter or gaseous residues such as formaldehyde that are especially irritating to delicate eye and respiratory membranes and usually occur as breakdown prod-ucts of synthetic building or decorating materials. Another major con-tributing factor would be the presence of certain volatile organic compounds from glues, paint solvents, corking materials, adhesives, sealants, foams, resins, and plastics. Adding to the air pollution would be fumes from air fresheners, office equipment cleaners, aerosol sprays, waxing compounds, strippers, polishers, scented toilet deodor-ants, toilet cleaners, furnaces, insecticides and fungicides, not to men-tion the scented deodorants, body lotions, hair sprays, and perfumes of the many occupants and all trapped in a very tightly sealed modern building. Even the photocopiers, fax machines, and other electronic equipment can create ozone and, when mixed with the above, may create a kind of invisible office smog.

These inhaled irritants in the air, especially if you are daily almost continuously exposed to them, could prolong a low-grade undiag-nosed and untreated sinusitis, rhinitis, or bronchitis almost indefinitely and produce many of the symptoms complained of by the sick-build-ing occupants. Many cases of mildly symptomatic ethmoid sinusitis in particular are not so easily diagnosed and may frequently be over-looked. A few building occupants may also be allergic to some of the contaminants such as mold, dust mites, and cockroaches, whereas oth-ers with very sensitive respiratory tracts may develop hyperreactive membrane disease from constant exposure to inhaled irritants. Similar exposures at home or in the car while driving to and from work, some-times for long distances, might add further irritation to a very reactive upper or lower airway.

In this kind of environment, residual symptoms from a viral head cold or flu might tend to linger for a longer period, thus adding some additional symptoms and exacerbating others. An infected postnasal drip and a dry throat in a drafty low-humidity environment might also cause nausea. Excessive fatigue and a lack of concentration is not unusual if you have with a persistent rhinosinusitis; and neither are hoarseness, coughing, and sometimes wheezing very uncommon if you have a persistent rather mild bronchitis. Headaches, nasal congestion, and sometimes nosebleeds may also be noted with a low-grade chronic rhinosinusitis.

The usually very open working areas of these office buildings make them more subject to draftiness from central air-conditioning and forced-air heat, especially since their ventilating duct fans probably have to run more forcibly and more constantly to satisfy their spaciousness and often inappropriately located thermostats. Outside-wall floor-to-ceiling glass in some buildings often creates convection currents in cold weather, thus adding more draftiness to the area. This draftiness tends to dry out the eyes and especially the protective mucous blanket of the respiratory tract, making it more vulnerable to irritation as well as to infection. This can occur even with central humidification, which is so often inadequate, especially in a large open area. In smaller areas, however, unless your desk is directly exposed to the draft from an air-conditioning or heating vent, the expired lung and body moisture that you tend to partially recover through inhalation appears to be more consistently available.

Proper humidity in your immediate environment is very important not only to your comfort but also to your health, especially as far as your sinuses and respiratory tracts are concerned. In most instances, humidity is also the most difficult environmental factor to regulate properly, especially in a large, drafty area. The drying effects on mucous flow from exposure to a continuous draft can render your respiratory tract and sinuses more vulnerable to infection as well as more susceptible to any irritating fumes or particle pollutants in the air. A lack of humidity can also cause a very unpleasant dryness of the eyes and skin, especially during the winter months. On the other hand, leaking roofs and pipes, as well as poor ventilation, may cause an accumulation of humidity in ducts, walls, behind bathroom tiles, and in ceiling spaces, as well as beneath floors and carpeting, which can lead to growth of toxic molds and bacteria. This can result in biological contamination of buildings by way of their central ventilating systems.

In sick building syndrome, the most difficult thing to explain is the statement by many of the sickened occupants that they feel fine and are asymptomatic as soon as they leave the building. Certainly no toxic effects or any symptoms due to chronic irritation of the respiratory membranes or persistent infection of the nose, sinuses, or lungs could be expected to disappear so quickly. Some doctors believe that exposure to sick buildings could lead to a condition of multiple chemical sensitivities where a person might begin reacting to almost anything in his or her environment, but so far there is no proof of this.

It would seem likely that there is more than one causative factor usually involved in sick building syndrome and that it may vary from building to building, from area to area, and possibly even from one country to another, although the effects on the occupants and especially their respiratory tracts appear to be somewhat similar. Until we have a broader knowledge of the many various noxious fumes and particle matter spread into the environment by the myriads of synthetic products and materials used in building construction as well as their effects on the human body and especially on the respiratory tract and sinuses, we may have considerable difficulty in correcting the problem or even in knowing who or what is to blame.

As one possible solution, new building construction and furnishings should have regulatory standards for all inside-air-polluting materials, including paints, stains, glues, adhesives, resins, solvents, sealants, building and duct insulations, plastics, wiring insulations, woods, particle boards, paneling, synthetic furnishings, carpeting, draperies, upholstery, and soundproofing. Regulatory standards should also take into consideration the various cleaning materials, air fresheners, perfumed soaps, fungicides, and pesticides as well as the quality and quantity of outside air exchange required to dilute and exhaust them. Here numerical consideration would also have to be given for the number of occupants using scented deodorants, body lotions, hair sprays, and perfumes as well as the number wearing synthetic clothing. Electronic equipment may even require special rooms with their own air exchange and exhaust mechanisms.

New gaseous compounds are constantly being developed and frequently discharged into the environment, and some will undoubtedly prove irritating to the nose, sinuses, and respiratory tract. We should also remind ourselves that whatever gaseous or water-soluble substance we breathe deep into our lungs, small amounts may often find their way, just as with inhalation anesthetics, into our circulating blood. The same thing might be said of soluble pollutants entering the nose, with its very rich blood supply, as noted in those who snort cocaine for a quick fix, and more recently Ritalin powder as a quick stimulant. Either of these may enter the bloodstream very rapidly in this way and occasionally produce serious complications and even cause death.

REDUCING EXPOSURE

As previously mentioned, not only the concentration and irritating qualities of an air pollutant but also the frequency and duration of exposure are all very important in determining its injurious effects on your respiratory tract and sinuses. Any potential damage may be minimized considerably by the air dilution of open spaces, by circulating air exchange, by wind direction, elevation, humidity, and temperature, as well as by the location and proximity of the polluting source with regard to the victim. Any one or all of these factors may determine whether a sinus-prone individual stays healthy or has a flare-up of sinusitis or bronchitis, and even whether he or she contracts a viral respiratory infection on the next exposure, since persistent irritation of the nose and lower respiratory tract, especially when accentuated by any membrane-drying effect, can break down the local body defenses of effective cilia activity and free-flowing mucus, thereby making the respiratory membranes and sinuses more susceptible to a bacterial or viral invasion.

PROTECTIVE SHIELDING

When you are working outside around irritating fumes, sprays, or powders, it is important to protect your nose and respiratory tract with proper masking, and unless the particulate matter is rather coarse, simple "dog masks" are not always enough. Even wood dust released by sawing and sanding contains some very fine particles that will pass through or around these masks, and you are only kidding yourself if you use them to protect yourself from fine toxic sprays, gases, and fumes. Mahogany, cherry, redwood, fir, and salt-treated wood dusts can be especially irritating to your nose, sinuses, and respiratory tract, as well as to the eyes. Simple glasses are not sufficient to prevent sprays, fumes, and fine dust from harming the eyes, and you must remember that any irritating matter entering the eyes, such as vapors, liquids, water-soluble powders, or very fine dust, will very rapidly reach the nose through the nasolacrimal or tear ducts and may cause a rhinitis or inflammatory irritation of the nose with possible involvement of the sinuses as well. Some eyedrops and especially their preservatives have been guilty of this, and some have even caused asthmatic attacks. Goggles with side shielding are important around sprays and dust, and even more so if the wind is blowing. With all such exposures to outside irritants, it is important to protect your respiratory tract as much as possible by working or standing with the wind at your back or by creating your own breeze from behind with an efficient fan.

You should be especially careful in breathing silicone or Teflon sprays, since they are insoluble inert substances that may sometimes act as a foreign body and could remain in your body or lungs almost indefinitely. When grinding metals, sandblasting, or sawing and sanding fiberglass or plaster, you should wear an effective filter mask and good eye protection. Otherwise such activities could be a major hazard to your health, especially later in life. Macrophages or phagocytes, as members of the body's Pac Man group, along with the help of the lymphatic system, may remove a foreign body such as silica dust from the alveoli, or small air sacs of the lungs, but inhaling excessive amounts could cause some accumulation within the very small cilia-deficient respiratory bronchioles leading to these air sacs and could produce irritation, swelling, and obstruction there.

OTHER METHODS

Inside the house and workplace, you should take great care to control dust and other airborne pollutants. Air conditioners and most circulating systems should have good filters, which you should check and change regularly. Special electronic filters and air cleaners in certain cases can be very beneficial. Only very necessary sprays should be used in the home or car or at work and when possible with adequate protection to the user. When spraying, the "hold your breath and walk away" routine is important to remember. Fresh paint fumes should be avoided by sinus-prone individuals at home or at the office, especially during the winter months, when windows are usually closed. The so-called odorless paints are just as irritating to the nose and sinuses, and sleeping in a freshly painted room or even next to one may often produce a protracted sinusitis. Some of my more stubborn sinus problems have occurred in patients who had slept in or next to a freshly painted room, even for a relatively short time. Freshly painted areas will remain very irritating to the nose, sinuses, and even the lungs for 10 days or more after painting depending on how thoroughly the room is aired out, and prolonged exposures on a daily basis during this period should definitely be avoided. When possible you should delay any inside house or office painting until warm weather, when windows can stay open and window exhaust fans may be used.

An exhaust fan to the outside should run constantly when you are using a home woodworking shop, and each dust-producing machine should be exhausted separately whenever possible. The floor dust should never be swept up but rather sucked up with a properly filtered shop vac. This very fine wood dust may get into the heating or air-conditioning ducts and travel throughout your house almost indefinitely. Whenever possible, special fine-particle filters should be used in the return ducts from a workshop.

I recall a particularly troublesome pollution problem that occurred when Sheetrock workers were sanding in a home with the air-conditioning turned on. The very fine plaster dust was subsequently introduced into the entire ventilating system and continued to be distributed throughout the house for some years thereafter. In this instance, using special filters and cleaning them frequently helped considerably once the occupants realized whence all the fine white dust on the furniture originated. (Here I should point out that a fine white dust deposit on the furniture may also sometimes occur from using a cool mist humidifier.)

A somewhat similar but far more serious problem occurred in some homes and buildings when it was popular to install air-conditioning and heat ventilating ducts made of plastic and lined on the inside, instead of the outside, with an exposed core of fiberglass for insulating purposes and noise reduction. In some instances, these liners would break down, releasing fine needlelike fragments of fiberglass into the ventilating systems, hopefully to be trapped by the filters. Many of these ducts were later removed, and the problem has now been corrected by specially sealed fiberglass liners, but people living in older houses with this kind of duct installation should check their filters often to make certain that their respiratory tracts are not being exposed to fiberglass particles in the air. The idea of vacuuming ventilating ducts sounds good but is not always very successful in removing all of the fine dust particles and may sometimes even disturb others. Careful selection of filters and changing them regularly seems to be just as important.

When you are using handheld sanding or sawing tools, individually attached vacuum units are only partially effective, and you should wear an efficient mask for additional protection. Even if you are not allergic, heavy concentrations of dust can be just as irritating and harmful to your respiratory tract and sinuses, and the greater the concentration, the more irritated and inflamed they may become.

SMOKE EXPOSURE

Also within the home, strong consideration should be given to the polluting effects of secondhand cigarette smoke, not only because of possible lung cancer, a reduced sense of smell, and its possible effects on vision in old age as well as on the heart and lungs, but also because of its potential significance in upper respiratory tract infections, including sinusitis. Smokers are generally not too concerned about harming themselves, but a smoker could be responsible for initiating or maintaining a respiratory problem for other members of the household. Cigarette smoke does diminish cilia activity in the nose, sinuses, and lungs. Add to that its irritating effects on mucous membranes, and you have an ideal setting for chronic rhinosinusitis and chronic bronchitis from repeated exposure. Breathing secondhand smoke may not always initiate a sinus infection, but once it develops from a cold or flu virus, the added irritation, depressed cilia activity, and a temporarily impaired protective mucous blanket may make it more difficult for the body to cast the infection off. Cigar smoking, which has increased 50 percent since 1993, may offer an even greater risk for lung cancer and puff-for-puff produce far more secondhand smoke. Breathing cigar smoke is even more irritating to the membranes of the nose and sinuses, and far more likely to cause mouth, throat, and esophageal cancers. Even a favorite pet may be unsafe from the harmful effects of secondhand smoke. In rare instances, your cat or dog could develop a rhinosinusitis, have it aggravated by secondhand smoke, and then pass the infection on to you. Moreover, secondhand smoke could increase the chances of your pet dog developing lung cancer.

Some individuals are hypersensitive to tobacco smoke, and even minimal exposure for them may result in an asthmatic attack, an episode of rhinitis, a sinusitis flare-up, and many times a rather intense headache. Even residual smoke in the rugs, clothing, draperies, bed linens, and upholstery could initiate such a reaction for some individuals. Cigarette and cigar smoke, like strong perfumes and certain chemicals, are more of a primary irritant to the delicate membranes of the respiratory tract and sinuses, rather than a true allergen. Breathing these irritating air pollutants, however, may not only aggravate an allergic rhinitis but might also bring it on.

Animal danders, molds, pollen, dust mites, cockroaches, latex residue, and newsprint are also some rather frequent contaminants or pollutants of many household environments. Some may be of particular significance for certain sinus-prone individuals with allergies, and each has been taken up separately under that subject.

Vacuum cleaners and wet mops should, however, replace brooms within the homes of most allergy or sinus sufferers. Vacuums should ideally have a very effective horsepower to limit dust from escaping after being stirred up by their brushes, and for small cleanups, a hand vacuum without a brush may be more sensible. Vacuum replacement bags should not be torn and not allowed to overfill. Great care should be taken not to squeeze the bag in removing or disposing of it. Fine-particle filters for vacuum cleaners are available and should be used when practical. When vacuum cleaners are being used, sinus-prone individuals should be out of the room and sometimes even out of the house if they are particularly sensitive to dust, molds, or dander. Vacuum cleaners usually remove only the very superficial dust from carpeting, their revolving brushes often dispelling much of it into the air, and their collecting bags frequently allowing very fine particles to escape back into the room air.

CHEMICAL IRRITANTS

Sinus sufferers may also have to give some concern to the occasional irritating fumes emitted by synthetic upholstery, carpeting, drapes, curtains, and some insulating materials not only in the workplace and car but also in the home. As previously mentioned, some of these emit formaldehyde fumes and other chemicals that can irritate the nose and sinuses as well as slow cilia activity. This is not something easily corrected, and since it is usually considered to be an infrequent occurrence in the home, chemical irritants should be given a fairly low priority. It is usually impossible to correct such factors in the workplace or in the car other than by diluting with more outside air, which may occasionally be even more polluting. Chemical irritants can be given occasional consideration, however, before you make any purchases or installations in the home, but if carpeting, drapes, or furniture is already installed, it may also prove less of a problem with the passage of time. Some synthetic carpeting may display a rather strong odor, which could be a warning to the sinus-prone individual or the patient with chronic lung disease.

If you are prone to acute sinusitis flare-ups or have chronic sinus disease, it is important to select a home and a working environment as free of irritating air pollutants as possible. Otherwise your acute or subacute sinusitis may become chronic, and your chronic sinusitis may never completely clear up as long as you live or work there. Since pollution anywhere in the environment can be a significant health factor for many people who have sinusitis, identifying its source or sources and avoiding it as much as possible could play a major role in a possible cure or at the very least in providing a better quality of life if you are a chronic sinus sufferer.

CHAPTER FIFTEEN

Household Heat
and Humidity

HUMIDITY, OR THE amount of water vapor in the air, is one of the least understood of the natural phenomena in our environment. It also seems to be given far too little attention and recognition when it comes to its effects on our respiratory tracts, our sinuses, and our health, as well as that of nearly all living things. Weather reports, fortunately, are now including the heat or comfort index in addition to the air quality or ozone count, the wind chill factor, the mold count, and the pollen count when revealing the true quality of the air we breathe.

The heat index (HI) takes into account not only the temperature but also the humidity or wetness in the air and is reported as the apparent temperature, which may be as much as 20 degrees higher than the actual thermometer reading on a very hot and humid day. When the humidity is high, your body is less able to dissipate or give off heat as effectively through the evaporation of sweat and by the exhalation of warmed moisture from the respiratory tracts and lungs. Dogs and cats are unable to sweat, so they usually pant to speed up loss of body heat, especially when the surrounding temperature equals or exceeds that of their own bodies, which would also lessen any further body heat loss through infrared radiation. Excessive panting, however, may involve considerable muscular activity, which in turn can increase body heat. This may be counterproductive in a closed car on a hot day, where temperatures may be far in excess of 100 °F and therefore fatal to a favorite pet.

As far as your own heat regulation is concerned, you generally lose

60 percent of your body heat through infrared radiation, 22 percent by lung and skin evaporation, 15 percent through air conduction, and 3 percent from surface contact with cooler objects. Of course, these percentages will vary according to the surrounding temperature, humidity, draftiness, and hot or cold contacts with your skin.

Dispensing of body heat by such means is important not only to your comfort but also to your health as far as heat exhaustion, heat-stroke, muscle cramps, excessive fatigue, and oxygen consumption are concerned. A good breeze or a fan can make a big difference in the sweat evaporation and the dissipation of body heat as well as your general comfort. If you have ever spent a hot Sunday afternoon on the water or at the beach and then tried to drive home for some distance that night, you already know the meaning of excessive fatigue from excessive humidity. It can make you drowsy and could be dangerous. A body of water on a very warm day gives off a very heavy layer of water molecules and, like a steam bath, may tend to overheat, dehy-drate, and exhaust your body rather than to invigorate it. Too much exposure for too long a time may even alter the body's chemical bal-ance. This can also be true of hot tubs, especially in enclosed areas. Molds, fungi, a treatment-resistant bacteria known as *Pseudomonas,* as well as the now famous *Legionella pneumophila* bacteria that caused the very serious outbreak of Legionnaire's disease at the American Legion convention in Philadelphia in 1976, all breed well in these excessively moist areas, may enter your respiratory tract and lungs on fine moisture droplets, and may even infect the sinuses.

Your joints, muscles, and sinuses, especially if previously damaged and scarred, will usually hurt more if the humidity is high. In older people, stiffness in muscles or joints is a common complaint on humid days, and even more if you live near the water. How often have you heard someone say, "It's not the temperature, it's the humidity"? In fact, it is both, since warm air will hold more moisture. Wood con-tracts and swells with changes in humidity and may give us a clue as to what goes on within our own organic structures. Since excess mois-ture in the air will dilute its oxygen content, an individual who has emphysema will experience more breathing difficulties on very humid days and will notice a welcomed relief in the reduced humidity of air-conditioning. Dry skin or xeroderma noted in cold, dry, moisture-defi-cient weather can be a great annoyance to some, especially the elderly and those with certain diseases prone to this condition such as hypothyroidism, AIDS, leprosy, and lymphoma, as well as those with an inherited skin condition known as ichthyosis.

The ideal relative humidity for the respiratory tract and sinuses, which seem to be the areas of the body more drastically affected by humidity changes, has been variously estimated to be somewhere between 45 and 65 percent. In cold weather, the relative humidity is usually well below that, not only outside but even in our homes, schools, and office buildings, where on many cold days the relative humidity may be in 25 to 35 percent range. A fall in relative humidity below the 30 percent level may cause a decrease in cilia activity and the rate of mucous flow in the nose, enhancing the chances of a nasal or sinus infection. On a cold winter day, it is difficult to raise the relative humidity in your home above 35 percent, whereas on hot, humid summer days it may rise into the nineties in a non-air-conditioned house. Therefore, if you live in a cold or temperate climate, your winter weather is mostly too dry, causing the nasal mucous membranes to dry out, become infected, and subsequently infect the sinuses, whereas midsummer weather (especially at low elevations) is generally too humid, causing the respiratory membranes to retain their moisture and to swell, resulting in sinus blockage. From this it is easy to see why vacationers and people with sinus or respiratory problems might prefer to spend time in the mountains during the humid summer weather. Moreover, too much humidity not only encourages the growth of dust mites, bacteria, molds, and fungi in household and working environments but also prolongs the survival of any viruses deposited there.

It is important to remember that in a cold environment, even if the relative humidity (RH) is high, which is usually not the case unless you add more moisture, the total moisture content of the air is still relatively low, since cold air can't hold much moisture. Furthermore, the drying effects on your respiratory tract and skin as well as on any plants or animals in the area are still significant, unless of course you can warm that air and add more moisture, which is what you should try to do in your home during the winter months—and also what your nose is trying to do for you as well.

The nose, your own built-in humidifier, works overtime to deliver a pint or more of moisture every 24 hours to the air you breathe, provided, of course, that you breathe through your nose and not through your mouth. The warmed, filtered, and moistened air provided by the nose is important to the health of your respiratory tract and lungs. The true moisture content of inhaled air when it finally reaches the lungs depends on the outside humidity, whether you are exposed to a wind or draft, are standing still or moving about, how much nasal breathing and therefore nasal humidification is involved, whether you have been drinking adequate nonalcoholic or noncaffeinated fluids and are therefore well hydrated, how much of the body moisture cloud is re-breathed, and finally how much re-breathed air and moisture remains behind in the tidal air each time you breathe out.

With so many variables affecting the moisture content of the air you breathe, it is not surprising that the estimated ideal relative humidity in the environment, as far as the respiratory tract and sinuses are concerned, covers a wide range, and especially when you realize that such an apparently simple act as breathing through the mouth will increase your need for more moisture in the air, since you are then bypassing your own built-in nasal humidifier. The amount of nasal humidification added to the air you breathe over a 24-four hour period will depend on whether the nose is always open, partially closed, or completely obstructed; whether you are mouth breathing only temporarily because of exercise, excessive talking, or singing; whether you mouth breathe for 6 or 8 hours at night because of nasal swelling and blockage during sleep; or whether you are a continuous mouth breather due to a permanently obstructed nasal airway.

Moreover, the amount of humidification available from a normal nose depends not only on the amount of recaptured moisture from exhaled lung air but also on your body fluid content. If you are taking a fluid pill, have diarrhea, or have been drinking alcohol or consuming an excessive amount of caffeinated products, both of which are diuretics, or even sweating profusely and neglecting fluid intake, then all of the body tissues, including the membranes of the nose, sinuses, and entire respiratory tract, will have lost some of their fluid content, and nasal humidification will subsequently be diminished. How much of the moisture given off by the lungs and body surface is re-breathed will depend on how much nasal breathing is involved, whether you are moving about or remaining still, and how much you are exposed to a draft, wind, fans, or air-conditioning. You should remember that central air-conditioning in the average-size house on a fairly humid day may remove as much as 4 or 5 gallons of water from the air you breathe.

All you have to do is to forcibly breathe on a slightly cool mirror or just breathe out on a cold day to see how much moisture is released each time you exhale. On a cold morning, runners will often cover their mouths partially to trap some of their warmed and moistened lung air for re-breathing, which is not a bad idea, provided the mask or face cover doesn't interfere with getting enough oxygen. If you have asthma or chronic obstructive pulmonary disease (COPD), you should not exercise outside on cold days anyhow because of possible secondary bronchial spasm, sometimes referred to as exercise asthma, and also because of thickening of the mucus in the lungs and respiratory tract from breathing the cold dry air. True exercise asthma with wheezing may occur in warm weather as well. Very serious bronchial spasms may also occur in a few individuals from a physical allergy to cold even without exercising.

When exercising, most of us are forced to breathe through the mouth to acquire sufficient oxygen, thus bypassing our nasal humidification, as well as the filtering and warming of the air normally provided by the nose. The mouth may perform some of these functions, but not so effectively as the nose. You may also notice that when you talk continuously or sing, you usually have to breathe through your mouth, which as a result may become very dry. An individual who breathes through a tracheotomy opening in the neck will often button the collar of an extra-large shirt over the breathing hole to entrap moisture on a cold day, especially since he or she doesn't have the additional warming and humidification of nasal breathing. This may also reduce the chances of bronchial spasm and helps to keep the mucus thin and free-flowing so that it may be easily coughed up. As previously mentioned, there is also some re-breathed moisture trapped within the lungs and respiratory tract in the so-called tidal air. Here the movement of air and moisture in and out of the lungs is like the ebb and flow of the tide, and each time you breathe out, some moist lung air is not completely exhaled but is left behind in the upper and lower respiratory tracts to be inhaled again with the next breath. This tidal air is usually very high in moisture content and helps to keep the nose and nasopharynx moistened as well. When you breathe out through your nose, the nasal turbinates also manage to capture a significant amount of this expired moisture for reuse.

Unfortunately, we are constantly overtaxing the body's nasal humidifier by living, sleeping, working, and traveling in air-conditioning, which by its nature removes moisture from the air during the cooling process. We are all aware of how much our home and car air conditioners drip on a hot and humid day. When the warm circulating air passes over the gas-cooled coils of an air conditioner, the relative humidity of this cooled air increases rapidly until it reaches the saturation point of 100 percent RH, and the excess moisture then precipitates or condenses out and turns to water runoff, since this suddenly cooled air is now unable to contain all of the moisture previously held by the warm air. A slower but very similar process takes place when the dew point temperature is reached on a cool evening or night after a warm day, and the next morning you may find the ground covered with condensed moisture or dew.

Even the kinds of heat you install in your home can influence the dryness of not only your body skin but also the mucous membranes of the nose and sinuses. With modern living, we have gravitated more and more away from the healthier radiant heat, such as that provided by old-fashioned radiators and baseboard radiation, to circulating forced air, stoves, heat pumps, and space heaters with blowers, all resulting in an almost continuous movement of air within a room as well as out of a room. This draftiness will tend to remove or disperse the moisture cloud usually surrounding your body and created by insensible skin evaporation, perspiration, and the constant exhaling of moistened air. This loss of moisture for re-breathing may tend to thicken the mucous flow in the nose, which in turn may slow the sinus drainage as well as the sinonasal cleansing action. A slowing of the mucous flow offers bacteria and viruses a greater opportunity to invade the underlying membranes and likewise encourages the spread of respiratory infections within the household, day care centers, schoolrooms, carpools, and the workplace.

Early in my medical career, I had the opportunity to investigate 70 medical families at Johns Hopkins, 35 living in a radiator- or radiant-heated environment, and 35 living in housing with drafty forced-air heat. Twenty-three families from each group also had one or two small children. Because of the nursery school contacts of some of the children and the variety of the patient contacts of the doctors in each household, it was not possible to determine if one type of heat made the occupants more susceptible to respiratory infections in their contacts outside the home, although it probably did. However, it was very apparent that whenever a viral respiratory infection was introduced into a forced-air-heated home by one of its occupants, the virus was much more inclined to make the rounds of all the occupants, who also seemed to have more trouble getting over it as well as over any lingering sinusitis or cough.

For 35 years after that, I made a serious effort to question every sinusitis patient I treated about the type of heat he or she had at home and at work as well as where the heat delivery and exhaust vents were located with regard to beds, desks, easy chairs, and primary working areas. Unfortunately, many of the heat and air-conditioning vents were located near the head of the bed or directly over it, exposing the individual to a rather constant draft. Time and again there was a consistent finding of more respiratory infections and more sinus problems with more difficulty preventing or clearing them up in people living or working in a drafty, warm-air-heated environment, and even more so when the heat vent arrangement was poor. Completely closing off a vent, deflecting its airflow away from a bed, or even rearranging the furniture was sometimes necessary to avoid sitting or sleeping in a draft. Some previously healthy people could even date the onset of their sinus problems to moving from a radiant-heated home with old-fashioned radiators to one heated by a heat pump or forced air. A similar problem with the nose and sinuses was also noted in those who sat or slept too close to an air-conditioning vent as well.

A drafty heating system at home or in the workplace, which may repeatedly disrupt or disperse the body's moisture cloud, is one of the main reasons why house occupants or office workers so often complain of never really feeling warm. You may note the same effect when a fan blows over your body. The fan is not blowing colder air; it is simply dispersing the moisture of evaporation away from your body, carrying heat with it and allowing more evaporation and heat loss to follow, thus making you feel not only cooler but drier, since it is also depleting your skin and respiratory tract of their much-needed moisture. Drying your hands with a warm air blast in the public restroom is fairly effective and saves paper towels, but it also leaves your skin very dry, and it may take awhile to recover. Using these public air dryers also leaves a moist bacterial or viral-laden hand smudge on the mutual turn-on button, which might present a problem, especially in flu season.

With any significant air-movement type of heat, its drying effects may also be transmitted to any pet animals, birds, flowers, and wooden furniture throughout the house. Under the circumstances, a piano may even find it more difficult to stay in tune.

A similar drying effect is created in the home by the ever popular woodstove. A stove's flue updraft can draw the cold outside air with its low moisture content into the house, mostly through another chimney flue, exhaust vents, soffits, or through cracks around doors and windows, while venting some of the inside warmer air with its higher moisture content up the stovepipe to the outside, thus creating a progressive fall in humidity within the home on cold days. Fireplaces may have a similar effect, as do furnaces, unless of course the builder was wise enough to provide the furnace room with an outside independent source of air. Some woodstoves are now being similarly constructed with their own independent air source for the same reason. Fireplaces can also be provided with an outside source of air, and at the same time, by using glass doors on the fireplace, you may greatly diminish the escape of heat and humidity from the room. Unfortunately, when closed, these glass doors will also reduce the room's radiant, convection, or reflected heat from the fire, but this can be used selectively, especially if you have another effective source of heat and most of the time just want to visualize the inner warmth of burning logs. Some people turn to gas logs as a possible solution for humidity loss from the home, but these too may present a similar problem if placed in an existing chimney with the vent open or possibly a carbon monoxide danger if no vent is installed.

On the other hand, unvented gas logs and propane heaters in small, tightly sealed rooms may gradually cause excessively high moisture levels. This in turn may produce an increased growth of harmful bacteria, molds, and dust mites with an increase in sinonasal swelling, sinus blockage, and sinus infections for its occupants. Too much continuous moisture in a room or house may also damage insulation, sheeting, and siding, as well as inside and outside painting. Excessively high moisture levels can also make it more difficult for people with heart and lung conditions to obtain enough oxygen.

If you can afford it, you may want to install baseboard radiant heat, usually electric, but better still, cast iron with circulating hot water, in addition to a heat pump, which may then be reserved for air-conditioning or as a backup heat to be used when you are away. Baseboard radiant heat will provide a more even type of heat throughout the room, especially under windows and glass doors, and with a great deal less air movement or draftiness as well. It does mean adding a second form of heat to the house, and radiant heat is often more expensive to operate than a heat pump, except when the latter is forced into electric supplemental heat at temperatures near 20 °F and below. For economic reasons and because the ducts are needed for air-conditioning anyhow, not many builders or developers will install a second form of heat on their own, and it is usually too late once construction is well under way. Some of the more expensive houses may have it, but that is usually due to a prospective owner's early request.

From this discussion, you can readily see that not only the inside and outside temperature but the type of heating and cooling systems you have can affect the moisture content of the air you breathe, which in turn can affect the health of your lungs, nose, and sinuses, the dryness of your skin and eyes, the static electricity in rugs and clothing, the condition of furniture, and your own general comfort, as well as that of your pets, plants, and flowers. It can also affect the performance of some musical instruments as well as any sensitive electronic equipment, including computers. Therefore, any true measurement of a healthy environment should include not only the temperature but also the humidity reading.

Humidity measurement devices, except for the more expensive ones, unfortunately are not always completely reliable. There are two principal indicators of environmental humidity, each of which affords a measurement of the water vapor present in the atmosphere or room air at a particular time and location. The one most commonly referred to on the radio and television or in the newspaper is the relative humidity, or RH. Relative humidity gives us a measurement in percent as to the amount of water vapor present in the air when compared to the greatest amount of vapor that same air could possibly hold at that particular temperature and at that particular altitude or atmospheric pressure. This measurement is important because it takes into consideration the temperature as well as the altitude and therefore is more relevant to your individual health and comfort wherever you are.

In other words, if the RH is 50 percent, then the air contains one-half the amount of moisture it is capable of holding at that particular temperature and at that altitude. Of these two variables, however, the atmospheric pressure or altitude is of lesser importance, since it has the least influence on the RH. This is especially true because the atmospheric pressure or barometer reading is much the same inside as it is outside a house, whereas the temperature will usually vary significantly from inside to outside as well as from attic to basement, and therefore so may the relative humidity. You can feel very dried out in your home on a cold winter day when there is much less moisture available anywhere, and the relative humidity even in a warm house will therefore be lowered considerably. Although this warm inside air is capable of holding much more water vapor than the cold air outside, unless moisture can be mechanically introduced into the home with a vaporizer or humidifier, the inside air will continue to draw water vapor from all available sources, including your body and respiratory tract as well as those of your pets and even from fish tanks, plants, and furniture.

The other less common form of measurement is specific humidity, which is totally independent of the other natural phenomena such as temperature and atmospheric pressure. Specific humidity simply compares the weight of the water vapor in a certain amount of air in grains to the total weight of that same amount of air in pounds. Since it does not take into account the other variables of temperature and altitude, it is therefore not so helpful as far as our comfort readings are concerned and also not so easily measured.

In understanding the relative humidity, it is important to remember that the colder the air, the less water vapor it is capable of holding; and conversely, the warmer the air, the more water vapor it can accommodate, but only if it is available. On a cool late-summer or early-fall morning after a rain the night before, the relative humidity can be very high, since there is plenty of moisture available from the rain, but the cooler morning air can't accommodate very much without becoming completely saturated. If the air is cool enough and there is sufficient moisture available from rain, melting snow, the wet ground, or a nearby body of water, then the relative humidity may easily reach a saturation point of 100 percent RH and will then precipitate from the air onto the ground and other cooler objects in the form of dew, somewhat against the old adage that the dew rises. The temperature at which the air can hold no more water vapor and is therefore considered saturated is called the dew point and is often reported on the television or in the newspaper. This is also the point at which clouds and fog form. As the day warms up, the relative humidity may drop to 50 percent or even lower, since the warmer air is capable of holding even more moisture, and this increase in temperature without a corresponding increase in available moisture lowers the percentage. Of course, a heavy shower during the day could raise the RH again, especially if it clouds over with a corresponding drop in temperature.

When you add moisture to your home environment with a steam vaporizer or humidifier, you are attempting to lessen the difference between the actual moisture content of the air and what the air is capable of containing at that temperature. More important, by doing this in cold weather, you are raising the relative humidity without lowering the temperature. This is important for people with sinusitis because they don't do as well in a cold, damp environment as they do in a warm, slightly humid environment. Too much humidity, however, may have an adverse effect on you, since your nasal membranes will then be unable to release enough of their own moisture and may therefore tend to swell and to further obstruct your sinus drainage openings.

Although the part that altitude or barometric pressure plays in humidity readings is usually rather minor when compared to that of the temperature, it may become a factor for the sinus-prone individual living in the usually higher humidity at sea level as compared to the lower humidity often found high in the mountains, or when exposed to the greatly reduced outside humidity introduced into the exchanged air of plane cabins at high altitudes. This almost continuous exchange of low-humidity colder air from outside the plane with the inside warmer air containing more humidity, most of which is supplied by the body moisture of the passengers, results in a persistent lowering of the cabin moisture content, often to the increasing discomfort of the occupants. It is not surprising that long-distance air travelers complain of respiratory problems and appear more vulnerable to respiratory infections and sinusitis as well.

It is most important to remember that humidity, either too much or too little, and air pollution and cold temperatures are your three main environmental enemies, and when extremes in all three occur together, your sinuses are bound to suffer. This statement is not meant to diminish the role of pollen in many cases of rhinosinusitis, since it too can be a very troublesome form of natural air pollution in its own right.

Relative humidity readings are generally measured by a wide variety of gauges commonly known as hygrometers and converted by mathematical formulas, graphs, and charts. Some of the earlier gadgets took into account the well-known effect of humidity on human hair, and consequently a fine hair was often used as the humidity gauge sensor. Blond hairs from which the oil had been extracted were considered to give a more accurate reading. The very good hygrometers on the market today are far more technical, much more accurate, and considerably more expensive. Their readings, however, may sometimes vary as much as ±5 percent, and the most accurate ones may have to be cleaned and calibrated often. One of the more accurate ones uses a chilled mirror device that works by measuring the dew point directly. Psychrometers work by comparing the dry bulb and wet bulb temperatures of the air and are fairly inexpensive. The sling type is used by many and considered very accurate. If your desires lean toward simple operation and less maintenance, a capacitive-type of sensor that measures humidity directly and is battery run, easier to operate, and usually accurate to ±2 percent is available but is often more expensive.

Since relative humidity is so dependent on the temperature, and therefore may vary considerably from outside to inside the home, from room to room, and especially from attic to basement, hygrometer readings may vary as much as 10 to 20 percent RH and occasionally as much as 50 percent in going from an extremely warm room to a very cold room in the same building. The heavier cold air will often settle into a normally damp basement area, and with it may go a rise in relative humidity, provided the moisture is available and not being drawn off by a dehumidifier. That is why cellar air is usually cold and damp, and attics are usually drier, or why cellars tend to grow mold, and attics usually don't. It is also why we are much more comfortable with central air-conditioning than with single-room air-conditioning when moving about from one part of the house to another where temperatures and therefore relative humidity might vary from room to room. It also emphasizes the point that larger rooms and rooms further from the central source of heat or cold air will require a larger or a greater number of ducts if the temperature, and therefore the relative humidity, is to remain much the same throughout the house. Good insulation, of course, can play an important role in this uniformity of temperature and humidity as well. Air leaks through chimney flues, exhaust ducts, cracks in and around doors or windows, improperly sealed soffits, and the frequent opening and closing of outside doors, especially during cold weather, can have very significant effects on indoor humidity as well as on the sinuses and respiratory tracts of the occupants.

Many of us fail to take into consideration the many sources of humidity replenishment we have in our homes as well as the many facets of modern living that also tend to take humidity away. Some sources that provide additional humidity, especially in cold weather, when the water evaporation in a warm houses with lowered humidity is most active, include refrigerators and fish tanks; running water from showers, tubs, and sinks; the soaking of clothes, socks, and stockings; wet washcloths, towels, and clothing hung up to dry; toilet bowls and toilet tanks; the traps of all sinks, showers, and tubs; dishwashers, washing machines, and dryers; coffee making and cooking; and watered plants and flowers. Even the plants themselves will give up moisture, and so will the bodies of any house occupants, including people and pets. Even some building materials such as wood, plaster, and especially concrete absorb moisture on damp days and release it on cold, dry days. Furniture does the same thing with swelling and contraction, sometimes resulting in the loosening of glued joints.

This inside moisture supply is in addition to any central or local room humidifiers, as well as any high outside humidity released by rain or melting snow and seeping into the house through cracks, ducts, and other openings and enhanced or sucked in by air being exhausted from the house through active chimneys, flues, and ducts. It is important to remember that the downdraft from an unused fireplace may feed the updraft of an active one even from a remote part of the house, even to some degree with the damper closed. You should always consider this in evaluating a drafty house or a house found to have an excessive loss of humidity in cold weather. Also helping to deplete household moisture are active exhaust fans from bathrooms, dishwashers, kitchens, stoves, and workshops, all of which may permit a reverse flow of cold, dry air into the house when their fans are not moving.

Again it should be emphasized that just as too much moisture in the air you breathe can cause nasal membranes to become swollen and spongy, thereby blocking sinus drainage, so too little moisture may cause thickening of the sinonasal secretions, also impairing sinonasal drainage; and both extremes offer a greater opportunity for bacterial or viral invasion of the nose and sinuses.

To keep the humidity at an ideal level for the nose, sinuses, and lower respiratory tract, I have always preferred hot steam vaporizers to the cool type. They may be more expensive to run and are more inclined to mar the finish of a floor or table if not cared for properly, but they have the advantage of being self-sterilizing to a degree and are therefore much less inclined to harbor bacteria and fungi, which tend to inhabit cool humidifiers and may be expelled into the air on their very large droplets. Steam vaporizers give off a very small molecule of water rather than the large droplet of a humidifier, and their vapor will remain suspended in the air for a much longer period, travel further on air currents, and may therefore be more available. The cool mist and ultrasound humidifiers will often leave powdery deposits on tables and furniture and conceivably within your respiratory tracts and lungs as well. Any contaminants in their water will also be blown around the room, whereas the hot steam vaporizer leaves most of that behind. The smaller vapor droplets or water molecules also have a better chance of transmitting moisture to the far reaches of the respiratory tract and lungs. One hospital in Baltimore felt so strongly about this that it replaced every one of its cool humidifiers with the steam type.

Both types, however, should be cleaned every week or two, often depending on the existing mineral deposits in their water reservoirs or their tendency to grow bacteria or mold. A fiberglass, ceramic, or metal tray will protect a floor or table from water spill, but the hot steam head should be carefully located well out of the reach of small children, since a burn could result. They do not have to be located directly beside the bed; placing them in a corner or almost anywhere in the room works just as well, provided they are not located next to a room exhaust vent. They should have the capacity to run for 10 to 12 hours without refilling so that they last through the night. A room vaporizer or humidifier, however, should be used sparingly if you have been told that you are allergic to dust mites, since they thrive and multiply in carpets, bed linens, mattresses, upholstery, and stuffed animals, especially in a damp environment. A room humidity reading above 65 percent might encourage more swelling of sinus orifices and even encourage the growth of mites, bacteria, mold, and fungi, as well as the survival of some viruses.

Some of the same problems also apply to central humidifiers, and even though they are intended to cover the entire house, they are usually not as effective locally as a single-room humidifier. A lot depends on the type, the duct structure within the house, and how well they are cleaned and tended. Unfortunately, they are often neglected for long periods, allowing bacteria and fungi to grow and sometimes permitting the water intake or injector nozzles to become completely clogged with mineral deposits. Cold spots in a central heat duct system may cause condensation, so proper duct insulation is important. To adequately reach distant rooms may require a stronger central fan or blower, but even then, many vapor droplets will cling to the duct walls. Central humidifiers should be completely shut off in warm weather to make the air-conditioning more efficient, and they should also be thoroughly cleaned then to avoid contamination of the environment with mold or bacteria. Except for people living at high altitudes, a basement apartment will seldom need a humidifier even in very cold weather, and its use may only encourage the growth of mold.

In general, even if you have central humidification, a child with a tendency to sinus, nasal, or lower respiratory infections, including croupe and bronchitis, will often benefit from the addition of a steam vaporizer in a corner of his or her bedroom on cold nights during the winter months, and this will usually be true for adults as well. This is especially true in houses with heat pumps or forced-air heat of any kind. Again, it should be emphasized that a steam vaporizer should always be located out of reach of any small children in the house.

CHAPTER SIXTEEN

Weather and
Cold Temperatures

OTHER THAN THE seasonal effects of pollen for some, the three factors in our general environment that seem to cause the most trouble for people who have chronic sinusitis are air pollution, cold temperatures, and extremes in humidity. If the pollution is minimal, if the humidity is neither too high nor too low, and if the weather is pleasantly warm, not too windy, and devoid of excessive temperature changes from day to night, then even if you have chronic sinusitis, if you use good judgment, you may be relatively comfortable much of the time. On the other hand, if you are someone with fairly healthy sinuses and you move to a damp, cold valley or a humid seaside town, and although you may never have been troubled by sinusitis before, you could soon begin to suffer. Even though you may be exposed to cold weather for only part of the year, there may be enough sustained sinus swelling and low-grade infection from persistent or repeated wintertime flare-ups to carry your sinus problems through the warmer spring months and into the summer, when the further addition of warm-weather smog, mold, and pollen might exacerbate it and keep it going. With the subsequent change to fall weather, with its closed-in living conditions, its cool nights accentuating pollution fallout, and drafty heating systems starting up in your home, at school, or at work, the same sinusitis symptoms may begin again often as a continuation of the infection from the previous winter, thus establishing a chronic pattern. The warm summer weather will nearly always diminish the symptoms of chronic sinusitis, often convincing you and sometimes your doctor that you are finally getting well, when in truth a low-grade chronic sinusitis with its cloudy discharge may continue to exist. If such is the case, you should seek prompt medical treatment, since it is much easier to clear up a lingering sinus infection before the arrival of cold weather, especially before the head cold or flu season begins.

Weather, the most formidable force on earth, can provide not only extreme temperature changes but also significant variations in humidity, in barometric pressure, and in wind currents that can chill the body, dry out the nose, and clog sinus openings, as well as pick up and direct the flow of pollen, mold spores, and pollutants along the ground, over the mountains, through the valleys, and into our respiratory tracts and lungs.

Not only will an increase in relative humidity accentuate joint pains for some arthritic patients, but many times a fall in barometric pressure, as noted with an approaching storm, may do the same thing, even though these inner body structures are sealed off from the outside by layers of tissue and skin and even though there is no good scientific explanation for the reaction. It is, therefore, not too surprising that a rise in humidity or a fall in barometric pressure can also influence the aches and pains of partially blocked, scarred, or chronically diseased sinuses, which normally contain air and are directly connected to the outside air. Some people who have obstructive sinus disease are extremely aware of rather mild changes in barometric pressure, often experiencing a pain or pressure feeling in the brow, behind the eyes, in the cheeks, or sometimes in the upper teeth, and not infrequently followed by a headache.

I recall many sinus patients who have experienced this, but one in particular stands out. She had noted obstructive sinus disease for 4 or 5 years and could detect even the slightest drop in the barometric pressure of an approaching storm with her built-in sinus barometer. This was true whether she was inside or outside the house. Each time a storm approached, she would develop fairly intense pains in her forehead, behind her eyes, and in her cheeks and upper teeth for an hour or two before the storm's arrival, with even earlier and more prolonged symptoms from a front moving in. Her symptoms would then disappear within minutes to several hours after the storm or front passed, when the barometric pressure stopped falling and began to rise. As the storm approached, however, her symptoms would nearly always intensify. When a hurricane moved up the coast, she would notice the onset of sinus pain 4 or 5 days before, gradually increasing in severity and gradually diminishing over a 24-hour period after the hurricane passed.

A much more dramatic effect occurred when a tornado went through her front yard. Although she wasn't aware of the tornado coming, she began to notice face, cheek, and upper teeth pains several hours earlier, apparently due to the approaching storm that later spawned the tornado. The discomfort in her sinuses gradually increased until the tornado hit and then disappeared entirely within 20 to 30 minutes. At the time the tornado struck, she was 1 to 2 miles away, having just left home to pick up her children, and she returned home immediately after it passed. Since this was a sudden and rather localized phenomenon, the effect on her sinuses was a very impressive and dramatic occurrence. An interesting sidelight was that her dog began to whine 15 to 20 minutes before the tornado struck and was immediately let into the house. The dog's reaction could also have been the result of the barometric pressure fall and its effect on the dog's ears or sinuses. However, it would seem more likely that it resulted from the sound of a whirling wind in the distance, since the dog quieted down as soon as he came in the house, where the barometric pressure would still be the same as outside.

Her house, incidentally, was located only 8 to 10 feet above sea level, where a barometric pressure change might be even more noticeable. However, what makes this difficult to explain is that we know from plane flights that the rather sudden increase in pressure during descent, and not the lowering of cabin pressure when climbing, causes most of the ear and sinus discomfort. Perhaps in cases such as hers it is the effect of pressure irregularities in an approaching storm on scarred and obstructed sinuses that makes the difference.

The drying effect of cold and windy weather on our lips, face, nose, and lungs is familiar to most of us and especially to those prone to sinus or lung disease. There is little doubt that warmth is of considerable benefit to the sinus-prone individual, especially since warm air holds more moisture and therefore has less drying effect on respiratory membranes than cold air. Warming the tissues of the face, nose, and nasal membranes will increase the circulation of blood through those areas as well as through their underlying structures, including the sinuses, and is similar to what hot compresses can do in a more exaggerated form. Improved circulation in the nose and sinuses would mean better tissue oxygenation with better cellular metabolism and, if sustained, should provide better mucus production, a more effective cilia sweep, an increased flow of mucus, a faster reduction in swelling, and presumably a better local enzyme, antibody, and cellular response to disease. Heat improves circulation, and good circulation is very important in controlling infection as well as for healing tissues. That is why, when you have an infection in a hand or foot, your doctor will recommend soaking it in very warm water, and also why for more than a century open infected war wounds have been treated with frequent or continuous application of hot, moist compresses.

On a cold day, your body may lose as much as 60 to 75 percent of its heat through the head and neck, depending of course on the intensity of the cold, how much is lost through body radiation, perspiring, and breathing, your exposure to drafts and to wind, the thickness and distribution of insulating hair, the kinds of head and body coverings you wear, the amount of insulating fat deposits beneath the skin, and the thickness of the skin's outer layer. Knowing this, you can easily understand why our ancestors wore a scarf, a hat, and a nightcap, even though they weren't aware of such statistics or always exactly why.

I have observed numerous instances in which the simple consistent wearing of a hat or head covering of some kind when outside in cold or windy weather, routinely from mid-September to mid-April in the middle temperate zone and for longer periods in a more northern climate, has made a very significant difference to the sinus sufferer. This recommendation should be followed religiously by the sinus-prone individual in cold weather even when going outside for just a few seconds to pick up a morning paper, bring in a bicycle, or retrieve a few logs for the fire. Sinus-prone individuals should keep a hat by the door in cold weather, use it every time they go out, and they'll have fewer sinus problems.

In a similar way, covering your throat or neck in bitter cold with a scarf, turtleneck, or dickey can make a difference if you are prone to throat and chest symptoms. This may even make a difference in the thyroid gland's hormone production in freezing weather, since it is located just below the Adam's apple in a very exposed part of the neck, and its carefully regulated secretions are essential to the health and metabolism of all body cells as well as to the regulation of body heat. This could even be significant to the sinus sufferer if his or her neck is openly exposed to very cold temperatures for a relatively long period, since a surprising number of people with diminished thyroid function seem to have sinus problems. A doctor in London many years ago observed that 80 percent of his patients with lowered thyroid function, even when fairly minor, and who also had a tendency to be over-weight, would develop swollen, pale, and spongy nasal membranes and that many of them would have an increased susceptibility to head colds. This finding has also been noted by others since then. It is like-wise interesting to note how many people in their late forties, espe-cially women, may show some depletion of thyroid function, which may also produce a greater intolerance for cold temperatures. It can also cause fatigue, lethargy, puffiness or edema, constipation, hoarse-ness, weight gain, thinning brittle hair, dry skin, depression, and inability to concentrate. A blood test for thyroid function is very sim-ple and could be worthwhile in evaluating the older chronic sinusitis sufferer. If diminished function is demonstrated, taking thyroid replacement pills might improve sinus problems as well as some other bodily functions.

Many of my own chronic sinusitis patients have benefited signifi-cantly from wearing a ski cap and even socks to bed in cold weather, since the feet are also a major source of body heat loss. Years ago it was noted that chilling the feet could significantly lower the temperature in the nose by constricting the blood vessels within its membranous lin-ing, and any reduced circulation there could affect the sinuses as well. For similar reasons, sleeping near an open window on a cool night is unwise, and even sleeping next to a closed double-insulated window on a cold night can be equally harmful due to the drafts created by con-vection currents, especially over the head of the bed. The inside glass can still be cooled by window frame conduction, causing the cooler inside air next to the glass to fall and the warmer air in the room to be displaced and to rise, thus creating a continuous up-and-down draft over the bed and around your head. If you feel compelled to open a bedroom window even slightly at night in cold weather, it should be done in an adjoining bedroom, bathroom, or hallway. Sleeping next to an open window in an industrialized area even when the weather is fairly warm will often cause respiratory and sinus problems due to pol-lution fallout from the cooler night air. This effect on sinus-prone peo-ple as well as on those with lung problems was noted frequently in the Baltimore area in the late spring, summer, and early fall.

The bedroom thermostat should not be set at a low temperature to try to save money. Warmth, like adequate humidity (and they often go together), is important if you are a sinus sufferer, and you should remind your spouse that any savings derived from a lowered thermo-stat will be quickly used up in drugs and doctor's bills. Too warm a bedroom is not good for the sinus-prone person either, since it can cause nasal congestion, swelling, and even sinus blockage. If you can't maintain a moderately warm, even, and nondrafty heat in cold weather, especially in the bedroom, then the heat vents should be closed off completely and replaced by one or two electric oil-filled radiators, which could very well reduce medical expenses and eventually pay for themselves. This will provide a less drafty and more even radiant type of heat, but you should take great care not to purchase one with a fan, as that would only cause more draftiness and would defeat the whole purpose.

Just as cold air causes constriction of surface vessels in the rest of the body, it has the same effect on the nose, the face, and, in all likelihood, some of the underlying structures such as the sinuses, especially those adjoining the front part of the nose and face; and as previously pointed out, impaired circulation can cause impaired tissue and glandular function. Vascular constriction in the nose from exposure to cold is usually followed by nasal congestion with the further possibility of sinus blockage. The temperature within the front part of the nose closely matches that of the outside air, which also makes the external nose much more vulnerable to frostbite, whereas the temperature in the back of the nose more accurately approaches normal body temperature. Lowering the temperature in the nose by getting your feet wet, and especially by immersing your feet in cold water, won't necessarily bring on a head cold or flu unless the virus itself is present in the respiratory tract and in sufficient numbers to overwhelm your body's defenses. Along the same line, Louis Pasteur found out years ago that he was unable to infect fowl with inhaled anthrax bacteria until their feet were immersed in cold water. Also, one of the many things AIDS research has taught us about viruses is that their numbers do count. The AIDS virus has been found in almost every body fluid and glandular secretion including tears, saliva, and even earwax, but it is almost entirely from the areas of heavy viral concentrations such as found in blood and semen that infectious transmissions occur. We also know that stasis or stagnation of mucous flow in the upper respiratory tract or nose makes it easier for organisms such as viruses and bacteria to invade the tissues beneath the protective mucous blanket. If on exposure to cold temperatures, the flow of mucous secretions within the nose is reduced due to impaired circulation and also from the drying effects of low-humidity air, thus rendering the membranes more susceptible to invasion, it might also give a smaller concentration of a cold or flu virus a better chance of success, and this could likewise be true for the rest of the respiratory tract as well. The same principle might apply to chronically scarred and diseased sinuses that have impaired circulation, diminished cilia function, and retarded mucous flow and are just barely managing to control or prevent a bacterial infection from developing. In such instances, further impairment of circulation from exposure to cold might very well trip the balance and precipitate an acute flare-up.

Anyone prone to sinus flare-ups, head colds, or even bronchial spasms such as noted in asthmatics should not jog outside on cold mornings, sleep in a cold room, or go to bed with a wet or damp head following a shower or hair washing; nor should you swim outside in cold weather, or even inside if you have to go outdoors immediately afterward.

The chlorine in swimming pools can also impair mucociliary flow in the nose and sinuses. Although chlorine is effective in killing most bacteria, in swimming-pool strength, it is ineffective against most viruses. The nasal and sinus irritation from weekly swimming in chlorinated water in the wintertime plus going outside into the cold immediately afterward with a damp head can be enough to keep a sinus infection going all winter, and I have found this true for many patients and especially for children. Chlorine fumes existing in the air over a pool as well as in the chlorinated water itself can be very irritating to the nose, causing inflammation and swelling of nasal membranes resulting in rhinitis, sinus blockage, and infection.

If you must swim in a chlorinated pool in the wintertime or dive in chlorinated pools in the summer, a nose clip may help to stave off some sinus attacks, especially for children who like to spend more time underwater than on the surface. A steroid spray after swimming may reduce the nasal irritation or hyperreactivity of the mucous membranes if you are particularly sensitive to chlorine, but it should not be used more often than prescribed. Sometimes under these circumstances an antihistamine immediately after swimming may be worth considering. If you take it before swimming, it should be the non-sedating kind, and you should take the same kind after swimming if you have to drive home afterward. Driving a car with the window open or a convertible with its top down can be a real threat to a sinus-prone person on a cool night. The same would apply to riding a horse, skiing, or riding a bike or snowmobile on a cold day or night without proper head covering and also for sleeping or sitting in a cold draft. If such situations can not be avoided, then you should use as much thermal protection as possible especially for your head, neck, and feet.

A particularly troublesome condition I sometimes encountered in very young children that seemed to predispose them to sinusitis is the tendency for some of them to sweat rather profusely on the backs of their heads and necks, especially when asleep. Moisture on the skin will conduct or transfer a greater amount of heat away from the body than air will. With a wet neck and head, sleeping in too cold a room or in a draft from a fan, air conditioner, or heat duct will accentuate the heat loss by evaporation, and the chilling effects on the head and neck could cause a reflex vascular constriction with diminished circulation in the rest of the head, face, nose, and sinuses. This situation seemed to encourage infectious sinus flare-ups as well as the persistence of an existing sinus infection. Fortunately, as children grow older, this problem seems to improve, but the associated sinus problems must be kept in check until then.

Another situation I encountered that seemed to promote sinus flare-ups in certain individuals, especially in cold weather, involved those who showered at school after athletics and would then go out into the cold with a damp head. I often found it difficult to persuade a young person to cool the shower water gradually in order to shrink the dilated surface vessels on the body and head, thereby reducing heat loss and helping the body adjust to the cooler dressing room and the cold outside air. I also met considerable resistance when asking youngsters to dry their hair thoroughly and not to go outside without first covering their heads with either a warm hat or hood. It may be true that a full head of long hair can provide some insulation to the scalp, but not if it is wet or even damp, which of course can make sinus problems even worse. Loosely woven or perforated baseball caps afford little or no protection against the cold, and they tend to compress and diminish hair insulation as well.

Most animals including humans have a very fine muscle attachment to each hair to make them stand up for better insulation and thermal protection when the body is chilled, and any tight-fitting cap you wear would naturally tend to reduce this. This automatic raising of hairs is called piloerection, and the porcupine as well as some blowfish also find it very useful as a protective mechanism. Even though our own hair insulation is greatly diminished compared to that of early humans, we can still see the hairs stand up on our arms when we are cold. Hoods on pullovers and jackets can be very helpful to sinus-prone individuals on a cold day if they would only use them, but hoods tend to obstruct side vision for runners and cyclists, which means that any advice along this line may go unheeded.

Exposing yourself to sudden temperature extremes such as going in and out of a meat refrigeration room can play havoc with your sinuses, just as grilling outside on a cold night and going back and forth from warm to cold without covering your head can precipitate a sinus flare-up, sometimes even if you have fairly healthy sinuses. Any sudden breathing of cold air may also, in some individuals, produce a temporary nonproductive cough and even bronchial spasm with wheezing when no other initiating cause can be demonstrated. The latter, as previously pointed out, could present a serious problem for the child being rushed to the emergency room on a cold winter's night with a serious breathing problem such as croup or epiglottitis.

The elderly and very young are usually more susceptible to cold temperatures as well as to sudden temperature extremes. In the elderly, this susceptibility is due mainly to their own tired, erratic thermostats, poor circulation, depletion of fatty insulation just beneath the skin, and loss of muscle mass for generating more heat, so that jogging in place, flailing the arms or involuntarily shaking, or shivering are all fairly subdued and no longer as beneficial. With children it is usually their increased heat production, its rapid dispersal, and their exaggerated heat loss that may get them into trouble. Small children, with their fast heartbeats and high metabolic rates, burn body fuels very rapidly, and their small, compact size and rich vascular network make it possible to quickly distribute the heat fairly uniformly throughout their bodies, which can also mean a more rapid heat loss. Their proportionately larger skin surface when compared to their total volume plus their rapid breathing also gives them a very effective heat exchange, provided it is not overdone. If you compare their body size to the number of BTUs or calories given off, it becomes apparent that children make rather effective little furnaces, except of course when the thermostat runs out of control, and then they may need a tepid bath to cool them down.

The internal body temperature of all warm-blooded creatures must be maintained within a very narrow range for their systems to function normally. Lower the body temperature too much, and you get dangerous hypothermia; raise it too high, and you get brain damage, with death a possibility either way. A body temperature elevation in the range of 107 °F or more can be fatal or at least permanently damaging to brain tissues, and death may often occur several days later. To provide the necessary regulatory heat, the body will burn about 2,000 calories a day, a calorie being a unit of heat content or energy. Two hundred fifty-two calories make 1 British Thermal Unit (BTU), a heat measurement used mainly by industry. The fuel to provide this heat comes from the food you eat, the liquids you drink, and any surplus fuel you may have stored in your body. Combustion of the fuel is aided by the oxygen you breathe. Heat loss from the body is facilitated by conduction to colder objects, by infrared radiation, by convection from moving about or exposure to drafts and the wind, and by heat evaporation loss through breathing, excreting, and perspiring. From this it is easy to see that you not only have to generate a lot of heat but also have to conserve it.

When you are exposed to cold, your surface heat loss is reduced by shutting down the circulation in the skin and by drying up the sweat glands, but of necessity you still have to breathe and to blow off heated moisture. However, some of this is captured and retained by the nose and nasal turbinates, provided you breathe through the nose. If this heat loss is not checked sufficiently, then your muscles will begin to quiver, and you may experience a shaking chill to generate more heat by which each quivering muscle gives off four or five times the amount of heat it would generate with normal activity. Food intake, especially carbohydrates comprising mainly sucrose and glucose, will give a quick boost of calories or heat, and protein ingestion, with its specific dynamic action, or SDA, will provide a sustained boost. Fats from food and body storage will also generate a very efficient caloric response.

For sustaining body heat in cold weather, you should preferably eat and drink warm foods whenever possible. Quenching your thirst by sucking ice or eating snow may sometimes be necessary, but if the body is already too cold, it may be counterproductive, since as ice or snow melts it will accentuate body heat loss.

In cold or windy weather, when the respiratory tract tends to dry out, thereby diminishing the sinonasal as well as the tracheobronchial mucous flow, it is important to drink more fluids. Under such circumstances, you would be wise to drink at least 8 full glasses of liquid a day and more when exercising, drinking alcohol, or taking fluid pills or too much caffeine, as all will increase urinary output. The perception of thirst tends to diminish with age, so that older people should force themselves to drink and not wait until they feel thirsty. Actually, the thirst sensation usually lags well behind the water deficit in everyone. Adequate water in your body tissues can act as a thermal buffer and helps to prevent overcooling as well as overheating.

When the elderly try to generate more heat by fast walking or running, they may invite exhaustion and even a heart attack, especially on a very cold day. They often eat less than others and have fewer calories to burn and usually less storage of body fat. Consequently, when anticipating exposure to the elements, the elderly should dress more warmly and insist on more bed covering. A bedroom thermostat set only as low as 65 °F can be an open invitation to life-threatening hypothermia for a sparsely covered elderly individual. Their peripheral structures such as fingers, toes, ears, nose, hands, and feet are especially vulnerable due to their diminished circulation. Some diabetics and anyone else with peripheral vascular disease, as well as those with spontaneous vascular spasms in the toes, fingers, or nose, often associated with Raynaud's disease, would seem especially vulnerable. Smoking and some antihypertensive drugs can complicate and confuse the body's peripheral circulatory response, and depressants, tranquilizers, narcotics, some antihistamines, and alcohol will sometimes suppress the shiver reflex, which is the body's emergency heat producer. Dilatation of surface vessels with excessive loss of heat may also result from alcohol consumption as well as from taking any belladonna products or nicotinic acid preparations. Older individuals generally have less ability to break down and metabolize or burn up alcohol. Even hot flashes can be responsible for some unexpected heat loss.

Years ago, dashing through snow in a one-horse open sleigh was no doubt very exhilarating, and the bottle of alcoholic spirits carefully tucked under the lap robe afforded great comfort and insurance against the bitter cold, or so people believed. With the wind chill index of the fast-moving sleigh very high, and the muscular activity of the occupants very low, with the heat loss from dilated surface vessels accelerated by the alcohol intake and the shiver reflex likewise depressed, the thin, poorly clad, inebriated, elderly reveler was extremely vulnerable. Hypothermia and pneumonia took their toll, leaving the grieving family to wonder why the heartwarming medicinal spirits had not warded off the fateful event, not realizing of course that it was probably a major contributor.

CHOOSING A PLACE TO LIVE

Since the Baltimore-Washington area, the Ohio Valley, and parts of the Mississippi Valley, as well as many of the industrialized seaside towns and river basins throughout the country, are known for locally indigenous sinus disease, I have been asked on occasion if moving from one of these areas to a warmer area with less humidity and less pollution would improve a chronic sinusitis problem. The answer is generally yes, but after listening to several unhappy patients who had tried it unsuccessfully, and since it is a major undertaking for a family to do this, I have been careful to recommend that they visit the area first to find out.

If you are considering moving to a new area to improve a chronic sinus problem, when possible, you should visit the area in different seasons or at several different times of the year before actually undertaking such a move. Some very warm slightly humid areas in the Midwest that once attracted many sinus sufferers now have too much humidity from extensive farm irrigating systems as well as too much pollution from industry and mining dusts, both of which can make sinus sufferers worse. Since warmth does seem to be of major help if you have sinusitis, and cold definitely a detriment, you should select an area where there are rarely any big changes in temperature from season to season and preferably even from day to night. Cold or even cool night air can, in some people, cause significant nasal and sinus problems, and you should therefore avoid sleeping near an open window on a cool night or even next to a closed double-insulated window on a very cold night.

Before purchasing a home or any building property in a new environment, you should determine the direction of the prevailing winds to make certain that engine emissions are not blowing in your direction from airports, parking lots, or nearby highways, and that pollution fallouts from incinerators, cement plants, tire factories, quarries, processing plants, refineries, generating plants, or mining projects are not enveloping the area. Running your finger across an outside windowsill on the prevailing-wind side of a prospective home will often give you a clue as to pollution fallout, especially if you wipe it clean and do it again a few weeks later to find out just how rapidly it accumulates. Air pollution from burn offs in marshes, bottomlands, or everglades should also be anticipated. Low valleys can act as settlement areas for heavy pollution particles as well as for particle fallout along with the cooler night air. Ground-level ozone, the primary pollutant in smog and a major indicator of unclean air, emanates from engine emissions as well as the burning of coal and other fossil fuels, often settling out in valleys or in low-country areas.

The site of your new home should also be evaluated as to the prevalence of pollen, types of trees, fields or orchards with possible crop dustings and fruit spraying, as well as the presence of barnyards, paper mills, dirt roads with excessive dust, automobile repair shops, printing shops, dumps, trash or landfills with their various gases and microorganisms, as well as golf courses and farms with their herbicide and pesticide sprays, all of which could possibly blow your way. At the same time, you should realize that a nose doesn't have to be allergic to become very irritated and chronically inflamed by a rather mild dose of an irritating inhalant on an almost daily basis.

The house itself should be inspected for damp, moldy basement rooms, types of heat, draftiness, kinds of insulation, sump pumps, air-conditioning and duct structure, as well as excessive wood dust, plaster dust, or animal dander that might have been left behind in the ducts as well as on the walls, ceilings, floors, and furnishings by previous owners and their pets.

Dehumidifiers are often needed in humid areas and help to limit the growth of molds or fungi, especially on exposed, unsealed concrete walls and floors. This is especially true in basements in warm weather, where the cooler air will usually have a higher relative humidity, causing moisture condensation on the cooler walls and floors. Molds or fungi growing there can cause allergic rhinitis and sinusitis. Once a mold, dust, or animal dander gets into a duct system, it may require a special effort and special filters to eliminate it and may take some time to accomplish this completely. Some knowledge of the previous owners, their hobbies, and their pets is therefore important. In evaluating a basement for dampness, remember that a dehumidifier has to drain and that emptying a pan of water once or twice a day can be quite a chore, especially if you are away for the weekend. However, the presence of a floor drain, sump pump, john, sink, or tub in the basement can of course obviate this.

Similar questions about living conditions and the environment have been raised by the parents of sinus-prone high schoolers who are considering where to go to college. This is always a difficult question to answer, since data of this type are not readily available from the school, and it is often impossible to predict what kind of housing facility the student will be assigned, be it a fraternity house, dormitory, housing project, basement apartment, farmhouse, or trailer. As previously noted, the three most important outside factors for the sinus-prone individual to consider in his or her selection are a warm climate year-round without temperature extremes, one with a moderate relative humidity most of the time, ideally somewhere in the 45 to 65 percent range, and, most importantly, one with as little pollution as possible. If these three requirements can be reasonably met, and if good judgment is exercised in arranging your living quarters, then things will probably go well, since the nose and sinuses can usually adjust if they can be kept moist for better mucous flow, warm for better circulation, and pollution-free for less irritation. Of course, pollution-free would also have to apply to molds and various pollens in the air if you are allergic to any of these, and that would usually mean avoiding basement apartments for the college student with mold allergy. Seasides and valleys with too much humidity or pollution and mountainous areas with too much cold and dryness in the air are not ideal for the sinus-prone person either, so you should look for an area with warmth, lots of sunshine, moderate humidity, and clean air.

When the sinus-prone student leaves for college, he or she should go early to select a bed well away from a window and not beside a radiator or even close to a heat or air-conditioning vent. A note from a doctor or better still his or her calling ahead might help the student avoid being close to a smoking area or having a roommate who smokes, since even secondhand cigarette smoke can impair cilia function in the respiratory tract, and cigar smoke can be even more irritating to the nose and sinuses. If a roommate uses too many scented sprays or deodorants, that may be taken up later when the bond of friendship is established. Perhaps a call by the student's physician to a general medical doctor in the area may also reveal the incidence of sinusitis there.

Once the decision is made, the college physician or student health clinic should be made aware of the student's sinus problem so that head colds and sinus flare-ups will be given prompt attention. Students away at college should, either directly or through their parents, keep their hometown specialist aware of their sinusitis status, mainly to prevent prolonged sinus infections with more permanent sinus damage. Doctors usually don't like to treat patients over the phone, but sometimes it is necessary and can be done when the college physician is not available and if the sinus doctor may talk directly with the student and be given the telephone number of a pharmacy near the college. I have found it necessary to do this on a number of occasions, thus avoiding more protracted sinus problems for some of my patients while away at college.

A prospective college student may have his or her heart set on a particular college in a certain location, and we, as their parents or physicians, hate to disappoint the student, but we should make him or her aware of any possible environmental problems early and remind the student as well as ourselves that a healthy student is a happier student—and many times a better student.

If you are prone to sinusitis, have chronic lung disease, or have an allergy to mold, or if you are troubled by frequent sinus headaches or by back, muscle, and joint aches or stiffness, and you still want to live near the seashore or beside a lake, pond, or river, you will have fewer symptoms and be far more comfortable if you select a home or building site on a high bank or hill where the breezes prevail. There is always a heavy layer of humidity over a body of water, especially in warm weather, not unlike a simmering pan of water on the stove, and always with the denser layers of water vapor closer to the surface. You have probably noted while driving along the highway on a clear day that you can usually detect a large body of water in the distance by a faint blue haze of water molecules or vapor extending fairly high into the sky but thinning out as it progresses upward. The higher up you are, the less exposed your body, nose, and sinuses are to this excessive dampness, and also to mold, since they usually go together. Too much humidity will prevent the nasal membranes from releasing their own moisture, which will tend to make them swell and block the sinus drainage openings. Moreover, the swelling and tightening of scar tissue or fibrosis around nerve endings in a nose or sinus as a result of swelling from excessive humidity may produce discomfort and can even initiate a sinus headache.

Not only will a gentle breeze tend to dispel the heavy humidity cap over a body of water on a warm day, but the movement of air around building walls and across rooftops may, especially on higher ground, tend to draw the excessive humidity away from houses, and when you are outside, to dispel it from your body as well.

So that you may further realize the importance of the environment and the air you breathe if you are sinus prone, I have included throughout this book further discussion of the many environmental factors that have to be considered, not only regionally, but also within the home, car, school, and workplace. These considerations are important because careful attention to them can affect your happiness and enjoyment of life in a very positive way, whereas ignoring them could in time convert a subacute sinusitis or even healthy sinuses to the status of chronic sinus disease, possibly for the rest of your life.

CHAPTER SEVENTEEN

Flying, Diving, and Sinus Barotrauma

SINCE THE PARANASAL sinuses are air-containing cavities normally connected to the nose and outside air through ducts or very small openings, they can easily be affected by significant changes in outside air pressure or water pressure. As long as this pressure change is not too sudden or too drastic, and as long as their openings are not significantly blocked, the sinuses can usually accommodate a not too sudden pressure change without any disturbing symptoms or unpleasant awareness on your part. If, however, there is a blockage of a sinus opening from a cold or hay fever, from a cyst or polyp in the nose, or from scarring caused by previous episodes of sinusitis or occasionally from surgery, any rapid changes in outside air pressure such as sometimes noted when skiing down a mountain, riding an elevator, skydiving, bungee jumping, going down in a balloon, diving, or flying can at times cause pain or tightness in a sinus area or in the upper teeth, sometimes followed by a headache.

Very sudden pressure changes, even for healthy unblocked sinuses, can at times be extremely unpleasant, especially for scuba or deep-sea divers, as well as for pilots, especially when flying in unpressurized planes. This condition, when applied to the sinuses, is called barosinusitis or aerosinusitis, and when a sudden pressure change results in an injury to the ears or sinuses, it is called barotrauma. German fighter pilots during World War II often asked that their ear drums be punctured to avoid this barotrauma, and their daily exposure to pressure changes would usually keep these eardrum holes from healing up. This seemed to solve their ear blockage, but they still had problems trying to keep the air pressure in their sinus cavities equal to that in the cockpit.

Most commercial planes usually cruise at an altitude of 33,000 to 39,000 feet, and their cabin pressure is usually maintained at 5,000 to 8,000 feet with a gradual raising or lowering of cabin pressure at a rate of 500 feet per minute going up and 300 feet per minute coming down to allow your sinuses and ears to adjust. With any sudden change in cabin pressure such as sometimes experienced when a plane drops too far too suddenly or dives too steeply, there may be an invagination, or sucking inward, of the mucous membranes lining the openings or ducts to the sinuses due to the sudden vacuum created within the sinus cavity and the rush of air to fill it. This can result in stretching of nerve fibers with sometimes rather sudden discomfort, or even tearing of the membranous lining of a sinus or its drainage duct or opening, often followed by bleeding. This problem is more likely to occur in the sometimes rather long drainage duct leading to a frontal sinus or even within the frontal sinus itself. This sudden pain and sustained obstruction followed by headache may persist until the hemorrhage is absorbed, the associated swelling subsides, and pressure equalization is restored.

This is one reason your doctor will advise you not to fly with a cold, even in a pressurized cabin, and why pilots are grounded when they have a cold or hay fever and permanently grounded should they develop chronic sinusitis. If you fly with a cold or sinusitis, the pressure changes may drive the infection deeper into your sinuses and may even force infected discharge into other sinuses that may so far have been spared. I learned early in my medical career that anyone who did fly with a cold, sinusitis, or an ear infection would require medications and especially antibiotics for two or three times as long a period as normally prescribed to get well and stay well. Shortening this course of treatment often results in a resurgence of the same persistent infection several weeks later, when it may be even more difficult to cure. I also recall treating many cases of subacute and chronic sinusitis that dated back to flying with a head cold followed by inadequate therapy.

People who fly with partially obstructed sinuses from old scarring, active allergy, or polyps, but with no evidence of a sinus infection, such as a cloudy discharge, should strongly consider following the same Valsalva inflation procedures for pressure equalization as those recommended for blocked eustachian tubes, since a sudden pressure change could convert a partially blocked sinus to a totally blocked sinus. With this maneuver, you clamp the nose with your thumb and forefinger, swallow, and then immediately blow into the nose without letting go. To protect the ears as well as the sinuses, you should generally do this three times a minute when climbing or descending and three times an hour, again at regular intervals, while aloft and flying at a fairly steady altitude. A sudden change in altitude, however, would require you to repeat the procedure immediately. I have taught this technique with very satisfactory results to hundreds of patients who fly regularly as well as to some who were afraid to fly because of previous ear or sinus discomfort.

Although this modified Valsalva maneuver for inflating the ears and sinuses is more important during a plane's descent, when a vacuum tends to form in a partially blocked sinus or ear, it should, as suggested, be carried out before that time to prevent subtle sustained blockage from making later inflations on descent more difficult to accomplish. In the past, I have been reminded by patients while draining and irrigating a sinus that any sudden vacuum or negative pressure created within a sinus cavity from drawing back on a syringe is much more painful than a sudden increase in positive pressure from pushing the plunger forward, and the same would apply to any sudden pressure changes during flight. Pain from positive pressure within a sinus cavity can take several hours to develop whereas pain from a vacuum or negative pressure may develop rather quickly. It would appear that some frontal sinuses, even those with rather long drainage ducts, can, when partially blocked, relieve themselves of too much positive pressure more easily and with much less discomfort than when a vacuum or negative pressure is present. For the same reason, it is much easier to blow through a partially collapsed drinking straw than to suck through one, and sucking hard may only lead to more collapse with further blockage. Also, with the sudden rush of air through a long frontal sinus duct to relieve a vacuum, the chances of membrane collapse, invaginations, tissue rupture, bleeding, and pain are greater. Any of these sudden pressure changes, particularly when diving or flying, seem more inclined to affect the frontal sinuses, and this is probably more likely to occur in the 20 to 40 percent that have elongated ducts rather than in those with just an opening into the sinus.

With regard to inflating the ears, it is especially important to swallow immediately before blowing, since the eustachian tubes are normally closed except when swallowing or yawning, and it requires a great deal more pressure and effort to inflate a middle ear through a closed eustachian tube. This modified Valsalva maneuver, when performed properly at regular intervals, requires very little effort and no real exertion. It is simply a matter of coordinating the swallow immediately before blowing, and it should not—and need not—be done forcefully. Blowing or exhaling too forcefully, such as during weight lifting, karate, strenuous jogging, or vigorous sex, may in rare instances cause temporary blindness due to very small hemorrhages in the back of the eye known as Valsalva retinopathy.

The same procedure for inflating the ears and sinuses on a plane would apply to scuba divers as well. For every 33 feet a diver descends, there is an increase in water pressure of 14.7 pounds per square inch, also known as 1 atmosphere. When you dive, the self-contained underwater breathing apparatus, or scuba, adjusts the air pressure within your nose, sinuses, lungs, and ears to this increase in outside water pressure as you descend so that you don't rupture your eardrums and so that you can expand your chest to breathe. Just as pressure equalization in the lungs when scuba diving depends on breathing regularly, pressure equalization in the ears and sinuses depends on inflating regularly. As would be expected, the pressure effects of the outside water on the lungs, sinuses, and eardrums in deep free diving without a tank can be especially severe and, because of the very rapid descent, will require even more frequent inflations.

If ear inflations are not done properly and at appropriate intervals, a diver could rupture his or her outer eardrum, thus allowing cold water to enter the thermal protective middle ear cavity and causing severe dizziness, nausea, and sometimes vomiting. The present generation of divers should be especially mindful of this, since some of them may have weakened eardrums from ear tube insertions in childhood. Following tubal removal or rejection, the hole in the eardrum may sometimes heal with a very thin and very weak layer of cells called a monomeric membrane, thus making the eardrum especially vulnerable to rupture.

Most divers agree that this modified Valsalva technique for ear and sinus inflations is safe and effective provided they do it frequently enough during rapid descent and even fairly often once they level off below. Since trapped air is gradually absorbed from any closed body cavity such as the middle ear or a blocked sinus, it must be replaced, or else a partial vacuum will develop in any closed-off cavity with rigid walls. If the vacuum or negative pressure is allowed to continue, membrane swelling with further sinus or eustachian tube blockage and eventually fluid accumulation will occur, often paving the way for an ear or sinus infection. The speed of descent, ear sensitivity, and degree of relief when inflating may sometimes help the diver to decide how often to inflate. Again, it should be emphasized that ear and sinus inflations can't be done too often, but they can be done too seldom, and this would be especially true when you are diving or flying.

Simply swallowing or just stretching the jaw muscles will work for a few individuals with exceptionally well-functioning eustachian tubes, but it won't relieve a partially obstructed sinus. A few individuals have permanently open eustachian tubes, and they will usually experience no ear blockage symptoms with almost any kind of outside pressure change. Some of them may even be aware of air moving in and out of their eustachian tubes when they breathe. However, if you are prone to ear or sinus blockage problems when you dive or fly, even if you have supposedly normal eustachian tubes, you would still be wise to use the swallowing and immediately blowing with the nose clamped-off technique. On gradual ascent from a deep dive, when your ears and sinuses have to release their excessive air pressure, frequent swallowing in addition to regular breathing is usually all you have to do.

Again, the sudden development of a significant pressure difference, especially a vacuum, in the ears and sinuses can cause damage, or barotrauma, to both of these structures and result in pain, hemorrhages, sinusitis, eardrum rupture, ear infection, mastoid infection, scarring, loss of hearing, vertigo, and even a rupture of the tiny membrane covering the window to the inner ear, causing severe vertigo and deafness. In some instances, severe vertigo in a diver could even be fatal due to vomiting and aspiration or even from the loss of a sense of direction as to which way is up, especially in dark, murky waters and particularly for the novice diver. Some of the merchant seamen who served in the North Atlantic in World War II and were blown overboard without a life preserver drowned almost instantly because the ice-cold water rushing into their ears created such violent vertigo that they couldn't tell which direction to swim in to reach the surface; many swam downward instead.

We have learned that a vacuum may begin to form from tissue absorption of air in a blocked noninfected middle ear within about 20 minutes after developing a blocked eustachian tube, and the same would apply to an uninfected, completely blocked sinus cavity.

However, the larger sinus cavities with considerably more air space may take longer to show the effects of a significant pressure increase or vacuum formation, since air, unlike liquids, can readily expand or compress.

Although no harm would normally be expected from inflating too often, a physician would be very reluctant to recommend this procedure to a person flying with acute sinusitis, an acute ear infection, or a cold, but no one with these conditions should be flying anyhow. Some of my patients who flew or dove professionally have informed me that on occasions when they did dive or fly with a cold or ear infection and therefore had to inflate their ears and sinuses, they often got away with it, but not always. Prophylactic decongestants by mouth before flight and a decongestant nasal spray during flight can be of considerable help, especially if you are already congested or have had trouble with your ears or sinuses when flying in the past. If you have no choice and must fly with an acute infection in your nose, sinuses, or ears, I would strongly recommend taking a broad-spectrum antibiotic as well as a decongestant well before embarking and for at least 2 to 4 weeks and sometimes longer after landing. Once the infection has departed, if an ear, especially, still feels blocked due to residual swelling, then repeated inflations may be necessary, preferably while you are still covered by an effective antibiotic, to further reduce swelling and to restore ear pressure dynamics, which are essential to the complete relief of eustachian tube blockage.

In such cases, any after-flight inflations of the ears by the modified Valsalva technique should be performed three or four times an hour at regular intervals when you are awake and continued until constant relief is obtained. That usually means continuing inflations until there is no longer any popping sound in the ears when inflating and until swallowing after successfully inflating results in an immediate release of the excess air trapped within the ear. To verify success with this, it is especially important that you do this the first thing in the morning in order to test it, when your head tissues and membranes are normally slightly swollen anyhow. In a few cases that fail to respond to conservative treatment, a temporary tube may have to be inserted through the eardrum to restore pressure dynamics in the middle ear.

As one can readily see, the middle ear cavity and a sinus cavity resemble each other in many ways. Both are mostly surrounded by bone, lined with a ciliated mucus-secreting membrane, and connected to our upper air passages by tubes or openings also lined with ciliated mucus-secreting membranes. They both require a fairly constant flow of air from the upper airway to function properly. If they don't have it or go without it for very long, both will develop a vacuum with retention of fluid, sometimes discomfort, and possibly infection. Both are normally fairly sterile cavities that try to keep themselves that way with their anti-infectious mucous secretions and by constantly sweeping themselves clean. Both can be blocked up and infected by respiratory infections such as colds or flu, and both are subject to chronic infection if treated inadequately or for too short a period. Both may develop drainage problems where blockage or swelling must subside before any infection will clear up completely and where any sustained blockage will cause it to recur and possibly to become chronic. Both are susceptible to any allergy problems involving the nose, and both are affected by external pressure changes in air or water such as noted when flying or diving. Both are occasionally subject to serious infectious complications, especially involving the central nervous system or brain if they go untreated, and both may sometimes require expert treatment to cure. Nowhere else within the body do two such functionally different bony cavities share so many important similarities.

Flying or diving during episodes of allergic rhinitis can sometimes cause serious blockage problems for the ears and sinuses. When it is necessary to do so, the allergic rhinitis should be controlled with steroid nasal sprays, decongestants and non-sedating antihistamines, each beginning far enough ahead of time to be effective during the flight or dive.

In planes with pressurized cabins, a second factor comes into play that directly affects the nose, sinuses, and respiratory tract of the air traveler, namely re-breathing each other's air as well as breathing a somewhat polluted and very dry air. Gathering a number of individuals from all parts of the country, and sometimes from all over the world, into a very small area such as a plane cabin can naturally introduce into the environment all kinds of clothing and shoe dust, bacteria, and viruses, as well as allergens such as dust mites, pollen, molds, and animal dander. All of these potential allergens may collect in the plane's carpets and seats and be propelled into the air every time someone shuffles his or her feet, walks down the aisle, or sits down. Pulling clothing, personal effects, and luggage from overhead storage spaces scatters dust and adds to the air contamination. That luggage may even have traveled a dusty road on top of a truck in some faraway place. When you add to that the germs coughed up, blown out, or sneezed into the air, plus the formaldehyde fumes from synthetic materials, the odors from heated food, perfumes, body deodorants, decontaminating sprays, air fresheners, and toilet chemicals, it is no wonder that many airline travelers develop temporary nose, throat, and lung problems.

In our global society, with long-distance air travel increasing every day and especially with previously closed countries opening their doors to emigrants and war refugees, a local endemic disease in one country now has the potential of becoming a worldwide epidemic. I have talked with many patients who contracted a head cold, flu, or sinusitis within 3 to 5 days of a plane flight, often the usual incubation period for respiratory viruses, especially during the winter months when rhinoviruses and influenza viruses are so prevalent. This problem probably occurred less often when the airlines were adding 100 percent outside air with a nearly complete air exchange in less than 5 minutes as compared to the 50 percent addition to recirculated air being practiced by most airlines today. More sophisticated air-filtering systems including high-efficiency particulate air (HEPA) filters have been added to justify this reduction in the circulated outside air. These filters are generally considered effective in screening fine particle matter and some bacteria as small as 0.3 micron from the circulated air. Because of the concentration of passengers in such a small area, and new passengers from different areas being added each time a plane lands, allergic individuals can expect a much greater exposure to allergens on a plane, brought in on shoes, clothing, hair, and carry-on luggage, than they might find in their own homes and therefore should contemplate some preventative care before flying—a problem that should also be of concern to sinus patients with nasal allergies.

A third factor that comes into play in pressurized plane cabins, and one that can also wreak havoc on your nasal passages, sinuses, and lower respiratory tracts, is the lack of humidity in the air. Apparently at the present time no additional humidity is introduced into the cabin air except from heating coffee and tea, or from the moisture vaporized and blown off by the lungs or evaporated from the skin of the plane's occupants. Their moisture loss is further accelerated by the progressive reduction in cabin humidity each time the very dry outside air is introduced and part of the stale cabin air is exhausted. The availability of additional humidity is very important in a dry environment if you don't want to give up too much of your own body moisture. The cold fresh air picked up by a plane at high altitudes is very low in humidity. As it enters the plane and is heated, it is then capable of holding a lot more moisture, but none is available except from the bodies and respiratory tracts of the passengers. It is my understanding that efforts to humidify this air have so far been impractical and unsuccessful.

This very dry air tends to thicken the protective mucous blanket of the upper and lower respiratory tracts of both passengers and crew, thereby slowing the flow of mucus and encouraging the penetration of viruses or bacteria into the underlying membranes of the respiratory tract and sinuses. A sluggish mucous flow, enhanced by a progressive lowering of the humidity, invites cross-contamination from other passengers who have an existing sinus, nose, or lung infection, and they can also expect their own infections to become significantly worse for the same reason. People with lower respiratory tract infections will usually be coughing more owing to the very dry air and further adding to the spread of disease.

A similar problem from the drying effects on the respiratory tract and sinuses can also be expected if you live at a high altitude, unless of course you make some effort to add humidity to your immediate environment. Normally healthy sinuses should have no apparent difficulty in adjusting to the reduced air pressure of living at a high altitude, but the reduced humidity, often drying out the nasal membranes and causing crusting and bleeding, can present a problem. However, many people eventually seem to adjust to it, provided sinus infections are not allowed to go untreated for an extended period. Deformities within the nose such as a deviated nasal septum, enlarged turbinates, nasal polyps, or even allergic swelling can, however, make such an adjustment much more difficult.

Even jet fighter pilots, who must fly at high altitudes and often have to breathe 95 to 100 percent oxygen to function efficiently, not only experience the marked mucus-drying effects of pure oxygen but will often notice vacuum headaches later due to the especially rapid absorption of concentrated oxygen from their sometimes temporarily blocked sinus cavities.

If you fly frequently or on long trips, you would be wise to drink plenty of water before embarking to counteract the dry-air effects on mucous membranes as well as to counteract the dehydrating effects of caffeine and alcohol often imbibed en route, since both tend to increase urinary output and dry out respiratory membranes.

Sterile saline nose sprays can be helpful as a fast way of maintaining and moisturizing nasal membranes on long flights. It should be pointed out, however, that sprays carried on planes should be tightly capped and carried upright, say in a breast pocket of a shirt or coat, to prevent them from emptying into your carry-on luggage, purse, coat, or trousers when the pressure in the cabin is lowered and the pressure of the trapped air in the upside-down spray bottle remains high. A similar problem from pressure change may develop with sprays or drops stored in a suitcase in the baggage compartment. Any extra sprays stored there should be tightly sealed and placed in a sealed plastic bag in case a leak should occur. Plastic bags should be emptied of their air in the process of sealing to prevent air expansion with interruption of their seals. It is also a good idea to carry any important medications that you take regularly on your person when you fly, just in case your luggage is lost.

If you consider that when you travel by air, you are forced to breathe an unnatural pressurized or depressurized air to which your sinuses and ears must adjust, a polluted air often containing multiple allergens sometimes collected from all corners of the world, a re-breathed and commonly shared air that often contains viruses and bacteria, and an abnormally dry air that can disrupt the protective mucociliary flow in the respiratory tract and thereby render you more susceptible to airborne diseases, there is little wonder that so many flight passengers develop sneezing, dry throat, nasal congestion, eye discomfort, fatigue, cough, ear symptoms, vertigo, respiratory tract infections, lightheadedness, headaches, and sometimes a temporary vague or detached feeling. You should also remember that inhaling soluble gases or finely vaporized substances collecting within the small space of a plane cabin is almost like injecting a smaller amount of the same thing into your bloodstream. That's how inhaled anesthetics work, and that is another reason why you should constantly protect yourself from breathing harmful sprays, fumes, and fine-particle matter.

To capitalize on a somewhat familiar quote, breathing while you fly could be hazardous to your health, especially if you are prone to sinusitis, allergies, ear problems, or lung disease.

CHAPTER EIGHTEEN

Polyps and Cysts

POLYPS

When I first tell my patients that they have a polyp or polyps in their nose or sinuses, their first question is usually "What are polyps?" and the next question is "Do they have to be removed?" Although many people have heard that intestinal polyps can be cancerous, the question of whether their own nasal polyps may be cancerous is usually avoided and seldom asked. Fortunately, with nasal and sinus polyps, this frightening possibility is not a cause for alarm.

Polyps may be found throughout the body wherever there is a membranous lining such as in the ears, throat, larynx, trachea, lungs, esophagus, stomach, intestines, glandular ducts, urethra, cervix, bladder, and uterus, as well as in the nose and sinuses. A polyp in the nose or a sinus is not a new growth such as a tumor, since it still maintains the same basic microscopic characteristics as its surrounding tissues. Its surface is also covered with the same kind of mucus-secreting ciliated membrane that lines the adjacent nose and sinuses, although sometimes the surface membranes of a polyp may thicken, flatten out, and lose their cilia in the presence of chronic infection or from constant exposure to the irritating and drying effects of the nasal airstream. Nor does a true polyp in the nose or sinuses change its basic microscopic appearance and become malignant or cancerous, as some do in other parts of the body such as the intestinal tract. Even though a polyp in the nose or sinuses doesn't become malignant, this soft pale grapelike structure may eventually enlarge to the point that it extrudes forward out of a nostril or backward into the throat. The pressure created on the surrounding tissues by nasal or sinus polyps gradually enlarging over a long period of time can, in some instances, partially destroy the bones of the nose, sinuses, or orbits. Some adults with long-standing nasal polyps may even develop a froglike nose, and children with extensive nasal and sinus polyps may develop elongated facial features, an open bite, sometimes a high arch to the palate, and in rare instances a wide separation of the eyes, especially when the ethmoid sinuses are extensively involved. Fortunately, very few people now wait until such extremes occur before consulting a doctor.

Nasal and sinus polyps are not an uncommon finding in individuals who have chronic sinusitis, and since polyps often obstruct sinus drainage very early in their development, they can be responsible for the infection's chronic state as well as for treatment failures. Polyps are also found in some allergic individuals with sinusitis but are more often noted in nonallergic sinusitis patients and even more so in nonallergic asthmatics over age 40. Polyps are especially common in asthmatics who have aspirin intolerance or sensitivity, although they may be found alone and without any signs of asthma in such cases. They are also frequently noted in conjunction with cystic fibrosis and with allergic fungal sinusitis. Approximately 14 percent of those who have nasal or sinus polyps will give a positive family history of similar problems, strongly suggesting a genetic predisposition in some cases.

With the introduction of newer and better fiber-optic nasal examining instruments as well as the CAT scan, doctors have become more aware of the significant role that even a very minute polyp can play in chronic obstructive sinus disease, and we now know that many times removing even a very small polyp blocking a sinus drainage opening is essential to the cure of the sinus infection. Since cysts in the nose and especially in the sinuses can sometimes be confused with polyps, they will also be discussed.

Since nasal polyps often begin in the sinuses, especially the ethmoid sinuses, and then gradually make their way into the nose, it is important to discuss nasal and sinus polyps together as part of a somewhat similar process.

Nasal polyps occur in about 1 percent of the population and were known as far back as 1000 B.C. Hippocrates himself supposedly suggested pulling a sponge through the nose as one method of removing them. Many theories as to the cause of nasal and sinus polyps have been proposed over the years, and it appears that there may be more than one reason for these rounded grapelike structures that show up in the sinuses or hang down in the nose. The fact that they are found in so many different disease states, including cystic fibrosis, Kartagener's syndrome, allergy, sinus infection, aspirin sensitivity, and allergic fungal sinusitis, would tend to support this theory. Even so, the frequent common denominator and the thing that so often makes a nasal or sinus polyp develop, continue to enlarge, and possibly to recur appears to be a localized area of membrane swelling, from whatever cause, possibly followed by a narrowing at its base that allows blood, lymph, and tissue fluid to flow into the swollen area but partially restricts their exit. There are also many different ideas as to the cause of this swelling, some simple and some very complex. Some have attributed it to a biochemical disorder resulting in increased leakage of fluid from blood vessels, some to allergens or histamine activity, some to nonallergic mediators such as found in aspirin sensitivity, some to the negative pressure dynamics in breathing, some to genetically inherent abnormalities of the mucous glands as in cystic fibrosis, and some apparently to persistent inflammatory changes as in chronic sinusitis. More recently, it has been suggested that the local release of inflammatory mediators, other than histamine, followed by an increase in tissue salt content may increase fluid absorption to the point of causing a protracted localized swelling.

Since nasal polyps are rather insensitive to pain, some feel that this apparent lack of nerve supply could cause venous congestion with leaking of clear fluid into the tissues resulting in a localized swelling and polyp formation. The diminished nerve supply, of course, could also be secondary to the constant pinching or pressure effect on the nerve supply of a developing polyp created by a constriction at its base. Some even attribute this narrowing at the base to the localized tissue accumulation of an adrenaline-like constricting substance known as norepinephrine.

Still others have attributed nasal and sinus polyp formation to a tiny spontaneous rupture or split in a surface membrane followed by a protrusion of the underlying soft tissues through this superficial membranous cleft. The same might also apply to a small area of membrane ulceration with a subsequent protrusion of soft tissue through its center, and in both instances a slight scarring or fibrosis at the margins or edges of the wound might act as a constricting band.

Most sinus doctors have on rare occasions observed a polyp developing in a nose or sinus as a result of postoperative scarring. However, if a slit in a nasal or sinus membrane is a frequent cause of nasal or sinus polyps, it is surprising that we don't see many more instances of polyp formation following surgery, especially from the numerous needle punctures used to irrigate maxillary sinuses, a very frequently performed office procedure over the past 100 years. With this procedure, a rather large needle is introduced through the inferior wall of the nose into the maxillary sinus cavity, causing a small slit in the membrane on both the nasal and sinus walls, and yet polyps are very rarely seen in either area. However, some polyps developing on the inside walls of the nose or sinuses, as well as on the turbinates themselves, might originate from a small dimple, crevice, narrow depression, or ulcerated pocket in the surface membrane, with swelling at the base and with a natural constriction also developing around the edges.

Many of the polyps found in the nose seem to arise from the anterior ethmoid sinus openings, especially polyps protruding from beneath the middle turbinates, where most nasal polyps are found and where they may also obstruct the frontal and maxillary sinus openings. Their development there may result from excessive swelling of the membranous linings of these very small anterior ethmoid sinuses due to one of the various causes already mentioned or even to some cause so far unrecognized. The poor circulation normally present in the anterior ethmoid sinuses also makes it a little more difficult for the body to reverse this swelling once it starts. When the ethmoid sinus cavity becomes completely filled with swollen membrane, a small membranous tag or nubbing may then push through the sinus drainage opening into the nose as the beginnings of a nasal polyp. This small sinus opening, usually only 1 to 2 millimeters in size, then acts as a constricting band or tourniquet partially restricting the return of blood, lymph, and tissue fluids from this membranous protrusion and causing it to continue to swell. Although this constriction at the base of the polyp in such instances may not be the initiating cause, it could certainly provide the impetus for the continuous progressive enlargement so characteristic of nasal polyps. The final result, however, is a nasal polyp that began at the sinus opening and now hangs down in the nose like a skinless grape. This may not only block your breathing, but you may sometimes feel the polyp moving back and forth in your nose with each breath. Other symptoms of nasal polyps often include a nasal tone to the voice, sneezing, sometimes drainage from the front of the nose, mouth breathing resulting in a dry throat, and an awareness of a postnasal drip as well as the usual signs of sinus blockage, including a cloudy discharge and sometimes a headache or facial discomfort.

I have observed a similar process in the formation of ear polyps protruding into the external ear canal through an existing hole in an eardrum and arising from a markedly swollen membranous lining of the middle ear due to an ear infection. These early ear polyps were noted on occasion to retract back into the middle ear cavity and out of sight when a shrinkage medication was applied to their surface, and in some instances not to reappear if the ear infection was thoroughly treated and cured.

In a similar manner, a sinus infection alone, if persistent, can cause enough sustained swelling of a sinus membrane to make it protrude through a sinus opening and produce a nasal polyp. However, in my experience, these infectious polyps are more often located on one side and usually limited to only one or occasionally two sinuses, whereas those thought to be related to cystic fibrosis, allergy, aspirin intolerance, allergic fungal sinusitis, or asthma are more often bilateral and tend eventually to involve most of the other sinuses as well. Furthermore, since the presence of a polyp at a sinus drainage opening usually causes sinus blockage with infection, it is often difficult to decide which came first or whether they both gradually developed together. Even more important, the sinus infection won't go away until the obstructing polyp is removed or shrunk down and adequate sinus drainage is restored.

Here it should also be apparent that removing the polyp should entail more than just snipping it off if you want a more permanent relief of sinus blockage and don't want the polyp to immediately start developing again from the remaining piece of stalk left behind. Ideally, for the best results, the constricting sinus opening should be opened up, enlarged, the sinus entered, and the polyp's membranous base excised along with the stalk. Occasionally, however, a nasal polyp may be grasped by a forceps or snare, and the polyp, its stalk, and base extracted or avulsed in its entirety. This would discourage a recurrence, provided, of course, that the reason for the polyp formation can be identified and treated. The same applies to maxillary sinus polyps, which may sometimes present beneath the middle turbinates or occasionally surface in the back of the nose as a choanal polyp. Posterior ethmoid and sphenoid sinus polyps may also develop in the back of the nose and should be treated in a similar fashion for more permanent results. Frontal sinus polyps, especially when they have to push through a narrow drainage duct to reach the nose, are less inclined to do so and will frequently remain within the frontal sinus cavity to cause blockage and infection. However, most frontal sinuses drain directly into the nose through a slit or opening rather than through an elongated duct, thus making a nasal polyp presentation more likely.

Nasal polyps arising from a sinus opening usually create a kind of dumbbell effect with some scarring or fibrosis developing in the narrow neck wedged into the sinus drainage opening. They are therefore usually reluctant to recede completely back into the sinus cavity, although some early ones with minimal scarring may disappear with medical treatment. If a polyp is wedged into a sinus opening for very long, pressure damage to the opening along with infection and ulceration may sometimes cause fusion of the polyp to the sides of the opening, thus making it sometimes appear that the polyp starts there rather than from within the sinus cavity itself. Occasionally, taking corticosteroid medications or using of steroid nasal sprays may make polyps smaller and when treated early before excessive scarring takes place may even make them disappear. Unless the basic cause of the problem can be found and treated, however, they will usually reappear, especially if the corticosteroid medications have to be discontinued.

Since these anti-inflammatory steroids by spray or by pill may occasionally prevent or relieve nasal polyp formation, you would have to assume that some kind of inflammatory mediator may be directly involved in some types of sinonasal polyp formation. Along this line, I have observed on a number of occasions a rather marked acceleration in nasal polyp growth with a viral upper respiratory infection such as a cold or flu as well as with recurrent acute flare-ups of chronic sinusitis, both of which would involve acute inflammatory processes. Although a slight to moderate increase in histamine as well as mast cells has been found in some nasal polyps, it would appear that histamine is an unlikely mediator for polyp formation, especially since Cromolyn nasal spray, a blocker of histamine release from mast cells, is totally ineffective in preventing or relieving polyp formation, as are the antihistamines. Moreover, the nasal polyps so frequently found in aspirin-intolerant individuals have generally shown no increase in histamine or mast cells over that found in normal nasal membranes.

Although polyps and nasal allergy have been found together in a number of people, it is now generally believed to be more of a coincidence and that the allergy is not directly responsible for the polyp formation but, when present, may tend to enhance their growth.

Nevertheless, if your doctor does suspect allergic rhinitis and if you have nasal polyps, especially on both sides of the nose, a complete allergic workup would be indicated, since early recognition and treatment of the allergy might also slow further polyp development. Surprisingly, except for the nasal polyps noted in people who have cystic fibrosis or Kartagener's syndrome, most of them show a high eosinophil cell count, which is so often indicative of allergy and may account for earlier beliefs that allergy played a major role in nasal and sinus polyp formation. The possibility that a toxic substance frequently associated with the presence and breakdown of numerous eosinophils could cause tissue damage with additional inflammation, localized swelling, and possible polyp formation has also been considered.

Since obstruction of a sinus drainage opening by a polyp nearly always initiates infection in that particular sinus, it is necessary to eradicate or remove the polyp to reestablish drainage and prevent chronic sinusitis. Taking antibiotics, without relieving the blockage, may temporarily clear up a sinus infection, but it will inevitably return once the antibiotics are discontinued. Therefore, in most cases, the blockage, the resulting infection, and any allergy that may be present should all be treated for a complete cure.

On a few occasions, I have seen allergic individuals with extensive nasal polyp formation blocking most of their sinuses and yet showing no positive evidence of a sinus infection, even after following them for a long period of time. Their only obvious symptoms were marked nasal blockage, sneezing, diminished taste or smell, clear drainage from the front of the nose, mouth breathing and a nasal tone to the voice, and usually not even a headache. Such cases are rare and difficult to explain. Normally a doctor would expect gross evidence of sinus infection from so much obstruction to sinus drainage. Also, no one knows why one individual will produce numerous sinonasal polyps that recur repeatedly even after careful surgical removal, and why others with multiple allergies, sinus blockage, and chronic sinus infection may develop no polyps at all.

Occasionally your doctor will see a cluster of nodular tissue, which is usually located in only one side of the nose, often extending into the sinuses, which may be mistaken grossly for a grouping of small polyps. This may turn out to be an inverting papilloma or nasal papillomatosis and should be identified by biopsy and completely removed, since they tend to invade the sinuses and can become cancerous. Unlike polyps, papillomas usually have little or no stalk, are more sensitive to touch, are more likely to bleed, and usually appear much pinker than the pale gray polyp. The human papilloma virus has been blamed for their development as well as for the formation of papillomata in other areas of the body.

In the nose, they start beneath the nasal membranes and usually leave the overlying mucous membrane intact early in their formation, which may account for their often delayed diagnosis. The use of magnified examining telescopes and the CAT scan have been most helpful in identifying them and determining the extent of their involvement of the sinuses as well as aiding in their complete removal. Since they too will block sinus drainage, they nearly always cause a unilateral sinusitis with a cloudy discharge. Consequently, whenever there is a finding of unilateral sinusitis with one or more small polyp-like growths in that side of the nose, it is necessary to rule out an inverting papilloma by a biopsy and sometimes with a repeated deeper biopsy. Because of the locally aggressive nature of these tumors, their tendency to invade bony structures, and their association with malignancy in up to 13 percent of cases, it is essential that they be diagnosed early and completely excised, since they can invade the base of the skull and orbit as well as the sinuses. Sometimes nasal polyps may be present in conjunction with nasal papillomatosis, thus making the diagnosis more difficult. Moreover, the presence of multiple nasal polyps often found in association with allergic fungal sinusitis may further confuse the picture.

Another new growth, which may occasionally resemble a cluster of polyps and is usually found in older children and particularly in male adolescents, is the juvenile angiofibroma. It is a benign, rather firm tumor that develops in the back of the nose or nasopharynx and often invades the sinuses and even the base of the skull in a very destructive manner. Since it often obstructs sinus drainage, it usually causes a persistent sinusitis and frequently bleeds. The diagnosis is usually made by fiber-optic exam, CAT scan, and biopsy. Fortunately, it too occurs rather infrequently.

When you accept the fact that sinusitis is primarily a disease of inadequate drainage and insufficient air exchange between the sinuses and the nose, and that the treatment or cure therefore has to be directed toward the reestablishment of adequate drainage and proper aeration of a diseased sinus cavity, it is easy to see that sinus blockage from a polyp can play an important role in the development of chronic sinusitis. Consequently, the proper and timely surgical removal of obstructive nasal and sinus polyps, and even an obstructive mucocele or cyst, in many instances can be a major factor in the prevention or cure of a potentially chronic sinus infection.

The introduction in recent years of delicate fiber-optic examining instruments with better lighting and magnification has made it possible to visualize very minute polyps tucked away in the small recesses of the nose, such as beneath a turbinate, yet completely blocking a sinus and totally unobserved on normal visual examination. Fortunately, CAT scans have also become very proficient in demonstrating even a very small polyp obstructing a sinus opening, although an occasional one may still be missed. A larger polyp that protrudes into the nasal airway and that you may be aware of as it moves back and forth when you breathe is usually easily visualized by the examining physician unless it is located too far back in the nose.

Occasionally a very large single polyp, usually of infectious origin and on a very long stalk, may arise in the large maxillary or cheek sinus and extend through a secondary sinus opening, or more often directly through a very thin or defective sinonasal wall, into the back of the nose and even into the upper throat. This ball-like structure will tend to lodge at the junction of the posterior nose and nasopharynx known as the choana and is called a choanal polyp. Sometimes these posterior polyps will break off and be swallowed or coughed up, which, for obvious reasons, could be dangerous, especially if it occurs when you are sleeping. On occasion I have had patients bring me some rather large polyps that they have either coughed up or sneezed out. A choanal polyp, like other nasal polyps, should be removed at its base, including its origin within the maxillary sinus, or it will tend to recur. Even a very large choanal polyp in back of the nose and nearly the size of a golf ball may be missed on routine superficial examination but should always be looked for if your nasal breathing is almost completely obstructed on one or both sides and your speech sounds very nasal with nothing else found to account for it. A nasal or sinus endoscopic examination should reveal a choanal polyp immediately, however, and a CAT scan will usually identify it as well as its usual site of origin within the maxillary sinus.

The very small polyps that may not affect your breathing at all and therefore go totally unnoticed can be just as obstructive to sinus drainage as a very large polyp. Unfortunately, they may go completely undetected for weeks and sometimes months in spite of a routine nasal examination, thereby promoting deep-seated chronic sinus infection and a failure to respond to treatment. Any time an infected sinus cavity fails to clear up with prolonged intensive medical treatment, your doctor should make a thorough search for a small obstructive polyp.

When nasal or sinus polyps are discovered, it does not necessarily mean that your doctor will recommend surgery first. Conservative measures with steroid nasal sprays and even in a few cases with systemic corticosteroids, as well as antibiotics, decongestants, and sometimes allergy treatment or occasionally aspirin desensitization shots, are usually tried initially. In some cases, however, early relief of sinus obstruction by surgical removal of a polyp or polyps, mainly to relieve infection, may be necessary, and your doctor may be reluctant to stop the antibiotic therapy until this is done. On more than one occasion, I have scheduled a patient for surgical removal of nasal polyps only to find that the polyps had disappeared with medical treatment; but unfortunately you can't depend on this happening. Nevertheless, some physicians have reported relief of symptoms and disappearance of nasal polyps in approximately 40 percent of their patients with medical therapy alone. However, once it becomes obvious that conservative measures cannot shrink away the polyps completely and reestablish adequate sinus drainage within a reasonable period of time, surgery in conjunction with medical and sometimes allergy treatment should be strongly considered.

Nasal polyps are more frequently found in men except when there is an associated asthma, and then they may show a preference for women. They are rarely seen in infants and children under age 10 and practically never under age 2. This is fortunate, since nasal or sinus surgery in children should be limited whenever possible. When one or more nasal or sinus polyps are found in a child or in a young adolescent, the doctor has to be highly suspicious of cystic fibrosis, although the diagnosis of this condition is now often made early and before any polyps are noted, usually from a history of repeated respiratory infections and a positive sweat test.

Nasal or sinus polyps, especially when found in adults with asthma, also make it necessary for your doctor to rule out aspirin intolerance, since you could have a syndrome consisting of aspirin sensitivity, asthma, and nasal polyps, usually with an associated rhinosinusitis. Aspirin, probably our most commonly used medication over the years, still has to be treated with a great deal of respect. It can help you in many ways, but it can also cause bleeding, stomach ulcers, esophagitis, Reye's syndrome, and ringing in the ears, as well as asthma and nasal polyps in certain aspirin-intolerant individuals.

People with aspirin intolerance, or the so-called Samter's syndrome, usually within a few minutes to a few hours after taking an aspirin or any other nonsteroidal anti-inflammatory drug such as ibuprofen may develop marked nasal congestion, sneezing, and a profuse clear watery nasal discharge, very much like a vasomotor rhinitis or an acute allergic rhinitis, and not infrequently followed by breathing difficulty, asthmatic wheezing, and sometimes GI upset with nausea, vomiting, abdominal pain, occasionally diarrhea, and in rare instances anaphylactic shock. Rather severe asthma, rhinosinusitis, and nasal polyps are usually found in a high percentage of these patients, although the polyps may be some years in showing up or may even be present for a long time without being recognized. The sinusitis problem, however, will usually become more persistent and more chronic once the polyps begin to form and obstruct the sinus openings.

Even though a few people may tend to outgrow this aspirin sensitivity, it could take a very long time. The nasal polyps, which are often bilateral and usually arise from the ethmoid sinuses, are nearly always accompanied by an ethmoid sinusitis, which has to be treated as well. Steroids by nasal spray, by mouth, or sometimes by shot have been used with good results, provided that they are covered by antibiotics in the infected patient. Aspirin desensitization has also been successful in some people. If treatment for the sinusitis is ignored, the accompanying asthma may become more difficult to control. Although aspirin-intolerant individuals may sometimes show a high eosinophil cell count in the blood as well as in nasal secretions, this is not considered to be an allergic condition. Those who have it will also show negative skin testing for the usual allergens known to precipitate asthma, unless by chance there happens to be a coexistent allergy to some inhalant or food. Immediate treatment for the acute reaction may sometimes require a rapid visit to the hospital emergency room for a shot of epinephrine as a lifesaving measure. Acetaminophen should thereafter replace aspirin products in the medicine cabinet. Of course, the other nonsteroidal anti-inflammatory drugs known as NSAIDs, which belong to the same family as aspirin, would have to be strictly avoided as well.

In recommending immunotherapy or any other prolonged allergy treatment for the allergic sinusitis sufferer who also happens to have nasal polyps, the doctor should not wait for a very extended period to evaluate the treatment results before going ahead with surgically relieving the sinus obstruction by removing the polyps. Otherwise the persistent sinus infection will not only create more scar tissue with a greater possibility of causing chronic disease but will also have the opportunity to infect other sinuses nearby even after the allergy may appear to be under control.

It is often surprising how many asthmatics with sinusitis already have, or eventually go on to develop, nasal or sinus polyps, and how much improvement in their asthma may sometimes result from removing the polyps and clearing up their obstructive sinus disease. Although some may notice no sustained improvement, very rarely will there be an increase in asthmatic problems as a result of the sinus surgery. Unfortunately, even after polyps have been removed, more than one-third of the patients with nasal polyps will have a recurrence of them, and this is especially true for those with superimposed allergy, frequent sinus infections, repeated colds, asthma, cystic fibrosis, or aspirin intolerance. Nevertheless, proper surgical removal seems to provide a slower rate of polyp recurrence than medical treatment alone, and often the two together will give the best results. Better surgical results can also be expected if any allergic rhinitis is brought under control and any associated sinus infection is treated before the surgical procedure.

It should also be mentioned that allergic people, especially healthy young adults in their twenties or thirties with bilateral sinonasal polyps and whose associated rather extensive sinusitis fails to respond to vigorous treatment, should be suspected of having allergic fungal sinusitis and investigated accordingly.

Occasionally, a polyp within a large sinus cavity, not yet obstructing the drainage opening and not producing a cloudy discharge, toothache, pressure pains, or headache, may be found accidentally on plain sinus X rays. These polyps need not be immediately removed unless they produce bleeding or look suspicious of a tumor or new growth on a CAT scan or MRI. If they should cause recurrent nasal bleeding, then they have to be regarded as possibly cancerous. If they don't cause symptoms, are smooth and rounded looking, and are not invading bone, they can usually be followed by an X ray in 3 or 4 months. To avoid excessive X rays, a single plain film or sometimes a very limited CAT scan will often suffice to see if the growth is enlarging, and if so how rapidly. If a polyp seems to be the likely diagnosis on X ray, the examiner should look very carefully at the nose and other sinuses for further confirming evidence of polyp formations.

CYSTS

If a CAT scan suggests that a smooth rounded structure within a maxillary sinus cavity is a cyst, namely, a membranous sac filled with fluid, then your doctor should check further, since sometimes a fairly thick-walled cyst arising from the floor of a maxillary or cheek sinus just above the roots of the upper teeth may be of dental origin. A dental consultation and dental X rays may sometimes be necessary to determine this. If, however, the CAT scan should identify it as a simple small rounded thin-walled mucous cyst arising from mucous glands and not obstructing the sinus drainage, not bleeding, and not causing any symptoms, it too need not be removed immediately but can usually be followed with a single plain X-ray film in a few months to see if the cyst is enlarging or about to obstruct the sinus drainage opening. If it is, it will have to be removed.

Both cysts and polyps are usually rounded smooth structures, and when discovered within a sinus on plain X rays, they may occasionally be difficult to tell apart, sometimes even with a CAT scan or MRI. On a number of occasions, I have seen small mucous cysts in a sinus completely disappear, apparently from spontaneous rupture, usually followed momentarily by a clear or pale yellowish drainage from the nose. Of course, you cannot depend on this to happen, and many cysts that do rupture will usually recur. Some cysts may enlarge, fill a sinus cavity, and continue to expand gradually under considerable mucus-secreting pressure to form a mucocele or thick-walled cyst, which may then compress and destroy the bony walls separating the nose, the orbit, and the brain from the sinus cavity. These have to be very carefully evaluated, treated early whenever possible, and either surgically excised or incorporated into the drainage process of the sinus itself, or sometimes into that of an adjoining sinus.

A permanently sealed-off sinus cavity, by continuing to secrete mucus under considerable pressure and over a fairly long period of time, can also become a mucocele, gradually eroding its own bony walls and any surrounding structures. These more often occur in the anterior ethmoid sinuses, which usually have the smallest drainage openings and are therefore more easily obstructed. As they erode, their walls may become thicker not only from their own linings but from acquiring the fibrous tissue coverings of any surrounding structures into which they expand. Occasionally surgery on the nose or sinuses may cause a cyst or a mucocele to develop should postoperative scarring succeed in completely sealing off a sinus cavity or a segment of mucus-secreting membrane, and yet they may not make themselves known until sometimes years after the surgery was performed.

As a general rule, cysts, especially in the smaller sinus cavities, may eventually obstruct sinus drainage and have to be removed. The same might be said for most polyps, although early ones may fairly often shrink away and disappear with proper medical treatment. Most cysts located almost anywhere in the body, because they are usually fed by a continuous flow of secretions under fairly high pressure, will gradually enlarge and may eventually erode or destroy adjacent bone if they have no room to expand. Nasal polyps, because they usually develop at a sinus drainage opening and cause sinus blockage symptoms early, will usually make their presence known long before most cysts, especially the thick-walled, fluid-containing mucocele, which may go virtually unnoticed along its destructive path for years.

Another cystlike structure, called a meningocele, which may sometimes develop from the meninges covering of the brain and erode or protrude through a defect in the upper part of the nasal cavity or sinuses, can sometimes be mistaken for an ordinary nasal or sinus cyst. It is usually found in only one side of the nose, may increase in size with lifting or straining, and will often momentarily reveal a slight pulsation commensurate with the heartbeat. The meningocele should be considered in the differential diagnosis of sinonasal cysts and approached with caution, as it connects directly to the brain area and contains cerebrospinal fluid. A CAT scan and MRI may often reveal the diagnosis, however, and should be obtained if your doctor is the least bit suspicious, since the treatment of a meningocele can sometimes be very complicated and even more so should it turn out to be an encephalocele containing brain tissue.

CHAPTER NINETEEN

Fungus Infections

Fungus infection of the sinuses, a fairly infrequent finding 25 years ago, is now more common due to new treatment modalities for malignancies, the increase in immunity-suppressing diseases such as AIDS, greater use of antibiotics for longer periods, and high-dose prolonged corticosteroid therapy, especially to avoid tissue rejection with organ transplants or grafts. People whose immune systems and their ability to control infections have been significantly compromised become more vulnerable to invasive organisms in their environment, including molds, yeast, and fungi. Disease-producing organisms that take advantage of this weakened bodily state are often referred to as opportunistic infections.

People who have undergone total body irradiation or chemotherapy in preparation for a bone marrow transplant for leukemia and certain malignancies are generally more susceptible to fungus diseases. AIDS has increased the incidence of opportunistic diseases, including fungal, rather markedly in the past 15 years, and therefore the possibility of fungal sinusitis has to be suspected in any immunocompromised patient with sinusitis symptoms. Years ago, diabetes was responsible for many of the incidental fungal infections in the sinuses, especially in the poorly regulated diabetics. Milder forms of fungal disease such as thrush in the mouth and fungal vaginitis, both usually due to *Candida,* began to show up fairly frequently with the increasing use of antibiotics and corticosteroid preparations. Although thrush is noted fairly often in the mouths of children as the so-called "milk spots," when it occurs spontaneously and unrelated to medications in older patients, it may indicate an immunodeficiency state and in a few cases could even suggest HIV infection. Candida may also cause fungal infections in the corners of the mouth, around the nail beds, beneath the nails, in the glans penis, under the breasts, in the ears, within the navel, in the anus, between the fingers and toes, and wherever there are folds of skin and moisture tends to collect. Even though thrush may be a normal inhabitant of the intestinal tract, weakened body defenses may allow it to spread from there to other body organs, sometimes with very serious consequences.

Very humid areas in our environment such as dark, damp basements or the proximity of a large body of water will encourage fungal growth, especially in the dark, constantly moist, and warmer areas of our bodies. During World War II, when troops would reach the hot and humid South Pacific, most of those on shipboard would come down with fungal infections, often starting in their ears, again a dark area of the body where moisture tends to collect, and especially from perspiring on a hot day. These fungal spores, often floating in the air but many times having preceded the troops onto the ships, would begin to flourish in the hot, moisture-laden South Seas. In some, the fungal infections involving their moist body areas became so bad and so difficult to cure that the troops began to refer to the condition as the Chinese rot, thus alluding to the South China Seas as its likely origin.

The more common fungi to invade these moist body areas are *Candida, Mucor,* and *Aspergillus,* with *Candida* usually being the milder one. Contamination by the *Saccharomyces* fungus found in baker's yeast and used in raw dough for bread and pizzas may in rare instances also lead to fungal or yeast vaginitis. Even some very small members of the mushroom family, similar to those that cause white rot in wood, have been known occasionally to invade the sinuses and to grow there. Molds, yeast, and mushrooms are all members of the fungi family and have been around almost forever. In 1845 a potato fungus was responsible for the starving deaths of millions of people during the Irish Potato Famine as well as the mass migration of Irish immigrants to America. Now, 150 years later, we have finally found a good-guy leaf-friendly fungus that can destroy the forest-devastating gypsy moth caterpillars that were brought to this country from France during the nineteenth century. Hopefully, this will also eliminate the extensive annual spraying now used for this purpose—and the resultant breathing of toxic pesticides.

Fungi present in moist body areas may be just passing through without involving the body tissues, or they may be saprobic and simply living on existing dead tissues and debris left behind by some other ravager; or in their potentially more detrimental form, they may be parasitic and therefore feeding on living, but usually rather sickly, tissues. In the latter case, a fungus becomes a disease-producing pathogen that may be perfectly content to remain a surface disease or may proceed further to invade and destroy any underlying or surrounding tissues, including vessels and bone. In either case, when fungi involve the sinuses, there is usually a significant bacterial sinusitis present as well, often paving the way for the fungus infection, which means of course that they both have to be treated. The sinuses seem to be less often involved with fungal disease than the lungs, possibly due to the sinuses' fairly secluded and well-protected location, the reduced nasal humidity (especially in the front of the nose when compared to the lower respiratory tract), and the rapid mucus clearance of the nose and sinuses when compared to that in the rather lengthy lower airway. Although persistent bacterial infections in the lungs may eventually involve the sinuses and vice versa, the same would appear less often true for fungal infections. Involvement of the mouth and esophagus by fungal diseases may exist as combined or entirely separate entities.

Early in my career, I saw a few cases of fungal sinusitis in habitual steam bath users, several of whom were also diabetics, and one case involving a man who worked in a corn canning factory where he was frequently exposed to excessive steam vapors as well as to the sometimes waste product of cooked cornstarch, no doubt an excellent growth media for fungi. These all appeared to involve primarily the maxillary sinuses. Another case also involving a maxillary sinus occurred many years after an apparent injection of a radioactive material into the sinus for a special X-ray study. Some of the radioactive material was retained and very likely encouraged the fungal infection as well as a subsequent malignancy.

Just as many individuals may be allergic to mold, some may develop an allergic fungal sinusitis, mostly due to the aspergillus fungus. Unlike fungal sinusitis in some others, these are usually not the unregulated diabetics, the immunocompromised, or the severely debilitated. They are usually young adults in their twenties and thirties, often with a history of being allergy prone or atopic, and usually having a history of allergic rhinitis or asthma. Most of them also have chronic sinusitis with polypoid changes in their nose and sinuses. Some will have a history of previous sinus surgery, especially for removal of polyps, and some for repeated surgical drainage of totally obstructed sinuses showing air-fluid levels on X ray. Some will show positive for skin and blood testing for specific fungal allergens as well as for the presence of eosinophilic cells in nasal smears suggesting an allergy, but some may have none of these allergic signs. Allergic fungal sinusitis is usually found in healthy individuals and is seldom a truly invasive condition, but this still has to be considered wherever there are signs of orbital or central nervous system involvement by a sinus problem, especially in an allergic person. Nonallergic invasive fungal sinusitis noted in an immunocompromised individual can be a much more destructive process and is far more likely to resemble a tumor invading the eye or the brain.

Some allergic fungal sinusitis patients will develop asthmatic wheezing similar to that sometimes seen in aspergillus fungal involvement of the lungs. Allergic fungal sinusitis should always be suspected in healthy young adults in their twenties or thirties with chronic sinusitis involving most of the sinuses on both sides, who have a history of nasal allergies as well as nasal or sinus polyps that keep recurring, especially if their sinusitis fails to respond to conventional treatment. Nonallergic and noninvasive fungal sinusitis is more inclined to involve a single sinus, usually one of the maxillary sinuses. However, if the fungus is the invasive type, it may spread to any of the adjoining sinuses but may still tend to remain on one side in most instances. When the fungus infection is confined only to the sinuses, there may be no suggestive signs within the nose of an underlying fungal sinusitis. However, in most instances, there will be nasal evidence of an associated bacterial sinusitis with a cloudy nasal discharge, and if it is the allergic type, there may be polyp-like changes in the nasal membranes or other suggestions of nasal allergy along with the usual symptoms of sinusitis. An MRI or CAT scan and nasal smears and cultures will sometimes help to make the diagnosis, but many times the fungus infection will first be discovered during an operation for a bacterial sinusitis or polyps, or sometimes following a puncture and irrigation of a maxillary sinus.

The more serious invasive fungal disease of the sinuses may occasionally reveal dead or devitalized tissue in the nose and turbinates due to vascular blockage of the blood supply to the tissues by the fungi. This is usually a very serious situation requiring a thorough medical workup and often surgical intervention before it has a chance to involve an eye or the brain. Since it is mostly found in unhealthy and immunocompromised individuals, it becomes even more serious, and early diagnosis with intensive treatment shouldn't be delayed. Because of this, it is often wise for those undergoing total body irradiation, or bone marrow and organ transplants or intensive chemotherapy to have their sinuses checked for chronic sinusitis before the procedure. Unfortunately, even when taken directly from an obviously diseased sinus, fungal cultures may still be negative. Moreover, since cultures may sometimes require a week or more for confirmation, such a delay may sometimes prove too costly. However, when fungal sinusitis is suspected, fungal cultures should still be obtained along with a culture and sensitivity studies for a possible bacterial infection, since it is usually present as well and will have to be treated also.

With the sophisticated sinus instruments doctors have today, it is fairly easy to enter a sinus under local anesthesia, inspect it, and obtain biopsies or samples of any suspicious tissue or foreign matter for immediate staining and for a more likely positive identification of fungal disease. Although still not always 100 percent informative, a tissue sample is usually much more accurate than a culture, and an immediate reading may make it possible for the doctor to then go ahead with definitive surgical treatment. The finding of a brownish to black granular material, a tanish brown puttylike substance, a greenish-brown to grayish gelatinous matter, or the suggestion of a fungus ball within a sinus cavity will also help with the microscopic exam and diagnosis. Irrigation of a large sinus cavity may also aid in demonstrating some of this foreign matter as well as provide a specimen for the laboratory. Occasionally a person with fungal sinusitis will have been aware of dark granular specs in his or her nasal discharge or sputum for some time.

X rays and especially a CAT scan will help in revealing the presence of chronic sinusitis and may also show any polypoid changes within the sinuses. In some cases of suspected fungal sinusitis, an MRI may be helpful in making the diagnosis. As already mentioned, skin and blood serum testing in allergic fungal sinusitis may also prove helpful.

Treating fungal sinusitis would include treating any accompanying bacterial sinusitis with antibiotics, decongestants, and possible irrigations. I also found it extremely important to correct any sinus drainage problems surgically and especially to establish the best possible air exchange between the nose and sinuses. This also includes excising diseased tissue, obstructive polyps, and devitalized tissue, including any dead bone within the nose or sinuses. Repeated irrigations before, during, and after surgery are very useful in removing fungal debris from hidden crevices within the sinus cavity and nose. In the case of allergic fungal sinus disease, allergy treatment and anti-inflammatory medications in the form of oral corticosteroids and steroid sprays sometimes even for a prolonged period can also be very effective. You might find this somewhat surprising, since cortisone or corticosteroid preparations may sometimes encourage fungal disease, but in this case, reducing the allergic inflammation and swelling, thereby encouraging better circulation, good aeration, and efficient sinus drainage, would seem to be more important for a successful cure. Since the picture of allergic fungal disease is usually one of chronicity and often involves other allergies, desensitization shots, usually omitting mold allergens that might cause more reactivity, may in some cases prove effective. Avoiding too humid an environment, where fungi or molds are likely to live, is also important, and you should avoid excessive use of humidifiers, and air out your bedroom or basement quarters frequently.

The antifungal medications, which can be very toxic to the body, can usually be avoided if you have allergic fungal sinusitis and are fairly young and healthy. However, these somewhat toxic medications may be necessary, especially when dealing with chronically invasive fungal disease in an immunocompromised individual, remembering, of course, that already unhealthy individuals may not tolerate toxic drugs without serious consequences. In my experience, antifungal medications were seldom necessary except in very advanced fungal disease, whereas surgically removing the diseased tissue, creating the best possible drainage, and providing the very best ventilation or air exchange for the diseased sinus seemed to give the best results. This usually meant not only enlarging the natural drainage opening of the sinus but, when the maxillary sinus was involved, also adding a window procedure for additional air exchange as well as easy access for frequent postoperative irrigations and endoscopic inspections. In any event, people with fungal sinusitis must be followed closely because of the likelihood of a recurrence, and this is especially true for the invasive types. In my opinion, most cases of invasive fungal sinusitis should be approached as a medical and surgical emergency, since it can be a deadly tissue-destroying disease that has usually been present for some time before ever being recognized, and especially since it usually occurs in an already unhealthy individual.

CHAPTER TWENTY

AIDS

SINUSITIS IS A common occurrence with HIV infection and even more so in the later stages of AIDS disease. Early on, sinusitis may be overlooked by the doctor and ignored by the patient often due to the grave concern of both for the many other problems caused by HIV infection. Also, the usual sinusitis symptoms of nasal swelling, congestion, inflammation, deep pressure pain, headache, cloudy infected postnasal drip, and morning sore throats may be somewhat diminished in many people with AIDS due to their lowered T cell counts and lack of immune response. Surprisingly enough, however, some may show an increase in allergy symptoms. As with other sinusitis cases, the incidence of sinus infection in a person with AIDS is greater during the winter months. A CAT scan and a fiber-optic exam of the nose may be necessary early in AIDS disease to identify the presence of a cloudy sinus discharge and to determine which sinuses may be involved. Sometimes even the mildest symptoms of sinusitis may mask an underlying very serious sinus infection and even a superimposed invasive fungal sinusitis. As the HIV infection progresses and the patient becomes even more immunodeficient, the sinusitis as well as other opportunistic infections may become more involved, more obvious, and usually more serious.

A study of 667 HIV-infected individuals admitted to the AIDS unit at the Johns Hopkins Hospital over a 3-year period revealed 68 with definite sinusitis and 4 with probable sinus disease. Other studies have shown this coincidence ratio to be much higher. In this study, however, those with T cell counts below 200 were generally found to have the more extensive bilateral sinus disease, usually responding poorly to treatment and far more likely to be chronic. In most instances, the lower the T cell count, the more serious the sinus infection.

The more common bacterial organisms involving the sinuses of people with AIDS early in the disease are generally the same as those found in most acute sinusitis patients, namely *Streptococcus pneumoniae* and *H. influenzae*, although secondary involvement by a fungus such as aspergillus, alternaria, or mucor may also occur. Finding an antibiotic-resistant organism or one of the rarer, more stubborn bacteria such as a *Pseudomonas*, sometimes a *Staph* or *E. coli*, and even anaerobic organisms that grow only in the absence of oxygen is not unusual, especially in a late-stage AIDS patient with chronic sinus disease. Even *Legionella*, the organism that causes Legionnaires disease of the lungs, has been found responsible for a sinus infection in an AIDS patient.

Although people with AIDS usually experience the same characteristic symptoms as other sinusitis patients but often in a milder way, a few seem to have more face pain, more sinus tenderness, and more facial swelling. However, the swelling in the cheeks or around the eyes may sometimes be more obvious due to emaciation and the loss of subcutaneous facial fat so often noted with AIDS. Since the maxillary sinuses seem to be more commonly involved, pain in the cheeks or upper teeth may be noted early in the disease. If you have AIDS, you should not delay in reporting pain in the upper teeth or sinus areas as well as any evidence of a cloudy discharge from your nose or throat so that early treatment of a sinus infection with antibiotics and possibly sinus irrigations might be started before chronic disease or even more serious consequences have a chance to develop. Physicians should be especially attentive to the fact that people with AIDS do very often develop opportunistic sinusitis and that their symptoms could be very minimal even in the presence of a very serious sinus problem. As disease progresses, and the patient's immune response to infection diminishes even more, all of the sinuses on both sides of the nose may gradually become involved, thus creating the condition of pansinusitis.

Some people with AIDS, even if they do not have sinusitis, may experience what seems like an excessive amount of clear, thick, rather sticky sinonasal secretions. These thick secretions not only make the sinuses more susceptible to infection and more difficult to clear once they are infected but also may confuse you as to whether you already have a sinus infection. Here the use of a mucus-liquefying agent such as guaifenesin is often effective and may even help the cough, which is not uncommon in the AIDS patient with sinusitis. On the other hand, the use of a first-generation antihistamine can cause further thickening of the mucous secretions with more sinus and lung problems.

Although bacterial sinusitis in the non-AIDS patient, unless accompanied by an acute viral infection such as a cold or flu, seldom produces a fever (this is especially true for adult subacute or chronic sinus disease), a person with AIDS with sinusitis will more often show a significant temperature elevation even with a chronic sinus infection. This fever may be partly due to the underlying AIDS disease and in some instances partly due to undisclosed opportunistic involvement of other areas not protected by bony walls like the sinuses, including the GI tract, the bronchi, and the lungs, possibly only mildly involved and producing no other symptoms except the fever. The immune system may have a difficult time warding off even small incursions by potentially infective organisms harbored in these very vulnerable areas. However, if you have AIDS and you suddenly develop a significant fever but your lungs are clear, your physician should carefully evaluate the sinuses as a possible source. The other systemic symptoms of chronic sinus disease—namely, fatigue, difficulty in concentrating, loss of appetite, and a sensation of weakness in the legs—may be accentuated in the AIDS patient due to the very debilitating effects of the HIV infection itself.

The AIDS patient with sinusitis will nearly always require antibiotics, often for several weeks longer than the usual treatment for sinus disease. This could be even truer for children with AIDS because of their normally small drainage openings and narrow nasal passages, which in the child may also tend to swell excessively with an infection and remain swollen for longer periods. In either case, the length of antibiotic treatment will depend on the duration of the sinus infection, the immune response and T cell count, how soon after onset of the sinus infection the antibiotics were started, how effective they are, how regularly they were taken, the general condition of the nose and sinuses, and the patient's previous history of success with antibiotic treatment for sinus problems. If you have AIDS with subacute or chronic sinus problems, you will naturally have to take antibiotics for much longer periods and may even have to take them indefinitely, periodically changing from one antibiotic to another, hopefully to elude antibiotic-resistant bacteria.

A few AIDS patients with sinusitis may need hospitalization for intravenous antibiotic or antifungal therapy on occasions, and some children with AIDS who have protracted sinus infections could occasionally require intravenous immunoglobulin therapy to bolster their immune response. As with nearly all cases of sinus infection, judging how long to continue antibiotic treatment will depend on how long it takes for the cloudy sinonasal discharge to become completely clear and preferably continuing treatment for several days to a week or more thereafter depending, of course, on how long the sinus infection has been present altogether. In any event, a person with AIDS will nearly always have to take antibiotics much longer to reach this point.

Nasal decongestants by spray or by pill may be very helpful, especially in the early stages of sinus infection as well as subsequently with any acute flare-ups. If you have AIDS, and have experienced or are experiencing unusually thickened sinonasal discharge, drinking additional fluids other than alcohol, using a saline spray, and taking a mucus liquefier such as guaifenesin might all be beneficial. Using a hot steam vaporizer, especially in the bedroom in cold weather, will also be useful in thinning the sinonasal drainage and protecting the membranes of the lower respiratory tract as well. Because hot steam vaporizers are mostly self-sterilizing and therefore less inclined to harbor fungi or other microorganisms than cool humidifiers, using hot steam would certainly be a wiser choice. For the same reason, your room should not be constantly and completely saturated with moisture but should be allowed to air out periodically. Regularly cleaning your vaporizer or humidifier is also very important.

Since corticosteroids are known to interfere with the body's own immune response to viral and bacterial infections, and may even tend to promote fungal infections, using a steroid nasal spray with sinusitis, unless there is also a significant allergic rhinitis, would seem to me to be a poor choice. However, corticosteroids have been used rather frequently by people with AIDS, and some studies have reported satisfactory results without any significant problems. Unfortunately, many of those who use them do so much too often, which could further depress the body's immune system. The proper use of manufactured saline nasal sprays and periodic decongestants when necessary would appear to be a safer approach.

Cultures for bacteria and fungi are important if you have AIDS and sinusitis, especially since you may be required to take an antibiotic for a much longer period and are also prone to fungus infections. Of course, a negative fungal culture does not rule out a fungal sinusitis, just as a negative culture for bacteria does not rule out a bacterial sinus infection. CAT scans, plain sinus X rays, and sometimes MRIs, along with periodic fiber-optic exams of the nose, would all be important in determining the extent of the sinus disease, its progress, and whether there are any sinus air-fluid levels needing operative drainage. If you have already had excessive irradiation exposure for some other problem, an MRI instead of a CAT scan of the sinuses may serve almost as well, especially when more follow-up studies may be necessary. An MRI can sometimes be especially helpful in identifying a superimposed fungal infection. Any acutely obstructed sinuses with air-fluid levels will have to be punctured and irrigated with normal saline solution, and this may have to be repeated periodically. If the obstruction to sinus drainage persists or continues to recur, surgery for a more permanent relief may be necessary.

Obstructive polyps or cysts may also have to be excised. Fungal involvement of the sinuses will require the usual treatment for the often accompanying bacterial sinusitis, with perhaps even more frequent nasal and sinus irrigations, as well as surgical establishment of good drainage and good aeration, both of which can easily be done under local anesthesia. In my experience, establishing exceptionally good air exchange between the nose and sinuses in a fungal sinusitis patient is just as important as establishing good drainage. Even though enlarging the natural opening of the maxillary or cheek sinus for better drainage makes more sense, since the cilia sweep will still be in that direction, creating an additional sinonasal window, especially for fungal infections, can afford an even better air exchange as well as an easier and less painful access for frequent postoperative sinus irrigations. In my opinion, both surgical procedures should usually be done in people with AIDS where indicated. The two openings may also afford better telescopic visualization of the sinus cavity for evidence of residual fungal disease and probably more successful flushing out of any retained clumps of fungal material. The additional use of systemic antifungal medications may be required for fungal sinusitis in a person with AIDS, especially for the invasive type, which can be devastating and should more often than not be approached as a medical and surgical emergency.

Up to 70 percent of AIDS patients may eventually develop chronic sinusitis, and its treatment in the advanced stages of AIDS can be discouraging both for you and your doctor. Not only will infectious flare-ups almost always recur very soon after you stop antibiotic therapy, but secondary involvement of the other sinuses, the nose, sometimes the ears, and even the lungs may develop and persist as well. A super-imposed fungal sinusitis may also spread to involve adjacent blood vessels and the surrounding bone, and thence to invade the orbits and the brain.

The prescribing of more and more antibiotics, changing them occasionally to avoid bacterial resistance problems or when cultures require it, plus frequent surgical drainage and repeated irrigations, may all be required on a fairly routine basis in the late-stage AIDS patient with pansinusitis. Daily prophylactic antibiotics on a continuous basis may have to be considered in some cases, once the infection has cleared, to prevent an almost immediate recurrence. These are sometimes prescribed in a reduced dosage on the theory that it takes less medication to prevent an infection than it does to treat it once it has occurred. Of course, the chances of developing antibiotic-resistant organisms may be significantly increased by a reduced-dosage regimen, and this should be kept in mind, since cross-contamination of a spouse or another family member with an antibiotic-resistant organism could prove troublesome.

Glossary

Words defined elsewhere in this glossary are italicized.

ABSCESS—a localized collection of *pus* usually surrounded by inflammation and swelling.

ACETAMINOPHEN—like aspirin, it is a nonprescription pain reliever and fever reducer sold in liquid or tablet form as Tylenol, Anacin III, etc. or often combined with certain other over-the-counter medications for relief of colds, flu, and sinusitis.

ACQUIRED IMMUNE DEFICIENCY SYNDROME (AIDS)—A chronic illness, so far incurable (although some seem to recover), caused by the human immunodeficiency virus (HIV), transmitted by exchange of certain body fluids and severely damaging to the body's immune system, thus encouraging *opportunistic infections* such as pneumonia, fungal infections, tumors, and sinusitis.

ACUTE SINUSITIS—a usually short lasting active infection of the lining membranes of the *paranasal sinuses* often associated with or following a viral respiratory infection such as a head cold or flu.

ADDISON'S DISEASE—usually a chronic condition caused by inadequate cortisone secretions by the two adrenal glands for mostly unknown reasons and requiring continuous hormonal replacement therapy for relief.

ADENOIDS—a collection of lymphoid tissue resembling a tonsil and usually about the size of a marble in a child, but often two or three times that size when inflamed, located behind the nose in the vault of the *nasopharynx* and contributing to the body's immune response to respiratory infections, especially in the first four years of life.

AEROSINUSITIS—an acute, sometimes painful blockage of an often partially obstructed sinus opening or duct, more often due to a sudden increase in outside air pressure as with rapid descent in a plane, a parachute, a bungee jump, or sometimes an elevator.

AIR QUALITY INDEX—also called the ozone index, is a measurement of outside ground-level *ozone* concentration and is used as the standard indicator of air pollution, including smog. The safety level has now been lowered to 80 parts per billion from 120 parts per billion. Abnormal elevations can affect the respiratory tract and sinuses.

ALLERGEN—a protein substance normally foreign to the body that on contact with the body may cause *histamine* release followed by an allergic response in someone previously sensitized to it.

ALLERGIC REACTION—a variable tissue response to excessive histamine release following contact with an *allergen* in someone previously sensitized.

ALZHEIMER'S DISEASE—usually a progressive mental deterioration, due to degenerative processes within the brain, beginning in late middle life and evidenced by varying degrees of confusion, memory loss, and disorientation.

ANAEROBIC BACTERIA—sometimes called anaerobes, these microorganisms live and grow in the absence of oxygen and therefore require special collecting and culturing methods.

ANAPHYLACTIC SHOCK—a severe, sometimes fatal body system collapse usually in a previously highly sensitized individual on reexposure to the same or a similar foreign protein substance and causing a massive histamine release often with tissue swelling, a precipitous drop in blood pressure, and a fast, usually very weak pulse.

ANEURYSM—usually a ballooning outward of the walls of a major or minor artery.

ANTIBIOTIC—a soluble substance often derived from a mold or bacteria in its natural state but now manufactured synthetically. In either form, it may inhibit or destroy certain microorganisms.

ANTIHISTAMINE—a medication used in the treatment of allergic reactions and having an antagonistic action against histamine, a substance released by the body in excessive amounts during an allergic reaction. It can be given by spray, liquid, ointment, pill, or shot.

ANTIVIRAL MEDICATION—a drug prescribed to suppress a viral infection and hopefully minimize its symptoms.

ASTHMA—a restricted breathing state of variable duration often caused by allergies, exercise, infections, or exposure to cold and characterized by difficult expiration, wheezing, shortness of breath, coughing, and a feeling of constriction in the chest. It is caused by muscular contractions in the walls of the bronchial air passages with narrowing and some swelling of their lining membranes as well.

ATELECTASIS—a condition of airlessness or lack of air in a whole or part of a lung usually due to bronchial obstruction from a foreign body, a growth, or a mucous plug followed by absorption of the entrapped air.

ATOPY—an allergic tendency or predisposition often with a familial history of similar problems and frequently in the genes.

ATROPHIC RHINITIS—a degenerative condition of nasal membranes including their hair cells, mucus-secreting glands, and underlying support tissues, sometimes including turbinate bones and nasal cartilage. The cause is generally unknown. As a result, the nasal airway is usually wide open, but the nose usually feels partially blocked and is very often infected.

BACTEREMIA—The presence of live bacteria in the circulating blood.

BAROSINUSITIS—is the same as *aerosinusitis* and indicates the sudden onset of sinus symptoms such as pain or headache caused by a sudden air pressure difference between the sinus cavity and the outside air, and the rush of air through a narrow sinus opening to correct it.

BAROTRAUMA—when applied to the sinuses implies an injury such as a hemorrhage or tear in the membranous wall, opening, or duct of a sinus due to a sudden change in air pressure and the subsequent rush of air.

BASOPHIL—a white blood cell that circulates in the blood and releases histamine in an allergic or hypersensitivity reaction.

CAT SCAN—stands for computerized axial tomography (often shortened to CT, or computerized tomography) and consists of a series of X-ray pictures taken several millimeters apart through a body organ or structure using a computerized process and with fairly minimal radiation exposure to the subject. It is the most effective way of visualizing the interior and bony walls of the sinuses.

CAVERNOUS VENOUS SINUSES—two reservoirs or lakes filled with venous blood lying at the base of the brain in back of the eyes and vulnerable to the spread of infection from the sinuses, which could be fatal.

CILIA—microscopic hairs that line the nose, sinuses, and lower respiratory tract for the purpose of sweeping them clean.

CHRONIC SINUSITIS—a sometimes irreversible condition in which repeated or prolonged continuous episodes of acute or subacute sinusitis have managed to cause enough permanent damage and scarring to the membranes, mucous glands, hair cells, drainage openings, or blood supply of a sinus cavity so that it can no longer sweep itself clean or flush out harmful substances.

CONCHA BULLOSA—usually an enlarged, somewhat rounded middle *turbinate* encompassing an ethmoid sinus cavity at its center and normally containing air. Like the other sinus cavities it may develop a *polyp, cyst,* or *mucocele,* continue to enlarge, and obstruct the nasal passage as well as any nearby sinus openings. It may also become obstructed and infected. However, when present, it does not necessarily invite disease or cause sinusitis.

CORTICOSTEROID—a hormonal secretion of the adrenal glands now synthetically produced in liquid, spray, pill, shot, and ointment forms often used to control inflammatory swelling caused by allergies, chemical irritants, sometimes infections, and burns of the nose, sinuses, and lower respiratory tract along with numerous other uses throughout the body. It is often called "steroid" for short.

CSF—abbreviation for the cerebrospinal fluid that surrounds, suspends, partly nourishes, and partly protects the brain and spinal cord.

CSF LEAK—an escape of cerebrospinal fluid from the central nervous system or brain into the nose, ear, or a sinus following head trauma, invasive diseases, ear or sinus surgery, and sometimes occurring spontaneously.

CYST—usually a sac of fluid, occasionally found in the nose or a sinus and usually lined on the inside with a mucus-secreting membrane causing it to gradually enlarge and block the nasal airway or a sinus drainage opening. Some eventually develop into *mucoceles*.

DANDER—consists mainly of deposits of saliva, dead skin scales, skin oils (sebum), and urine, all clinging to shed animal hairs or fur.

DECONGESTANT—a spray, drop, or pill frequently used to relieve membrane swelling of the nose and sinuses for better drainage, better sinonasal air exchange, and better breathing.

DEW POINT—the temperature at which the air will be completely saturated with moisture (100% RH), resulting in fog or cloud formation in cooler air or collecting on cooler objects and the grass as dew.

EMPHYSEMA—a chronic destructive lung disease causing a progressive loss of the lung tissue responsible for oxygen absorption and gaseous exchange.

EMPYEMA—a sealed-off body cavity containing infected matter or pus, or a totally blocked and infected sinus cavity containing pus and usually under pressure.

ENDOSCOPIC SINUS SURGERY (ESS)—delicate sinus surgery performed with the aid of magnified fiber-optic telescopes and special instruments primarily to eradicate the disease and restore sinus function, also known as *functional endoscopic sinus surgery,* or *FESS.*

ENZYMES—also known as *organic catalysts,* enzymes are numerous complex proteins within the body that are produced by living cells to promote, enhance, activate, reduce, convert, transfer, condense, digest, or otherwise affect various biochemical reactions or changes in other body substances, and at the same time remaining essentially unchanged in the process. They are usually identified by adding "ase" to the end of the reaction or to the end of the substance activated.

EOSINOPHILS—are white blood cells circulating throughout the body, often attracted to allergic tissues and certain infectious processes, especially parasitic infestations. They are readily identified in the laboratory with an eosin stain, hence their name.

EPINEPHRINE—a powerful stimulant also secreted by the adrenal glands but now manufactured synthetically. It is used in the treatment of shock, acute asthmatic attacks, laryngeal obstruction, cardiac arrest, and severe life-threatening allergic episodes. It is also sold in a bee sting kit as EpiPen.

ETHMOID AIR CELL—often shortened to ethmoid cell, to include the Haller cell in the anterior ethmoidal group and the Onodi cell in the posterior ethmoidal group, is frequently used to refer to a single ethmoidal sinus cavity.

FRONTAL ETHMOID—is an ethmoid sinus cavity initially belonging to the anterior ethmoidal group but during development may separate from the rest of the group and locate high in the brow area, often close to the frontal sinus drainage opening. When diseased, it sometimes blocks frontal sinus drainage.

EUSTACHIAN TUBES—two tubes each measuring 1 1/2 to 2 1/4 inches in length in the adult leading from the nasopharynx to the ears, lined with mucus-secreting membranes containing hair cells, normally collapsed except in the act of yawning or swallowing, and responsible for air exchange between the nasopharynx and middle ears as well as for middle ear drainage.

GASTROESOPHAGEAL REFLUX (GER)—the regurgitation of stomach acid and food up the esophagus occasionally as far as the mouth and sometimes to the nasopharynx and nose, usually due to a deficiency in valvular function at the gastroesophageal junction. If it occurs repeatedly, it may cause esophagitis, laryngitis, bronchitis, rhinitis, and sinusitis.

GOBLET CELLS—millions of mucus-secreting microscopic cells lining the nose, sinuses, and tracheobronchial air passages. They provide most of the mucus for the outer thicker layer of the protective mucous blanket covering the respiratory tract.

GRANULATION TISSUE—is also called proud flesh and may develop in any open, potentially infected wound in the body, especially following open surgery on a nose or sinus.

HALLER CELL—a large anterior *ethmoid air cell* or sinus cavity located just under the eye at its inner margin and above the maxillary sinus where it joins with the other anterior *ethmoid cells.* Infection in this sinus cavity may sometimes inflame and obstruct maxillary sinus drainage.

HAY FEVER—a poor choice of a name for seasonal allergic rhinitis, which causes sneezing, nasal congestion, watery eyes, and a runny nose due mainly to grass, weed, or tree pollens and rating the more accurate name of *pollinosis,* since it is not due to hay allergy, although an allergy to moldy hay may sometimes simulate it and may have instigated the name.

HEAT INDEX (HI)—a measurement of outside temperature that also takes into consideration the humidity reading, which on a hot, humid day would be considerably higher than the thermometer reading.

HISTAMINE—a powerful body stimulant normally released in small, regulated amounts mostly by the *mast cells* in body tissues but sometimes released in accelerated amounts with tissue injury or an allergic reaction. Overstimulation by histamine may produce unpleasant and sometimes very unhealthy body changes.

HIVES—also called urticaria or wheals, hives are small, rounded raised areas on the skin usually pale in color and often itching profusely. They may appear anywhere on the body surface and are usually the result of an allergic reaction.

HODGKIN'S DISEASE—a chronic tumor or nodule-forming malignant disease of the body's lymphatic system mostly involving the lymph nodes, spleen, and liver. The prognosis is guarded, but modern treatments have given very favorable results.

HYDROCORTISONE—also known as cortisol and similar to cortisone. It is secreted by the adrenal glands and is the most potent of the naturally occurring glucocorticosteroids or *corticosteroids.*

HYGROMETER—a device for measuring the water vapor or humidity in the air.

HYPERREACTIVITY—a state of heightened nonallergic sensitivity in which the nasal membranes may continue to react with varying degrees of inflammatory swelling, watery discharge, and sometimes sneezing to minimal amounts of irritating air pollutants, sometimes long after the original stimulus has departed.

HYPOTHYROIDISM—depressed body metabolism due to reduced thyroid hormone secretions by the two thyroid glands in the neck and affecting all body tissues, including the sinuses, if it goes untreated.

ICHTHYOSIS—a dry thickening sometimes fishlike scaling of the skin.

IMMUNE DEFICIENCY—a deficiency in the body's ability to ward off or subdue viral, bacterial, and fungal invaders, often manifest by a reduction in antibody production or T cell formation.

IMMUNOTHERAPY—a series of allergy desensitizing shots beginning with small doses of a specific allergen once or twice a week and gradually increasing the dosage as well as the intervals between shots with the idea of making the immune system more tolerant of the allergen.

INFLAMMATION—a fairly localized tissue reaction to an often harmful body stimulus such as injury, burn, allergic reaction, chemical irritation, or invasion by bacteria, viruses, or fungi and resulting in redness, swelling, and increased heat, mostly due to an increase in blood supply to the area.

INTERNAL CAROTID ARTERY—a very important branch of the common carotid artery in the neck. It penetrates the base of the skull on each side of the sphenoid sinus to supply blood and oxygen to the front part of the brain and eyes. Sinus surgery involving the posterior ethmoid and sphenoid sinuses could subject it to injury.

LARYNGITIS—inflammation of the larynx usually with swelling of the vocal cords and hoarseness, which the term is now often used synonymously. It can result from anything that interferes with the proper function of one or both vocal cords, including infections, benign growths, cancers, burns, lacerations, hemorrhages, allergic swelling, paralysis, trauma, chemical irritants, lung infections, excessive talking, repeated coughing, gastroesophageal reflux, low thyroid function, and even from an infected sinus drip.

MAO INHIBITORS—refers to monoamine oxidase inhibitors, which are mainly antidepressant medications.

MAST CELLS—individual cells found mostly in the connective tissues that bind together the supporting framework of the body. Like their blood circulating cousin, the *basophil,* mast cells are responsible for the release of histamine in an allergic reaction.

MECONIUM—a somewhat greenish semi-liquid matter representing the first intestinal discharge of the newborn infant and sometimes aspirated into the nose or lungs at birth.

MENINGITIS—inflammation of the meninges, or protective membranous covering of the brain and spinal cord.

MICROORGANISMS—usually an independent viable living substance of microscopic or ultra-microscopic size often used to designate a disease-causing bacteria.

MRI—magnetic resonance imaging. Like the *CAT scan,* an MRI takes a series of sectional pictures several millimeters apart through a body organ or structure. Unlike the CAT scan, it does not expose the patient to radiation, and since it is more useful in demonstrating soft tissues than bone, it is usually not as helpful in evaluating the sinuses. It is also more expensive. However, in certain patients where radiation must be avoided or where fungal sinusitis is suspected, and MRI can be of considerable help.

MUCOCELE—usually a fairly thick-walled cyst developing from the mucus-secreting lining of a sinus or from complete blockage of a sinus cavity, gradually expanding due to its continued internal mucous secretions and capable of eventually destroying the bony walls of the sinus and any other nearby structures. If it should become infected, it is known as a *pyocele.*

MUCUS—a clear, slippery secretion coating the entire respiratory tract and sinuses as well as certain other delicate membranes in the body. It is secreted by millions of microscopic glands and forms a protective coating or mucous blanket shielding these delicate membranes from injury or invasion by microorganisms.

MUCOUS MEMBRANES—the mucus-secreting membranes lining and protecting the respiratory tract, sinuses, GI tract, urinary tract, tear ducts, middle ears, eustachian tubes, and saliva ducts, as well as most of the other body canals and channels, including those responsible for reproduction. In the nose, sinuses, and lower respiratory tract, these membranes are often referred to as *respiratory epithelium* and contain cilia and mucous glands.

NASAL CYCLE—the spontaneous congestion and decongestion alternating between the two nasal passages in most of us every few hours and of which we are usually totally unaware unless one has a narrowed nasal passage, which will then make any nasal congestion more obvious on that side.

NASAL SEPTUM—a thin, normally midline partition in the center of the nose separating the two nasal passages. It is composed of cartilage in front and a very thin wall of bone behind. It is covered mostly by mucus-secreting membrane and provides some support to the nose, especially in front.

NASAL TURBINATES—(also called "concha," for shell-like) are three longitudinal structures on the outer walls of both nasal passages. They are approximately 1 to 2 1/2 inches long, with the largest and longest below and the smallest and shortest above. They each have a rolled-up scroll-like appearance from which they get their name. Each consists of a curved bony shelf covered by thickened ciliated mucous membrane containing many mucus-secreting glands. They shield and protect the tear duct and sinus drainage openings; filter, collect, and supply moisture to the air we breathe; warm the inhaled air; and, as their name would suggest, create turbulence in the airstream, thus involving a larger area of nasal membrane in the filtering process. Sometimes a higher, much smaller supreme turbinate is also present.

NASOPHARYNX—the rather large space behind the nose and above the palate containing the adenoids as well as the opening to the eustachian tubes on each side. Unlike the rest of the pharynx or throat below the palate, the nasopharynx is always open. It serves as a passageway to the throat for sinonasal discharge as well as for the flow of air between the nose, lower throat, and lungs. It acts as a resonance chamber in speech and by contracting its muscular floor and walls prevents regurgitation of food and liquids into the nose when swallowing, thereby also protecting the sinuses.

NON-RAPID-EYE-MOVEMENT SLEEP (NREM)—there are two types of sleep, NREM and REM (rapid-eye-movement sleep), both occurring in everyone and alternating throughout the night. NREM occupies about 80 percent of our total sleeping time, usually starting off in the beginning and representing the deeper sleep, especially in stages 3 and 4, which are known as delta sleep. REM sleep is lighter and follows NREM sleep in five or six cycles during the night, usually for shorter periods, often becoming more apparent after midnight, especially in younger people. The rapidity of eye movements while asleep and the changes in electrocardiograms, breathing times, and muscle tone vary with each type of sleep, and their recordings will identify which kind is active. Dreaming and body functions usually increase in REM sleep whereas most sleepwalking, sleeptalking, and nightmares occur during later-stage NREM delta sleep.

NSAIDS—or nonsteroidal anti-inflammatory drugs are pain-relieving and fever-reducing over-the-counter medications very similar to aspirin, and derived mostly from ibuprofen, naproxen, indomethacin, ketoprofen, etc. They are used to treat various inflammatory conditions and are often combined with other over-the-counter medications to treat colds, flu, and sinusitis symptoms. In some instances, they can cause GI bleeding, ulcers, esophagitis, and liver and kidney damage.

ONODI CELL—usually a fairly large posterior ethmoid air cell or sinus cavity located high in the back of the nose near the sphenoid sinus and very close to the optic nerve to the eye. When a doctor surgically explores this sinus cavity, optic nerve damage with loss of vision can sometimes occur.

OPPORTUNISTIC INFECTIONS—these occur when certain microorganisms in our environment take advantage of our depressed defenses or inadequately functioning immune systems due to AIDS or other immunity-suppressing conditions and seize the opportunity to invade our bodies and to infect us. Some common invaders are fungal infections, viruses, tuberculosis organisms, a *protozoa* called *Pneumocystis carinii* that causes lung infections, and also those causing shingles, herpes, salmonella, septicemia, certain tumors, and sinusitis.

OPTIC NERVE—the second in line of the 12 paired cranial nerves leading from the brain. It, along with its matching nerve on the opposite side, is responsible for our sense of sight, which in rare instances could be endangered by a sinus infection or by sinus surgery, especially in the posterior ethmoid–sphenoid area.

ORBITAL CELLULITIS—inflammation of the orbital tissues surrounding the eye usually resulting from an ethmoid sinus infection extending beyond its bony confinement and causing redness and swelling around the eye and sometimes bulging (proptosis) of the eye with the distinct possibility of harming vision.

OSTEOMA—a benign growth arising from bone almost anywhere in the body, but especially from the flat bones of the skull and jaw as well as from the bony sinus walls, where it may enlarge to obstruct sinus drainage, causing a persistent sinus infection.

OSTIOMEATAL COMPLEX (ANTERIOR OMC)—an area or space beneath the anterior part of the middle turbinate where the drainage openings of the anterior ethmoidal, frontal, and maxillary sinuses are in very close proximity and where an infection or blockage of one may involve all three.

OSTIOMEATAL COMPLEX POSTERIOR—also called the sphenoethmoidal recess (SER), is an area at the posterior end of the superior turbinate where the sphenoidal and posterior ethmoidal sinus drainage openings are in close proximity and where infectious drainage from one may involve both.

OTOLARYNGOLOGIST—(Otorhinolaryngologist) a medical and surgical specialist who is trained to treat diseases, conditions, and abnormalities of the ears, nose, throat, and larynx, as well as other associated problems in the head and neck, including sinus disease.

OZONE—a gaseous ground-level pollutant in our environment capable of irritating and inflaming respiratory membranes to cause bronchitis, rhinitis, and sinusitis. It is formed when *volatile organic compounds* (VOCs) from gasoline fumes, industrial chemicals, and solvents react with nitrogen oxides from burning coal, gas, and oil in the presence of hot overhead sun rays. A level of more than 80 parts per billion is now considered unsafe. Stratospheric ozone that protects us from ultraviolet rays is from a different source and it is the lack of this kind of ozone that can harm us.

PANSINUSITIS—a condition resulting when all the sinuses are infected.

PATHOGEN—a microorganism, virus, protozoan, fungus, or other viable substance capable of causing disease.

PILOERECTION—hairs standing on end due to contraction of a tiny erector muscle attached to each hair and controlled by the sympathetic nervous system. It may be seen on your arms as a response to cold temperatures and a body chill, but it can also occur in some cases of fear, fright, anger, and rage, especially in the lower animals, where it can also reduce body heat loss by thickening their furry coats.

PITUITARY GLAND—lies at the base of the brain directly over the sphenoid sinus and in rare instances may be involved with sphenoid sinus disease. It is one of our principal hormone-secreting glands, and because of its influence over other glands such as the adrenal or thyroid, it used to be referred to as the maestro or master gland. Because of its location, tumors of the pituitary gland are often surgically approached through the sphenoid sinus cavities.

PNEUMONIA AND PNEUMONITIS—these two words are often used interchangeably to denote inflammation of lung tissue that is often fairly localized to a segment of the lung but can involve the whole lobe, the entire lung, or both lungs. Most cases are due to bacteria or viruses but can result from a fungal or protozoan infection, from aspiration of foreign matter, from physical trauma, or from inhaling a caustic chemical or membrane-scorching heat.

POLYPS—usually rounded grapelike structures that can arise from membrane linings almost anywhere in the body. In the beginning, they are not considered new growths, since they initially maintain the same cellular characteristics as their tissues of origin. Although they may continue to enlarge, those located in the nose, sinuses, or ears will remain benign, whereas elsewhere in the body, especially within the GI tract, some may undergo malignant changes.

PROSTAGLANDINS(PGS)—a wide group of natural body chemicals found in nearly every cell of the body. They play multiple roles in cell function from pregnancy and delivery to protecting the walls of the GI tract from noxious substances, helping to regulate blood pressure as well as blood flow to the lungs and kidneys, and enhancing the body's inflammatory response to infection. They may be inhibited, especially in the latter role, by anti-inflammatory medications such as the NSAIDs.

PROTOZOA—a single-cell, sometimes lung-infecting member of the animal kingdom capable of causing pneumonia in immunocompromized individuals. It is a fairly frequent cause of opportunistic lung infections in AIDS patients under the name of *Pneumocystis carinii* pneumonia.

PUS—also known as purulence or purulent discharge, pus is a liquid product of infection containing microorganisms, white blood cells, dead or dying tissue cells, and digestive enzymes, frequently of a creamy consistency, usually varying from white to yellow to green in color, often collecting in an infected wound or cavity and many times eventually draining from it.

PYOCELE—is an infected *mucocele,* or thick-walled cyst, usually developing in a sinus cavity and initially containing uninfected mucus under pressure from the mucus-secreting glands.

RAYNAUD'S DISEASE—an unexplained usually intermittent spasm or constriction of small arteries or arterioles causing diminished blood flow to a finger or toe and occasionally to the nasal tip or tongue, easily recognized as a recurring paleness, blanching, or grayish color to the skin or membrane overlying the area. It is more common in younger women, each time lasting several minutes to hours, and is often precipitated by exposure to cold.

REBOUND PHENOMENON—(rebound swelling) a significant increase in nasal membrane swelling and congestion occuring within an hour or so of using a decongestant nasal spray or drops that should normally improve nasal congestion for a period of at least 3 or 4 hours or longer depending on the duration strength of the medication. The cause of this phenomenon is unknown, but there seems to be a localized neurovascular sensitivity to the medication that will nearly always increase with its continued use or the use of a similar product.

RELATIVE HUMIDITY (RH)—the ratio of the amount of water vapor or moisture in the air compared to what that same air at that same temperature is capable of holding when completely saturated. RH is expressed as a percentage. Cold air can't hold as much moisture as warm air, but its RH can still be very high, especially if additional moisture is available such as following a heavy rain or melting snow.

RESPIRATORY SYNCYTIAL VIRUS (RSV)—a viral respiratory infection very similar to flu. It may attack the upper and especially the lower respiratory tracts, particularly in children, but is seen fairly often in older individuals and the elderly. It can be very serious in infants or those with chronic lung disease, sometimes with fatal results. It may be accompanied or followed by varying degrees of sinusitis or bronchitis and especially by severe wheezing in very young children.

RESPIRATORY TRACT—the passageways connecting the nose with the alveoli or air sacs in the lungs. After passing through the nose, nasopharynx, and pharynx, or upper airway, air enters the larynx and is distributed to the lungs through the trachea, bronchi, and bronchioles forming the lower airway. The mouth, on the other hand, is our secondary upper airway, usually of no help in breathing at birth or even shortly thereafter, and mainly used later for added support to nasal breathing when talking, sobbing, crying, singing, and exercising or when the nasal airway is obstructed.

REYE'S SYNDROME—a very serious sometimes fatal febrile illness occurring in children or adolescents, very rarely in adults, and mainly involving their livers and brains. The exact cause is unknown, but it seems to be initiated by taking aspirin during a viral febrile illness such as chicken pox or flu.

RHINITIS—inflammation of the nasal mucous membranes, which may be acute or chronic and usually the result of an infection, allergy, or breathing some irritating chemical or dust. Local medications to the eyes or nose may also cause it.

RHINITIS MEDICAMENTOSA—a state of irritated and inflamed nasal membranes from excessive or improper use of various nasal ointments, drops, and sprays including steroids, Cromolyn, drying agents, and antihistamine nasal spray and decongestants as well as from nonsterile, improperly mixed salt solutions for nasal sniffing and irrigations. Also included would be nasal membrane irritation from use of eye ointments, eyedrops, and especially their preservatives, which enter the nose through the tear ducts, as well as membrane inflammation from other unsavory practices such as glue sniffing or dipping snuff as well as Ritalin, crack, or cocaine snorting.

RHINOSINUSITIS—inflammation of the mucous membranes of the nose and sinuses, which so often occur together.

SAMTER'S SYNDROME (ASPIRIN TRIAD)—a condition found in those with asthma and a sensitivity to aspirin, and who usually begin to develop nasal polyps within 5 to 10 years after onset of the asthma. Obstructive sinusitis symptoms will usually accompany the development of nasal polyps.

SEPTICEMIA—a serious sometimes fatal acute febrile illness requiring immediate treatment with blood cultures followed by intense antibiotic therapy and due to invasion of the bloodstream by mostly disease-causing bacteria or their toxins.

SEROMUCINOUS GLANDS—numerous microscopic glands located just beneath the surface of the mucous membranes lining the respiratory tract and sinuses that secrete both a thicker mucoid substance and a thinner watery fluid to form the inner layer of the protective mucous blanket covering the walls of the respiratory tract and sinuses. The outer thicker mucous layer is fed mostly by millions of microscopic *goblet cells.*

SEROTONIN—a naturally occurring blood vessel constrictor, or *vaso-constrictor,* found in most body tissues and especially in the brain. It also serves as one of the body's many nerve transmitters, or NTs, and among other things stimulates the smooth muscle in the walls of arteries to contract to narrow their channels and reduce blood flow.

SIDS (SUDDEN INFANT DEATH SYNDROME)—the sudden, unexpected death of an infant or small child, usually with no apparent cause found either before or at postmortem examination. Various things have been blamed including sleeping position, secondhand smoke, cold weather, prematurity, smoking during pregnancy, poverty, and genetics. SIDS is the most common cause of infant death between 2 weeks and 1 year of age, with the peak between the second and fourth month, and always seems to occur during sleep.

SINONASAL WALL—the common wall or partition separating the nose from the sinus cavities, usually containing a very thin layer of bone covered on both sides by mucous membranes and through which the drainage openings of the sinuses pass.

SINUS—a cavity, channel, or hollow space in the body. There are more than 40 sinuses located in the head alone, and most of them have their own special names. However, the word "sinus" or "sinus infection" refers to our paranasal sinuses. They consist of four paired hollowed-out structures in bone lying mostly adjacent to each side of the nose, into which they drain. The larger ones, namely, the frontal, maxillary, and sphenoid, are singular, paired cavities whereas, the ethmoids are a group of 7 to 15 separate smaller cavities on each side, each usually having its own separate drainage opening into the nose.

SJÖGREN'S SYNDROME—a chronic dryness of the mucus-secreting membranes, mostly of the eyes and mouth but often involving the respiratory and GI tracts as well as other body organs. The cause is unknown, but it is believed to be related to an autoimmune response in which the immune system treats these secretory tissues as foreign to the body and therefore reacts with an antibody-like response, shutting them down.

SUBACUTE SINUSITIS—the in-between state of acute and chronic sinusitis where the sinus symptoms, although still present, are usually milder than the acute stage but haven't reached the often irreversible state of chronic sinus disease, a fact that makes it extremely important to recognize this condition early and treat it vigorously.

SUBCUTANEOUS EMPHYSEMA—an infrequently occurring very temporary condition usually of no serious nature but somewhat shocking to the patient when bubbles of air may suddenly appear under the skin of the cheeks or around the eyes sometimes following maxillary or ethmoid sinus surgery and usually after sneezing or blowing one's nose. It resolves spontaneously and usually within 24 hours.

T CELLS—lymphocytes, or white blood cells, that fight foreign protein invaders of the body including bacteria, viruses, fungi, and molds. They are derived from the thymus gland (T), which is located in the upper chest and plays an important role in the early development of our immune systems. They have specific duties such as those assigned to the T killer cells and the T helper cells. The latter are sometimes called the Paul Reveres of the immune response, since they alert the killer T cells to the foreign invader. The B cell lymphocytes, on the other hand are derived from bone (B) and are responsible for forming antibodies to neutralize these invaders.

THROMBUS—a blood clot that forms in the heart or in one of the blood vessels of the body and may partially or completely obstruct blood flow. It may sometimes become infected to cause a septic thrombosis.

THRUSH—or oral candidiasis, is an infectious involvement of the membranes of the mouth by a yeastlike mold or fungus called *Candida albicans*. As the last part of the name would indicate, it produces white spots in the mouth, especially on the inside of the cheeks, but also on the tongue, palate, and gums. It is a benign condition but is occasionally indicative of an immune deficiency problem.

VALSALVA INFLATION MANEUVER—a technique used by divers, pilots, mountain climbers, and plane passengers to inflate their ears and sinuses in order to prevent a vacuum from developing within them or membrane injury from a too sudden rush of air to fill that vacuum (*barotrauma*). It consists of clamping off the nose between the thumb and forefinger, swallowing, and immediately blowing air into the nose without releasing it through the nostrils. The swallowing will momentarily open the eustachian tubes, allowing the increased nasal pressure from blowing to inflate the ears as well as the sinuses. This of course

THE SINUSITIS HELP BOOK

may have to be done repeatedly to keep up with any changes in out-side pressure and also with the body's spontaneous absorption of air from a closed ear or sinus cavity.

VALVULAR HEART DISEASE—impaired heart and possibly lung function due to a defective or damaged heart valve. A damaged heart valve will also attract bacteria traveling in the bloodstream and become infected, possibly causing more scarring.

VASOCONSTRICTOR—usually a medication in nasal drop, spray, pill, or shot form that causes narrowing or constriction of blood vessels with a more effective blood flow to the area and mobilization of excess tissue fluid resulting in a reduction in membrane swelling. When applied to the nose as a decongestant spray or drop or taken systemically by pill, it usually relieves nasal congestion, improves nasal breathing, and enhances sinonasal drainage, sometimes also relieving a sinus headache.

VASOMOTOR RHINITIS—a nasal condition usually characterized by an excess of clear nasal discharge, nasal membrane swelling, nasal congestion, and sometimes sneezing. It may be chronic or intermittent and may involve one or both sides of the nose and sometimes alternate from one side to the other. It is not caused by allergies, infection, occupation, chronic irritant exposure, or topical medications introduced into the nose. A psychological factor creating a localized nerve imbalance has sometimes been blamed in the past and may be a factor. It could also be due to a localized neurovascular dysfunction in non-allergic hyperreactive membranes. It is a diagnosis often made when no other cause for the rhinitis can be found.

VOLATILE ORGANIC COMPOUNDS (VOCs)—vaporized, rather toxic chemicals found in gasoline fumes and other petroleum distillates including the solvents in printer's inks, paints, glues, sealants, degreasers, corking compounds, certain cleaners, wax removers, as well as in most containers that say "Caution—use in a well ventilated area." VOCs not only are toxic to the body, especially the liver and brain, but also combine with nitrogen oxides in hot sunlight to form ground-level ozone, which can irritate the nose, sinuses, and lungs.

References

BOOKS

Bailey, Byron J., M.D., *Head and Neck Surgery,* J. B. Lippencott Company, 1993.

Ballenger, John Jacob and Snow, James B., *Otolaryngology: Head and Neck Surgery,* 15th Edition, 1995, Williams and Wilkins, Baltimore.

Bluestone, Stool and Kenna, *Pediatric Otolaryngology,* W. B. Saunders Co., 1996.

Bull, P.D., M.D., B.Ch., F.R.C.S., *Lecture Notes on Disease of the Ear, Nose and Throat,* Royal Hallamshire Hosp. And Childrens Hosp., Univ. Of Sheffield, Seventh Edition, Oxford, Blackwell Sc. Publications, 1991.

Cole, Philip, M.D., F.R.C.S. *The Respiratory Role of the Upper Airways,* Mosby Year Book Inc., St. Louis, 1992.

Cummings, M.D., Charles W. *Otolaryngology—Head and Neck Surgery* (Vol. 1), Mosby Year Book Inc., St. Louis, 1993.

Druce, Howard M., ed., *Sinusitis: Pathophysiology and Treatment,* Marcel Dekker, Inc., New York, 1993.

Kennedy, David W., MD, Paul A. Greenberger, MD, eds., *Rhinology and Nasal Allergy Year Book 1996,* Ocean Side Publications, Providence.

Kennedy, David W. , MD, Paul A. Greenberger, MD and Michael S. Benninger, MD eds. *Rhinology and Nasal Allergy Yearbook 1998,* Ocean Side Publications, Providence.

Lusk, Rodney P., ed., *Pediatric Sinusitis,* Raven Press, New York, 1992.

McCaffrey, Thomas V., *Systemic Disease and the Nasal Airway,* Thieme Medical Publishers Inc, New York, 1993.

Negus, Sir Victor, *The Comparative Anatomy and Physiology of the Nose and Paranasal Sinuses,* E & S Livingstone Ltd., Edinburgh and London, 1958.

The Otolaryngologic Clinics of North America, Vol. 22, No. 6, Dec. 1989, Philadelphia: W. B. Saunders Co.

The Otolaryngologic Clinics of North America, Vol. 29, Feb. 1996, *Pediatric Sinusitis,* W. B. Saunders Co.

Ritter, Frank N., *The Paranasal Sinuses,* The C. V. Mosby Co., St. Louis, 1973.

Schatz, Michael M.D., Robert S. Zeiger, M.D., Ph.D., and Guy A. Settipane, M.D., eds., *Nasal Manifestations of Systemic Diseases,* Ocean Side Publications, Providence, R.I., 1991.

Scott-Brown, W. G. C.V.O., M.D., B.Ch., F.R.C.S. Surgeon, Royal Free Hospital, ed., *Diseases of the Ear, Nose and Throat,* Vol 1 (1952), London, Printed in Great Britain by Love and Malcomson, Ltd.

Selye, Hans, *The Mast Cells* Butterworths, Washington, D. C. 1965.

Settipane, Guy A., M.D., ed., *H1 and H2 Histamine Receptors,* Ocean Side Publications Inc., Providence, 1988–1989.

Settipane, Guy A., ed. *Rhinitis* (second edition), Ocean Side Publications, Inc., Providence, 1991.

Settipane, Guy A., Valerie J. Lund, Joel M. Berstein and Mirko Tos., eds. *Nasal Polyps: Epidemiology, Pathogenesis and Treatment.* Ocean Side Publications, Inc., Providence, 1997.

Stewart J. H., ed. *Analgesic and NSAID Induced Kidney Disease,* Oxford, England: Oxford Univ. Press, 1993.

Takahashi, Dr. Ryo, Director, Dept. Of Otolaryngology, Jikei Univ. Sch. of Med., *A Collection of Ear, Nose and Throat Studies,* Tokyo, 1971.

Wolff, Harold G.: *Headache and Other Head Pain*, Donald J. Dalessio, M.D. and Stephen D. Silberstein, M.D., eds., Oxford Univ. Press, New York, Sixth Edition, 1993.

ARTICLES

Apter A., Bracker A., et al. "Epidemiology of the Sick Building Syndrome." *J. of A. and Clin. Immunol*, Aug. 1994, 277–88.

Baker, Susan P., Kopl Halpern. "Death from Balloons." *JAMA* 13 Dec.1995, Johns Hopkins Sch. of Public Health.

Bernstein JM, Gorfien J, Noble B, Yankaskas Jr. J. "Nasal Polyposis: Immunohistochemistry and Bioelectrical Findings (a hypothesis for the development of nasal polylps)." *Allergy Clin. Immunol* 99:165–175, 1997.

Bollinger, Mary E., DO, Peyton A. Eggleston MD, Elizabeth Flanagan, BS, and Robert A. Wood, MD. "Cat antigen in homes with and without cats may induce allergic symptoms." *J. Al Clin Immunol*, Vol. 97, No. 4, 907–14, Apr. 1996.

Carpenter, Kevin M., MD, Scott Graham MB, and Richard J. H. Smith, MD. "Facial Skeletal Growth After Endoscopic Sinus Surgery in the Piglet Model." *Am. J. Rhinol.* 11, 211–217, 1997.

Dockery, Douglas W., Sc.D., C. Arden Pope III, Ph.D., Xiping Xu, M.D., Ph.D., John D. Spengler, Ph.D., James H. Ware, Ph.D., Martha E. Fay, M.P.H., Benjamin G. Ferris, Jr., M.D., and Frank E. Speizer, M.D. "An Association Between Air Pollution and Mortality in Six U.S. Cities," *N Engl J Med* 1993; 329:1753–9.

Drettner B. "Pathophysiologic relationship between the upper and lower airways." *Am. Oto Rhino Laryngol.* 79: 499–505, 1970.

"Effects of Ozone Exposure: A comparison between oral and nasal breathing." *Arch. Of Envir. Health*, 43:357–360, 1988.

Eghrari-Sabet, Jacqueline S., MD and Jay E. Slater, MD. "Latex Allergy: A potentially serious respiratory disorder." *J. of Resp. Diseases*, Vol 14; No. 3: 473–82, Mar. 1993.

Falk, Jan E., MD, Jan E. Juto, MD, PhD, Goran Stridh, PhD, Gunnar Bylin, MD, PhD. "Dose-Response study of Formaldehyde on Nasal Mucosa Swelling." Dept. Of Otolaryngology, Søder Hospital, Stockholm, Sweden.

Findley, Larry J., Mark E. Unverzagt and Paul M. Suratt. "Automobile Accidents Involving Patients with Obstructive Sleep Apnea." *Am. Rev. Respir. Dis.*, 138:337–340, 1988.

Freeman, Geraldine L., MD. "Concurrence of Latex and Fruit Allergies." *Allergy and Asthma Proceedings.* Vol 18; No. 2: 85–88, Mar. Apr. 1997.

Fried, Marvin P., et al: "Intraoperative image guidance during endoscopic sinus surgery." *Am. J. of Rhinol.* Vol 10; No. 6: 337–342, Nov. Dec. 1996.

Godofsky EW, Zinreich J, Armstrong Michael, Leslie JM, Weikel CS. "Sinusitis in HIV-infected patients: a clinical and radiographic review." *Am. J. Med.* 93(2): 163–70, Aug. 1992.

Goldwyn BG, et al. "Histopathologic Analysis of Chronic Sinusitis." *Am. J. Rhinol* Jan.–Feb. '95, Vol. 9, 125–30.

Guntheroth, Warren G., MD and Philip S. Spiers PhD. "SIDS and near-SIDS: Where we stand in 1992." *J. Respir. Dis.*, 13(9):1280–94, 1992.

Gwaltney JM Jr., Phillilps CD, Miller RD, et al. "Computed tomographic study of the common cold." *N Engl J Med;* 330:25–30, 1994.

Haight JSJ and Cole P. "Nasal resistance after lateral recumbrancy." *J. Otolaryngol.*, 15 (Suppl 16) 9–13, 1986.

Haight JSJ and Cole P. "Topographical Anatomy of Pressure Points that Alter Nasal Resistance." *J. Otolaryngol.* 15 (Suppl 16) 14–20, 1986.

Hartwick RW, Batsakis JG. "Sinus aspergillosis and allergic fungal sinusitis (Review)." *Ann. Oto, Rhinol, Laryngol.* 100 (5 Pt 1): 427–430, May 1991.

Hilding A. "Experimental sinus surgery: Effect of operative windows on normal sinus." *Ann. Otol Rhinol Laryngol* 50:379–392, 1941.

Hilding A. "Physiology of drainage of nasal mucus. Experimental work on accessory sinuses." *Am. J. Of Physiology* 100:664, 1932.

Hinderer KH. "Effect of Air Currents on the Nasopulmonary Mucosa." *Rhinology* 13:1–5, 1975.

Hodgson M, Levin H, Wolkoff P. "Volatile Organic Compounds and Indoor Air." *J. of Al. and Clin. Immunol.* Aug. 1994, 296–303.

Kalinger, Michael A., MD, J. David Osguththorpe, MD, Philip Fireman, MD, Jack Anon, MD, John Georgitis, MD, Mary L. Davis, MA, Robert Naclerio, MD and David Kennedy, MD. "Sinusitis: Bench to Bedside Current Findings, Future Directions." *Otolaryngology-Head and Neck Surgery Suppl.* Vol. 116; No. 6: Part 2, June 1997.

Kane, Kevin J. FRACS (Australia) "Recirculation of mucus as a cause of persistent sinusitis." *Am. J. Rhinol.* Vol. 11, No. 5, 361–369, Sept. 1997.

Kennedy DW, Zeinreich SJ, Rosenbaum AE, Johns ME, Functional "Endoscopic Sinus Surgery," *Arch Otorhinolaryngol* 111:576–582, 1985.

Lanza D, Kennedy DW. "Current concepts in the surgical management of chronic and recurrent acute sinusitis." *J. Allergy Clin Immunol.* 90:505–511, 1992.

Lee, Dennis, MD, Robin Brady, MD and Gady Har-El, MD, "Frontal Sinus Outflow Anatomy." *Am. J. of Rhinol.* Vol 11, No. 4, July 1997.

Lew, Daniel, MD, Frederick S. Southwick, MD, William Montgomery, MD, Alfred L. Weber, MD and Ann S. Baker, MD. "Sphenoid Sinusitis." *N. Engl. J. Med.;* 309:1149–54, 1983.

Master D., Hess Longe S.H., Dickson H. "Scheduled Hand Washing in an Elementary School Population." *Family Medicine* 29, Issue No. 5, 336–339, May 1997.

Menzies, Richard, MD, M. Sc., Robyn Tamblyn, PhD, et al. "The effects of varying levels of outdoor air supply on the symptoms of sick building syndrome." *N. Engl. J. Med.,* Vol. 328:821–826, 1993.

Mirza, Natasha, MD, Kathleen T. Montone MD, Edward A. Stadtmauer MD, and Donald C. Lanza MD. "A schematic approach to pre-existing sinus disease for the immunocompromised individual" *A. J. Rhino* Vol 12; No 2:93–98, 1998.

"Nasal Polyp Update." *Allergy and Asthma Proceedings.* Vol. 17, No. 5, Sept. Oct., 1996.

Nillson, Gunnar, PhD and Dean D. Metcalfe, MD. "Contemporary Issues in Mast Cell Biology" *Allergy and Asthma Proceedings,* Vol 17; No. 2:1996.

Nordlee, Julie A., MS, Steve Taylor, PhD, Robert Bush, MD. "Identification of Brazil Nut Allergen in Transgenic Soybeans." *N. Engl. J. Med.*, Nov. 14, 1996, 688–692.

Nordstrom K, Norback D, Akselsson R. "Effect of air humidification on sick building syndrome and perceived indoor air quality in hospitals: a four month longitudinal study." *Occupational and Environmental Medicine* 51 (10): 683–8, Oct. 1994.

Pearlman, Steven J., MD; William Lawson, MD, DDS; Hugh Biller, MD; William H. Friedman, MD; Guy D. Potter, MD. "Isolated Sphenoid Sinus Disease." *Laryngoscope* 99; July 1989.

Puig, Christine M,. MD, Colin L.W. Driscoll and Eugene B. Kern, MD. "Sluder's Sphenopalatine Ganglion Neuralgia, Treatment with 88% Phenol." *Am. J. Rhin*, 12, 113–118, 1998.

Perneger, Thomas V., MD, PhD, Paul K. Whelton, MD, M.Sc., Michael J. Klag, MD, MPH. Risk of kidney failure associated with the use of acetaminophen, aspirin, and nonsteroidal antiinflammatory drugs. *N. Engl. J. Med.*, Dec. 1994; 331:1675–1679, Johns Hopkins School of Medicine & Public Health, Univ. Of Geneva.

Pommer W, E Bronder, E Greiser, et al. "Regular analgesic intake and the risk of end-stage renal failure." *Am. J. Nephrol*; 9:403–412, 1989.

Pope CA III, Thun MJ, Namboodiri MM, Dockery DW, Evans JS, Speizer FE, Heath Jr CW. "Particulate air pollution as a predictor of mortality in a prospective study of U.S. adults." *Am J Respir Crit Care Med* 1995; 151:669–74.

Rosen, CA, MD, Laurene Howell, MD, and James D. Smith, MD. "Efficacy of Different Surgical Approaches in Patients with the Aspirin Sensitivity, Asthma and Nasal Polyposis Triad." *Am. J. of Rhinol.*, Vol. 10, No. 4, 207–210, Aug. 1996.

Rosenthal J, Katz R, DuBois DB, et al. "Chronic maxillary Sinusitis associated with the mushroom Schizophyllum commune in a patient with AIDS." *Clin. Infectious Disease* 14(1):46–48, Jan. 1992.

Rothman, Glen B., MD, David E. Tunkel, MD, F.M. Baroody and Robert M. Naclerio, MD. "Pediatric Functional Endoscopis Sinus Surgery." *Am. J. of Rhinology*, Vol. 10, No. 6:343–46, 1996.

Sakakura Y., et al. "Reversibility of reduced mucociliary clearance in chronic sinusitis." *Clin. Otolaryngology* 10:79–83, 1985.

Sakakura Y., et al. "Nasal Mucociliary Clearance Under Various Conditions." *Acta Otolaryngol* (Stockh) 96: 167–173, 1983.

Sandler DP, Burr FR, Weinberg CR. Nonsteroidal anti-inflammatory drugs and the risk of chronic renal disease. Ann. Intern. Med.;115:165–72, 1991.

Schlanger G, Lutwich L.I., Kurzman M, Hoch B, Chandler FW. "Sinusitis caused by *Legionella pneumophila* in a patient with acquired immune deficiency syndrome (AIDS)." *Am. J. Med.*; 77:957–960, 1984.

Schwartz J., Marcus A. "Mortality and air pollution in London: a time series analysis." *Am. J. Epidemiol* 131:85–94, 1990.

Slavin, Raymond G., MD. "Recalcitrant asthma: Could sinusitis be the cullprit?" *J. Resp. Dis.*, 12(2):182–194, 1991.

Steinman, Harris A., M B Ch B, Capetown So. Africa. "'Hidden' allergens in foods." *J. Al. and Clin. Immunol.* Vol. 98, No. 2, 241–50, Sept. 1996.

Torkkeli, Tommi, MD et al (Finland) "Ciliary ultrastructure and mucociliary transport in upper respiratory tract infections." *Am. J. Rhinol.* Vol. 8, No. 5.

Wald ER, Guerra N, Byers C. "Upper respiratory tract infections in young children: duration of and frequency of complications." *Pediatrics*; 87l: 129–133, 1991.

Wheatley, Lisa M. and Thomas A. E. Platts-Mills. "Perennial Allergens and the Asthma Epidemic." *Science and Medicine*, May/June 1996: 6–13.

Whitcomb, David C., MD, PhD, Geoffrey D. Block, MD, MPH. "Association of acetaminophen hepatotoxicity with fasting and ethanol use." *JAMA*, Vol 272; No. 23:1845–1850, 1994.

Winther B., Brofeldt S., Christensen B., et al. "Light and scanning electron microscopy of nasal biopsy material from patients with naturally acquired common colds." *Acta Otolaryngol* (Stockh) 1984; 97:309–318.

Winther, Brigit, Jack M. Gwaltney, Jr., et al. "Viral Induced Rhinitis." *Am. J. of Rhonol.* Vol. 12; No. 1:17–20, 1998.

Yunginger, J. W. "Lethal Food Allergy in Children," *N. Engl. J. Med.*; 327:421–22, 1992.

Zinreich, S.J., MD, Kennedy D.W., MD, et al. "Fungal Sinusitis: Diagnosis with CT and MR Imaging." *J. Radiology* 169; 439–44, 1988.

Index

molds, 265–266
nasal hyperreactivity, 267–269
nonallergic, 256–258
pregnancy and, 258–260
reactive lower airway disease, 267–268
vasomotor or nonallergic hyper-reactive rhinitis, 260–261
rhinosinobronchial reflex, 33–34
rhinosinusitis
defined, 48
rimantadine, 123

S

Saccharomyces, 348
saline nasal sprays, 162
manufactured vs. home-made, 23
prevention and, 161–162
salivary nitrite, 27–28
Samter's syndrome, 202, 343
saunas
prevention and, 162–163
scar formation, 154
after surgery, 230
length of infection time for scarring, 49
obstructive sinus scarring, 49–50
scarlatina, 127
Schneider, Conrad Victor, 19
Schneiderian membranes, 19
secondary drainage openings, 17
benefit of, 17
indicating previous sinus disease, 17
percentage occurrence of, 17
secondary salivary glands, 25
nasogustatory reflex, 26
septal abscess
after surgery, 227
septal perforation
after surgery, 227–228
septicemia, 64, 143–144
seromucinous glands
function of, 19, 25
location of, 19, 25
nasogustatory reflex, 26
sick building syndrome
characteristics of building, 280
formaldehyde, 280–281
humidity in, 283
possible causes of, 281–282, 284
symptoms of, 280
volatile organic compounds, 282

sinonasal cleansing action, 26
benefit of, 24
defined, 21
during head cold, 29–30
obstruction of, and infection opportunity, 46
sinonasal mucous glands
secretion of in first days of cold, 26
sinonasal reflex, 33
sinus blockage, 47–49
causes of, 47
sinus cultures
diagnosis and, 72
difficulty in reading results from, 153
sinus drainage
promoting as prevention, 161
sinuses
additional sinus openings, 17
drainage of, 13, 17
frontal, 14–15
inflammation in, 47
interconnection to nose and lungs, 33–36
location of, 12–13
maintenance of nasal mucous blanket, 43
maxillary, 14
mucus from, 29
normal function, 11, 14
pollution's effect on, 275–277
protective role of, 22
purpose of, 21–23
secondary drainage openings, 17
sinonasal air exchange function, 44
structure of, 11–21
swelling of, and sleeping position, 34–36
sinus headache, 73–74
barometric pressure and, 95–96
biological clock and, 95
causes of
alcohol, 90–91
children and, 61
conditions that improve or worsen, 75
diagnosis and meticulous history of, 81
ethmoid sinus, 87–88
frontal sinus, 87–88
information about and diagnosis of sinusitis, 61